Mediterranean Rhinoplasty

Pier Giorgio Giacomini
Editor

Mediterranean Rhinoplasty

Springer

Editor
Pier Giorgio Giacomini
Department of Clinical Sciences and Translational Medicine
University of Rome Tor Vergata
Rome, Italy

ISBN 978-3-031-05550-8 ISBN 978-3-031-05551-5 (eBook)
https://doi.org/10.1007/978-3-031-05551-5

This Springer imprint is published by the registered company Springer Nature Switzerland AG
The registered company address is: Gewerbestrasse 11, 6330 Cham, Switzerland

This book is dedicated to my wife Antonella and to my children Giorgio and Livia, to whom I owe much for their patience and understanding over the years, when the passion for my job took me away too often.

Foreword

Rhinoplasty has always been a difficult operation requiring a high level of skill and artistry not usually demanded to the same extent in many other facial plastic procedures. The outcome must produce a nose that not only fills the aesthetic goals of the patient but must also breathe well, and the effort to achieve one of these goals cannot be allowed to compromise the other. So form and function must be balanced. The aesthetic rhinoplasty surgeon must also be a master airway surgeon as many maneuvers to achieve a pleasing cosmetic result can lead to a smaller intranasal airway; even a small deviation of the septum can be a larger problem when reduction rhinoplasty is done, unless it is addressed at the same time of surgery.

Aesthetically, in rhinoplasty there is no dotted line that tells the surgeon when the maximum aesthetic goal has been reached; there must be a learned sixth sense, as well as knowledge of nasal proportions that tells the surgeon when enough has been done and it's time to put on the nasal splint. And there must be the learned knowledge of following patients post-operatively for years that tells the surgeon what to expect long term after the nose has settled and all swelling has subsided.

Also challenging the nasal surgeon are the expectations of the patient on a surgery with very many psychological overlays. Will improvement be accepted over a desired perceived perfection? Does the patient have realistic expectations?

And so, as the rhinoplasty surgeon approaches the patient with all these challenges, wouldn't it be least stressful and easier for the surgeon to only have to change or modify one limited anatomic area on the nose, say a dorsal hump? But indeed, if Mediterranean noses do have fairly consistent characteristics as described herein, they must be one of the most technically challenging and complex types of noses to tackle because so much must be done in one setting. Not just a dorsal hump, but also a droopy tip that must be rotated and supported through a myriad of techniques and grafts, a thick skin envelope and wide tip that weigh heavily and fight against definition and refinement, weak lower and upper lateral cartilages that, if trimmed too much, may cause nasal valve collapse, alar retraction, or tip bossae.

It is precisely for that reason that the esteemed Prof. Pier Giorgio Giacomini has brought together world-renowned nasal experts to contribute to this masterful work—surgeons who deal with Mediterranean noses in a large percentage of their operations and who are respected for their great ability to teach, for their innovative techniques, and for their consistently reproducible pleasing results. On a personal note, I've had the distinct pleasure to both operate and/or share the lecture podium with many of the authors, with whom I share a great friendship. Readers of this text will benefit from discussions on the anatomy, function, aesthetics, and common characteristics of problems encountered in Mediterranean noses. They will be treated to multiple techniques in both endonasal and external rhinoplasty that preserve anatomic structures but modify them considerably while still maintaining and reinforcing support and produce natural looking outcomes.

May all of you, by reading this text, add to your armamentarium of nasal surgery knowledge and gain an understanding and appreciation of the nuances of the Mediterranean nose that will guide you in future surgeries. It is my honor to provide these introductory comments, and I congratulate Prof. Giacomini and his contributors on a great addition to the rhinoplasty literature.

With best wishes for great surgeries and happy patients.

Russell W. H. Kridel
Department of Otorhinolaryngology/Head and Neck Surgery
McGovern Medical School, University of Texas
Health Science Center
Houston, TX, USA

Preface

The approach to such a difficult task as remodeling the nose with rhinoplasty has changed overtimes. Current policy is to include the choice of different approaches and techniques to pursue and fulfill the aesthetic needs of the single patient, maintaining or restoring the correct nasal function. These different goals vary depending on the culture, anatomy, and age of each patient, but also of each surgeon. In this scenario, the geographical area where both patient and surgeon live has a considerable impact in terms of cultural background and anatomical cues related to racial characters.

Contemporary surgeons must therefore consider all the aforementioned topics when planning aesthetic rhinoplasty. This is the reason that prompted us to realize the present work. Achieving this goal has been possible only with the precious contribute of re-known and experienced authors daily facing the specific problems and solutions posed by rhinoplasty in patients dwelling the Mediterranean area.

To all of them, my deep and respectful thanks are due for their friendship, support, and cooperation and in the realization of this project.

Rome, Italy — Pier Giorgio Giacomini

Contents

Shape and Function of the Nose

1

Mariapia Guerrieri, Goran Latif Omer,
Rekawt Hama Rashid, and Stefano Di Girolamo

1.1 Anatomy and Function of the Nose

The nose represents the first tract of the upper respiratory ways. It has a complex external and internal structure which has evolved to serve several vital functions, first of all breathing. Nasal passage, though, is far from being a simple, static corridor for inspired air; on the contrary, it plays an active role on filtering, warming and moisturizing air, delivering it to the lower respiratory tract, well prepared to participate to gas exchanges. In addition to breathing, air conditioning and defensive filtering, the nose also possesses on its roof a delicate neuroepithelium responsible for the perception of olfaction. Moreover, thanks to its intricate internal structure, comprehensive of turbinates, meati and paranasal sinuses, the nose also joins the upper vocal tract as a sounding board, allowing human beings to produce specific sounds and modifying every individual unique vocal timbre. Voice isn't the only way the nose helps built a person's identity; being it a central feature of the face, in fact, its external shape is fundamental when it enhances someone's perception of self, playing a pivotal role in the construction of personality, self-esteem and self-expression through facial expressions and, eventually, together with other facial landmarks, the nose participates to one's awareness of his/her own beauty, ethnical background and culture.

Surgical rhinoplasty, therefore, is not only meant for functional or reconstructive purposes, but also and especially for aesthetic ones.

Rhinoplasty, both functional and aesthetic, aims to modify nasal shape and function acting on both the external and internal structures of the nose; therefore it's paramount for the facial plastic surgeons to know the anatomy.

M. Guerrieri · S. Di Girolamo (✉)
Department of Otorhinolaryngology, University of Rome "Tor Vergata", Rome, Italy

G. L. Omer · R. H. Rashid
ENT and Skull Base Surgery Department, Faruk Medical City, Sulaymaniyah, Iraq

P. G. Giacomini (ed.), *Mediterranean Rhinoplasty*,
https://doi.org/10.1007/978-3-031-05551-5_1

1.1.1 External Nose

The external nose can be subdivided in three aesthetical and functional units (Fig. 1.1):

- **Nasion region** (the upper third): Comprehensive of the two nasal bones that correspond to the radix of the nose [1].
- **Cartilaginous vault region** (the middle third): It is formed by the two upper lateral cartilages (ULCs). These are fused together superiorly with the nasal septum (keystone region), in order to give support to the middle dorsum of the nose, but they separate from the septum as they descend toward the external lateral triangle of the piriform aperture, where the sesamoid cartilages are. Moreover, superiorly the ULCs overlap with the caudal portion of the inferior surface of the nasal bones.
- **Lobule region** (the lower third): It is divided into supra-tip, immediately cephalic to the pronasale; tip or pronasale region, infra-tip, located between the pronasale and the base of the nostrils (Fig. 1.2). The lobule region is formed by the two lower lateral cartilages (LLCs), also called alar cartilages. These take contact with the caudal part of the ULCs, creating the scroll region [2]. LLCs have a

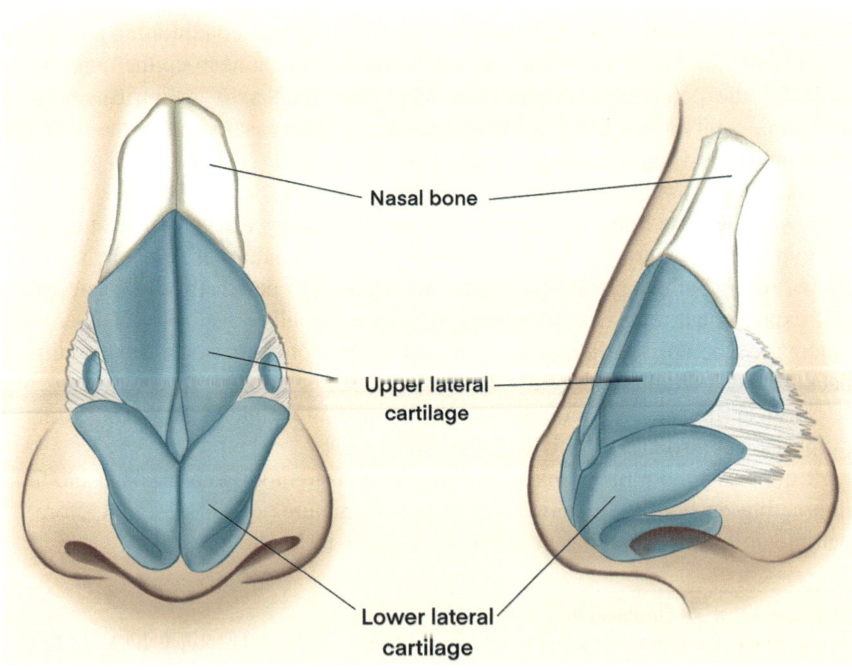

Fig. 1.1 External anatomy of the nose: the upper third (nasion) is formed by the nasal bones, the middle third (cartilaginous vault) is formed by the upper lateral cartilages (ULCs), the lower third (lobule) is formed by the lower lateral cartilages (LLCs)

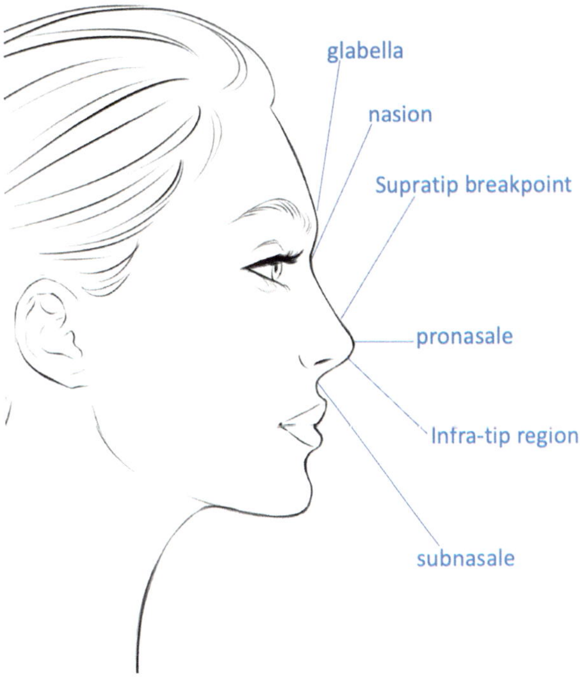

Fig. 1.2 Lateral nasal view

roughly "U" shaped form and can be divided into three units: *lateral crus*, the largest and strongest part that gives support to the lobule and shape the alar side wall. *Middle or intermediate crus*, divided into domal and lobular segments. Left middle crus is attached to the right one by a fibrous transverse thickening called interdomal ligament. The domal segments of the LLCs define the nasal tip. At this level, there is also a vertical oriented bundle of fibers, called Pitanguy or dermocartilaginous ligament, which contributes to the elevation of the tip and to its physical support [3, 4]. *Medial crus*, divided into columellar and footplate segments. These, together with the caudal portion of the nasal septum, form the nasal base.

These osteo-cartilaginous structures are covered by an intricated superficial musculoaponeurotic layer (SMAS) [5]. According to Saban, the nasal SMAS consists in a unique layer that goes from the frontal SMAS (frontalis muscle), to the internal nasal valve, where it divides into a lateral and a medial portion. Both these portions show a deep and a superficial layer. It is formed by nasal muscles (transverse nasalis muscle, procerus, compressor naris major and minor). Laterally the superficial layer continues from the dorsal portion of the nasal SMAS, passes over the LLC and it inserts on the skin of the alar margin (supra-alar layer). The deep layer originates from the nasal SMAS at the level of the INV, on which it inserts (valve layer). Medially the nasal SMAS divides into a deep medial layer, which runs between the anterior septal angle and the interdomal ligament, then it descends into the membranous septum, between the caudal border of the septum and the medial crura of the LLC, toward the anterior nasal spine. This anatomical structure corresponds to the Pitanguy ligament and its section determines nasal tip rotation and improvement of nasal tip definition. The superficial layer runs above the caudal border of the medial crura of the LLC to reach and intertwine with the depressor septi nasi muscle. Both the deep and superficial layers of the medial SMAS act lowering the nasal tip [6].

Soft tissues covering the osteo-cartilaginous scaffold of the nose consist in five layers: skin, superficial areolar layer, fibromuscular layer (SMAS), deep areolar layer and perichondral (periosteal) layer. The surgical dissection of these tissues can be performed in the subcutaneous, sub-SMAS and subperichondral planes [6].

1.1.2 Internal Nose

The nasal cavities are separated on the medial line by an osteo-cartilaginous septum. Its anterior part is formed by the quadrangular hyaline cartilage, which takes contact posteriorly with bony structures: the perpendicular plate of the ethmoid bone and the vomer. Inferiorly the nasal septum is inserted on the maxillary and palatine bones and it extends from the anterior nasal spina to the palatine crest, posteriorly [7].

The lateral nasal walls host the turbinates: inferior ones are made of a single bone, while the middle and superior ones are extensions of the ethmoid bone [8]. The three turbinates divide the nasal passage in three meati, respectively inferior, middle and superior ones. Here, the natural ostia of the anterior and posterior paranasal sinus can be found and also the output of the nasolacrimal duct. Turbinates host cavernous tissue that plays a pivotal role in the nasal cycle, warming the inspired air and creating a turbulent flow that gives the right sensation of breathing through the nose. This is also possible thanks to trigeminal branches that are particularly concentrated on the turbinates mucosa, namely, on the inferior one. Several studies have in fact showed how a surgical over-resection of the inferior turbinate may reduce this trigeminal sensation and alter the physiological turbulence of the air flow, resulting in a paradoxical sensation of nasal obstruction despite a wide nasal passage. This condition is known as Empty Nose Syndrome (ENS) [9, 10].

The mucosa covering the nasal cavities is classified as a respiratory pseudostratified columnar epithelium, made of several types of cells, namely, ciliated cells and mucinous cells. The latter are responsible for the production of a mucous biofilm able to trap air particles and microorganisms, while the cilia of the former move in a metacronal beat that sweeps the mucus toward the rhinopharynx.

1.1.3 Nasal Valves

Nasal valves, internal and external, are pivotal functional structures of the nose that must be acknowledged when performing a rhinoplasty (Fig. 1.3).

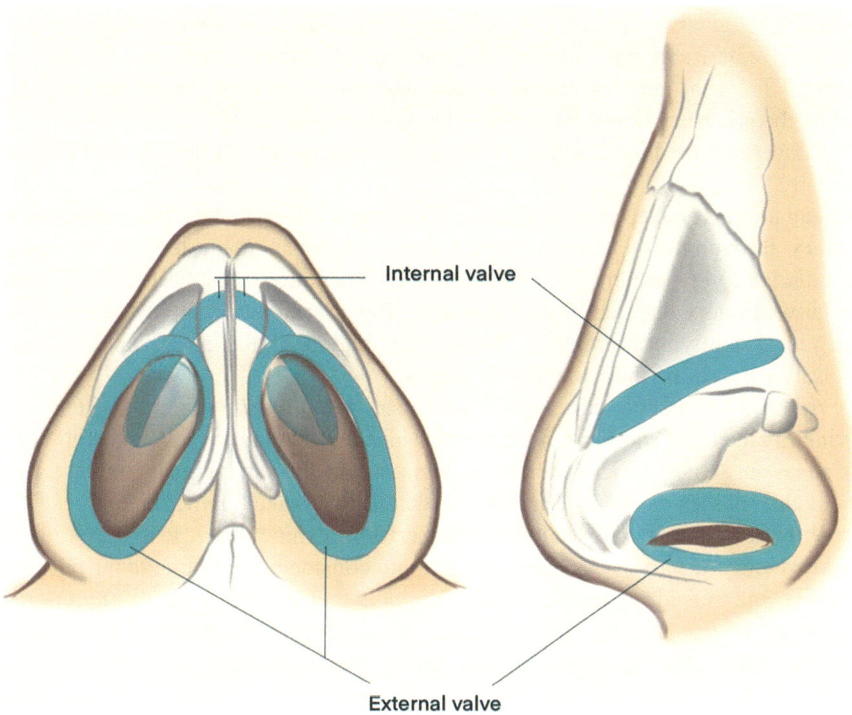

Fig. 1.3 External and internal nasal valves

The **internal nasal valve** (INV) area is bordered by the caudal septum, caudal portion of the upper lateral cartilages (ULCs), the head of the inferior turbinate and the remaining tissues of the surrounding pyriform aperture [11]. The INV is the narrowest portion of the nasal passage and therefore creates the greatest resistance to airflow [12]. The internal nasal valve angle should normally measure between 10° and 20°, albeit its shape and size depend on an individual's ethnicity. The middle vault, or the nasal valve area, is the most critical region for nasal breathing and small changes to the valve's cross-sectional area can exponentially increase airflow resistance [1].

The **external nasal valve** (ENV) is the region surrounded by the caudal septum and the lateral and medial crura of the lower lateral cartilages. It is located caudal to the INV [12].

1.1.4 Nasal Innervation and Blood Supply

The nose receives sensitive branches from the **trigeminal nerve** (V), specifically from the ophthalmic division (V1) and the maxillary division (V2). V1 divides into three main terminal branches: *lacrimal nerve, nasocilliary nerve* which ends in the external nasal nerve, and *frontal nerve* (supraorbital branch and supratroclear branch). V2 gives six branches: maxillary, sphenopalatine, zygomatic, superior posterior alveolar, superior anterior alveolar, lateral external nares and infraorbital nerve. The nasal muscles receive motor innervation from the **facial nerve** (VII), while the **olfactory nerve** (I) provides the sense of smell [1].

Concerning the blood supply, the nose is served both from the **internal carotid artery**, through the *ophthalmic artery* that gives the anterior and posterior ethmoidal arteries and terminates with the dorsal nasal artery, and the **external carotid artery**, through the *facial artery,* which ends with the angular artery, and the *sphenopalatine artery,* which divides into the nasoseptal artery (medial) and the lateral nasal wall artery directed to the turbinates. The arterial blood supply of these two carotid systems anastomize on the anterior region of the nasal septum (locus Valsalvae), forming the Kisselbach's plexus.

Albeit these anatomical cues are universal in the human race, facial features, primarily the nose, show specific characteristics that distinguish different ethnicities (Caucasian, Asian, African-American, etc.) and, in the same ethnic context, every individual possesses peculiar anatomical details that make him/her unique.

When evaluating a nose in order to perform a rhinoplasty, it is important to contextualize it into the face, taking into due consideration ethnic identity of the patient, and to analyse aesthetical and functional nasal units from different points of view. The *frontal view* allows the evaluation of nasal alignment, alar and nasal bridge width, nasal tip characteristics and tip rotation. *Side view* shows level and depth of the nasion, maximal dorsal projection, position of the pronasale, nasal length and nasal height, columellar show, tip rotation, extrinsic tip projection (defined as the nasofacial angle) (Fig. 1.4) and intrinsic tip projection, measured by drawing a line (parallel to the Frankfort horizontal line) from the centre of the alar crease to the pronasale. Then, a vertical line is drawn through the labrale superius (the most projecting part of the upper lip). Intrinsic tip projection is adequate if between 50 and 60% of the horizontal line lies anterior to the vertical line [13]. *Three-quarters views* allow a better evaluation of the profile line, tip rotation and projection. *Base view* is used to evidence alar base configuration, length and width of columella and alar flare. Dynamic views are also useful to understand the way the nose reacts during facial expressions (smiling and tilting the upper lip down) [13].

The combination of all these nasal measures gives place to countless possible nasal types, though some patterns are more common in specific ethnicities. Even if modern globalization, characterized by new pathways of migrations and more frequent interracial admixture, has made the attempts to define a clear racial facial morphology more and more difficult. In the past, there has been the tendency to divide noses into three groups [14]: **platyrrhine**, with small nasal bones, low radix and wide dorsum, flat midvault, decreased tip support and projection, acute nasolabial angle and thick soft tissue envelope (typical of African population); **leptorrhine**, with higher nasal radix, narrower dorsum, well projected tip and slightly obtuse nasolabial angle, thin soft tissue envelope (typical of Caucasian people); **mesorrhine**, which shows intermediate characteristics between leptorrhine and platyrrhine (typical of Hispanic population) [15].

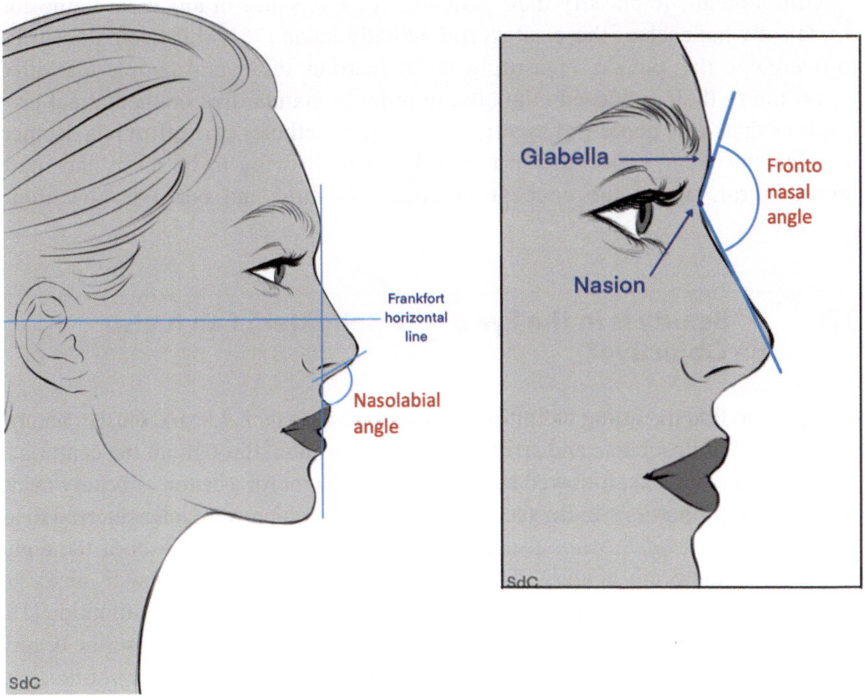

Fig. 1.4 Nasolabial angle and frontonasal angle

1.2 The Concept of Race and Ethnicity and Its Limits

Rhinoplasty is nowadays one of the most common facial plastic surgery procedures, required not only for functional restoration of the nose but also, and namely, for aesthetic purposes.

When it comes to the pursuit of beauty, though, many factors influence both the patient's desires and the surgeon's attitude to fulfil them. First of all, beauty is far from being a universal concept; even if we all subconsciously recognize it, in fact, it's paradoxically hard to confine it to strict objective definitions. The very notion of beauty changes from different cultures and even in the same cultural context, perception of it remains deeply subjective.

In this area of tension between what a person perceives as normal or beautiful and the need to conform to some ideal appearance stands the concept of race and ethnicity. These terms refer to one of the most elusive and mysterious aspects of social structures yet one of the most fundamental variables in defining mankind. While race is considered an objective term, ethnicity has a more subjective meaning; it tends to include race, but it also depends on culture, language, religion and nationality. Nasal surgeons widely accept the concept of race and commonly use racial categories such as "Asian", "African-American", "Caucasian" and

"Mediterranean" to classify their patients, in the absence of any clear definition or idea of what each of these categories actually mean [16]. Many scientists tried to overcome this puzzle, measuring facial features of several people classified according to their supposed ethnicity, in order to standardize mathematical proportions that were perceived as attractive [17], nonetheless the effort has deemed to be inconsistent, especially in a world that is growing to be more and more multicultural, where the concept of beauty is fluid and peculiar now more than ever.

1.3 If "Beauty Is in the Eye of the Beholder", Can It also Be Objective?

The quest to find the fitting definition of beauty, despite its fickle and elusive nature, has engaged philosophers and artists first, scientists later, throughout the centuries.

The ancient Greeks, followed by the Romans, sought for a canon of beauty made of harmonic proportions in the face and in the body, which were later referred to as the classical or *golden ratio*, also called *phi*, by the European artists of the eighteenth and nineteenth century. This canon of attractiveness seemed to apply to Caucasian population, even if later scientific studies denied such an assumption [18, 19]. This ideal canon of beauty, moreover, was even more unfitted to describe beauty in non-Caucasian subjects, despite the attempt to adapt the so-called *phi-mask* to different ethnicities [20].

Anthropologists in the nineteenth century were then interested in describing the various shapes of the nose they encountered in different populations around the world and so they developed what is known as the *nasal index* as a means of describing the pyriform aperture of the skull. It was a ratio of the maximum breadth of the anterior orifice (pyriform aperture) of the nose to its maximum length [21]. This kind of index soon proved to be unable to describe the shape of the nose, beautiful or not, since it was based on cephalometric measures, on the skull, and not on the soft tissues that actually compose the most of the aesthetic part of the nose and the face itself [16]. These tissues were instead taken into consideration by *anthropometric measures* of the nose and the face, which are commonly used nowadays to describe the shape of the nose and to predict the outcome of surgery [17, 22, 23].

Given the failure of most objective measurements to describe ideal beauty, especially in a multiethnic context; current trends in rhinoplasty are prompted towards the concept of beauty as *averageness*. In 1979 Symons carried out a study where multiple single faces were artistically melted into a composite face. The more faces were used, the more the composite one became increasingly closer to the average and was perceived as more attractive across multiple cultures [18, 24]. This can be explained with the fact that composite figures tend to eliminate the most peculiar details, increasing symmetry and, therefore, attractiveness. In other words, beauty and symmetry increase with increased averageness of facial features [18]. This would suggest that facial beauty is an objective and cross-cultural concept and even more interesting data reveal how slight deviation from the average on some individual characteristics can actually increase beauty and attractiveness [18].

1.4 Mainstream Beauty and Globalization

Never before occidental society has experienced the same tendency to cultural and ethnic admixture as nowadays. The increased frequency of interracial exchanges in a globalized multicultural context has made the concept of beauty and attractiveness somehow fluid and ever changing under the influence of a storm of continuous aesthetical inputs that come from the extensive use of social media. Beauty is now mainstream, multiethnic and desirable, thus both men and women of every age and status are pushed to seek for surgical facial remodelling, often nasal shape correction, in order to reach a receding ideal of attractiveness and self-satisfaction.

1.5 Patient's Expectations in the Mediterranean Area

The modern demand for beauty has increased the frequency of aesthetic surgery, namely, rhinoplasty. Therefore, facial plastic surgeons operating in different geographical areas are nowadays facing an augmented request for nasal shape correction, coming from a more variegated population. While the same surgical techniques could apply for every nose in the past, the current tendency is to customize surgery to the individual request, taking into account primarily the patient's expectations but also giving due consideration to his/her ethnical and cultural background, in order to obtain a satisfactory, ethnic preserving outcome. It must be told that specific geographical areas most frequently show recurrent patterns of nasal defects and, therefore, corrections (Figs. 1.5 and 1.6). Thus, the attempt to identify archetypes of nasal imperfection, so to develop the most fitting surgical solution for each. Palma et al. [13] focused their attention on the Mediterranean area, codifying four nasal archetypes:

- Drooping nose: It's basically a long nose with convex dorsum and normal nasal bridge width. Alar ridge may go lateral to the medial cantal lines.
- Strong, prominent nose: It's characterized by a significantly convex dorsum with wider nasal bridge and deep nasion. Nasal length is normal, but nostril asymmetry is common, due to caudal septal deviation. Tip is overprojected and columellar base is generally wide.
- Heavy nose: It has thick skin, dorsal hyperprojection, tip ptosis and hypoprojection, wider alar width, short and wide columella.
- Northern nose: It is a long and high nose, with narrow nasal bridge, dorsal convexity and thin alae.

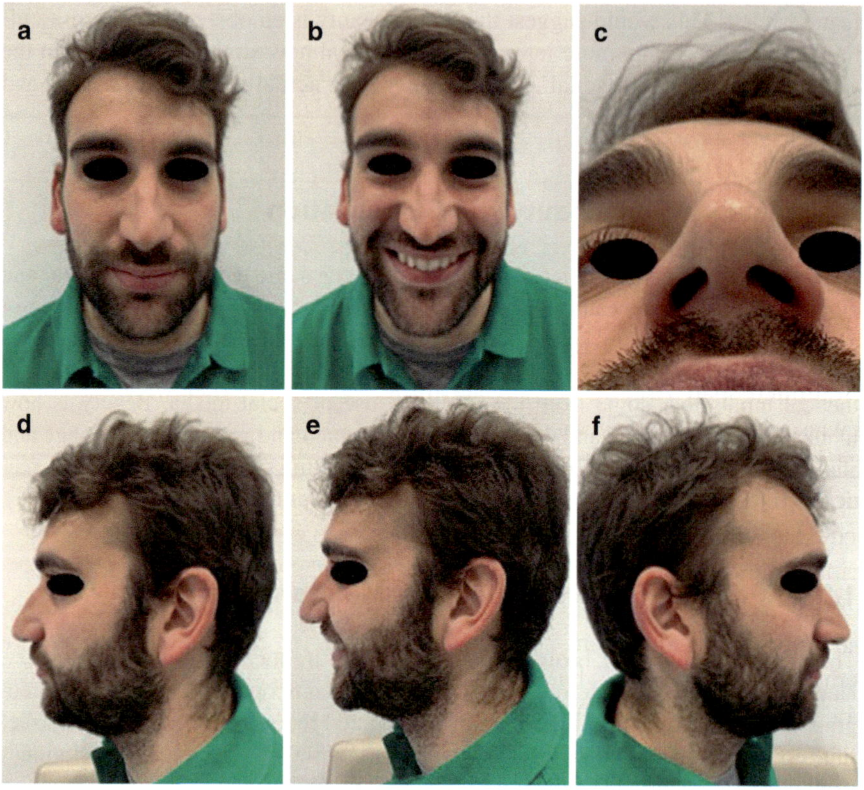

Fig. 1.5 Typical case of Mediterranean nose, with strong and prominent nasal bones (**a**), osteo-cartilaginous convexity of nasal dorsum, augmented alar width, reduced nasolabial angle and tip rotation (**d**–**f**) and dynamic tip ptosis, which is more visible during smile (**b**–**e**)

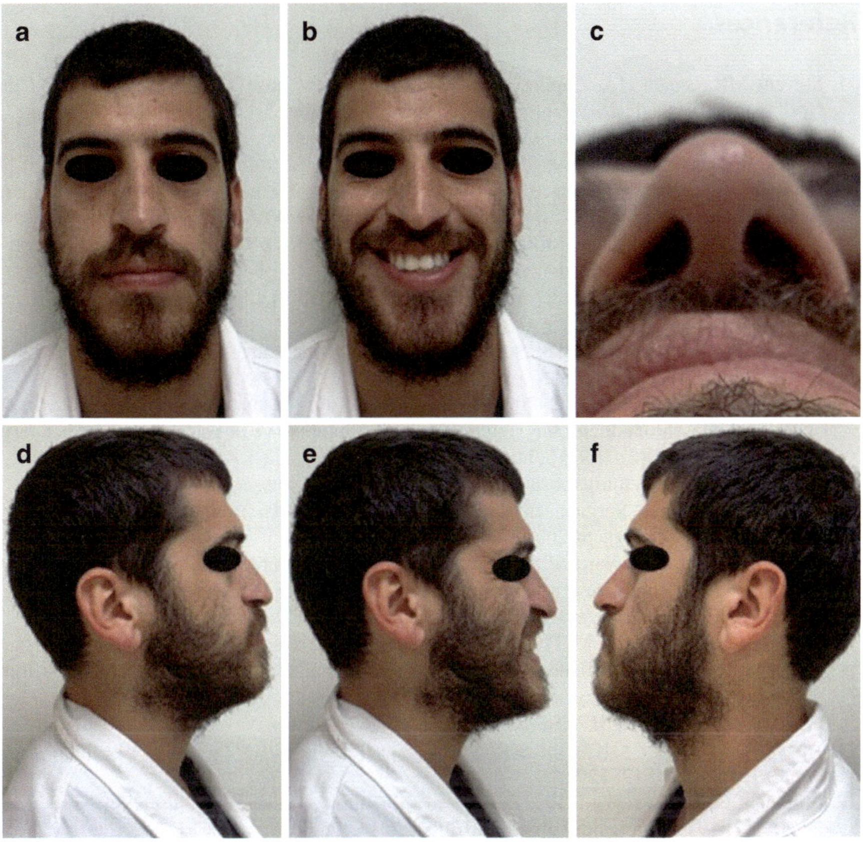

Fig. 1.6 Typical case of Mediterranean nose with acute nasolabial angle, reduced tip rotation, static tip ptosis (**a**–**f**)

1.6 Conclusions

The requests of patients seeking for cosmetic surgery are changing day by day, as the society we live in becomes increasingly multiethnic and multicultural, leaving old facial beauty standards behind. Thus, facial plastic surgeons approaching patients who ask for a rhinoplasty must learn to explore patient's ethnic, racial and cultural background, in addition to the patient's personal desires and expected outcomes. Current trend in rhinoplasty is to preserve a more natural look and to harmonize one's peculiar facial features, seeking for symmetry without affecting one's ethnic identity. A thorough consultation between surgeon and patient is key to tailor every intervention on the specific individual, with clear premises and defined surgical goals that are to maximize the chances of both patient and surgeon postoperative satisfaction.

References

1. Stevens MR, Emam HA. Applied surgical anatomy of the nose. Oral Maxillofac Surg Clin North Am. 2012;24(1):25–38. https://doi.org/10.1016/j.coms.2011.10.007.
2. Kasperbauer JL, Kern EB. Nasal valve physiology. Implications in nasal surgery. Otolaryngol Clin North Am. 1987;20(4):699–719.
3. Pitanguy I. Surgical importance of a dermocartilaginous ligament in bulbous noses. Plast Reconstr Surg. 1965;36:247–53. https://doi.org/10.1097/00006534-196508000-00014.
4. Giacomini PG, Boccieri A, Moretti A, Rosati V, Flora B, Di Girolamo S. Nasal tip rotation by exclusive superficial musculoaponeurotic system deep medial ligament management: an objective evaluation. Ann Plast Surg. 2020;85(1):12–7. https://doi.org/10.1097/SAP.0000000000002319.
5. Letourneau A, Daniel RK. The superficial musculoaponeurotic system of the nose. Plast Reconstr Surg. 1988;82(1):48–57.
6. Saban Y, Andretto Amodeo C, Hammou JC, Polselli R. An anatomical study of the nasal superficial musculoaponeurotic system: surgical applications in rhinoplasty. Arch Facial Plast Surg. 2008;10(2):109–15. https://doi.org/10.1001/archfaci.10.2.109.
7. Hollinshead WH. Anatomy for surgeons: the head and neck. Subsequent edition. Harper; 1982.
8. Oneal RM, Beil RJ. Surgical anatomy of the nose. Clin Plast Surg. 2010;37(2):191–211. https://doi.org/10.1016/j.cps.2009.12.011.
9. Gill AS, Said M, Tollefson TT, Steele TO. Update on empty nose syndrome: disease mechanisms, diagnostic tools, and treatment strategies. Curr Opin Otolaryngol Head Neck Surg. 2019;27(4):237–42. https://doi.org/10.1097/MOO.0000000000000544.
10. Di Girolamo S, Guerrieri M, Flora B, Passali F. Surgical treatment of empty nose syndrome: inferior turbinate reconstruction using intranasal mucosal flaps. In: Atrophic rhinitis—from voluptuary nasal pathology to the empty nose syndrome. 2020. pp. 117–125. https://doi.org/10.1007/978-3-030-51705-2_11.
11. Apaydin F. Nasal valve surgery. Facial Plast Surg. 2011;27(2):179–91. https://doi.org/10.1055/s-0030-1271298.
12. Friedman O, Cekic E, Gunel C. Functional rhinoplasty. Facial Plast Surg Clin North Am. 2017;25(2):195–9. https://doi.org/10.1016/j.fsc.2016.12.004.
13. Palma P, Bignami M, Delù G, De Bernardi F, Castelnuovo P. Rhinoplasty for the Mediterranean nose. Facial Plast Surg. 2003;19(3):279–94. https://doi.org/10.1055/s-2003-43163.
14. Cobo R. Ethnic rhinoplasty. HNO. 2018;66(1):6–14. https://doi.org/10.1007/s00106-017-0452-7.
15. Patel PN, Most SP. Concepts of facial aesthetics when considering ethnic rhinoplasty. Otolaryngol Clin North Am. 2020;53(2):195–208. https://doi.org/10.1016/j.otc.2019.12.001.
16. Leong SC, Eccles R. Race and ethnicity in nasal plastic surgery: a need for science. Facial Plast Surg. 2010;26(2):63–8. https://doi.org/10.1055/s-0030-1253505.
17. Farkas LG, Katic MJ, Forrest CR, et al. International anthropometric study of facial morphology in various ethnic groups/races. J Craniofac Surg. 2005;16(4):615–46. https://doi.org/10.1097/01.scs.0000171847.58031.9e.
18. Weeks DM, Thomas JR. Beauty in a multicultural world. Facial Plast Surg Clin North Am. 2014;22(3):337–41. https://doi.org/10.1016/j.fsc.2014.04.005.
19. Pallett PM, Link S, Lee K. New "golden" ratios for facial beauty. Vision Res. 2010;50(2):149–54. https://doi.org/10.1016/j.visres.2009.11.003.
20. Sturm-O'Brien AK, Brissett AEA, Brissett AE. Ethnic trends in facial plastic surgery. Facial Plast Surg. 2010;26(2):69–74. https://doi.org/10.1055/s-0030-1253496.
21. Williams RI. The nasal index; anthropological and clinical. Ann Otol Rhinol Laryngol. 1956;65(1):171–89. https://doi.org/10.1177/000348945606500116.
22. Farkas LG, Hreczko TA, Deutsch CK. Objective assessment of standard nostril types—a morphometric study. Ann Plast Surg. 1983;11(5):381–9.

23. El-Hakim H, Crysdale WS, Abdollel M, Farkas LG. A study of anthropometric measures before and after external septoplasty in children: a preliminary study. Arch Otolaryngol Head Neck Surg. 2001;127(11):1362–6. https://doi.org/10.1001/archotol.127.11.1362.
24. Symons D. The evolution of human sexuality. eweb:26542. 1979. https://repository.library.georgetown.edu/handle/10822/782278. Accessed 20 Apr 2021.

2 Nasal Biotypes in the Mediterranean Area

Antonio Moretti

2.1 Introduction

The Mediterranean area includes a heterogeneous and large variety of ethnic groups with an even wider variability of features considering the different traditions, customs, language, religion, and social status. The main feature that the various populations have in common can certainly be found in a singular anthropological origin, which is universally known as the Caucasian race [1]. Despite the melting pot and the ethnical differencies, throughout the evolving ages this common denominator has led to identify some physiognomic aspects which have become distinctive features and peculiar traits of the Caucasian ethnicity. The facial phenotype represents one of the somatic traits which identify the races of Caucasian origin; in particular the nose has been widely examined by anthropologists and ethnographers due to its specific morphology. Throughout the evolving ages, the nose, being described and represented within the figurative arts in the work of various writers and artists such as painters and sculptors, has been also the subject of study for medical disciplines eventually becoming an interpretative aspect to identify the character and personality of the individual [2, 3].

The classical paradigm of the Mediterranean nose is represented by the general concept of beauty, embodied by the masterpieces in the Greek sculptural arts, in the European Renaissaince arts and in the Neoclassical arts. Although currently there is no single standard model of reference for beauty, in the facial plastic surgery as well as in modern rhynoplasty, the canons of beauty are increasingly shifting from the neoclassical parameters to become more and more dependent on the patient's wishes and personal satisfaction [4, 5]. Although this direction can lead to justify a

A. Moretti (✉)
Department of Innovative Technologies in Medicine and Odontoiatrics, ENT Section, "G. d'Annunzio" University of Chieti-Pescara, Chieti, Italy
e-mail: amoretti@unich.it

P. G. Giacomini (ed.), *Mediterranean Rhinoplasty*,
https://doi.org/10.1007/978-3-031-05551-5_2

trajectory of analysis and a surgical approach that are linked to the personal satisfaction on the part of the patient, it is not possible to ignore certain specific rules and principles based on anthropometric, racial, ethnic, and gender parameters deemed necessary to obtain a result which has to be harmonious, natural and proportionate with the rest of the face. Globalization has imposed a standardized model of beauty but in rhinoplasty surgery it is essential to take into account the physiognomic and ethnic characteristics of the individual.

In the Mediterranean Basin, it is possible to distinguish three geographical areas: the European region in the north, which includes Spain, France, Italy, Greece, and a small part of Turkey, the Asian region in the east including Turkey, Lebanon, and Israel and the African region in the south including Egypt, Lybia, Algeria, and Morocco. In the present report, therefore, the pathognomic morphological typologies of the Mediterranean nasal biotype will be analyzed, stigmatizing the most frequent anatomical-structural disharmonies such as a prominent nasal dorsum, a bulbous tip, and a rinomegalia that usually represents the main demand for modification.

2.2 Historical Overview

Since ancient times the nose, in particular, has been a subject of significant interest in the Mediterranean area. In fact, it is known that the first documents that report news on the nose surgery are traceable to the Egyptian civilization and date back to 3500 years B.C, as reported in the papyrus found by Edwin Smith, which is now kept in the room of rare books of the New York Academy of Medecine [6]. However, from an historical point of view, the most relevant anthropometric studies on the nose are mainly ascribed to the evaluations of proportions and morphology of Leonardo da Vinci and Albrecht Dürer, to the physiognomic evaluations of Giovanni Battista della Porta contained in his work "*De Humana Physiognomonia*" written in 1598 and to the biometric evaluations of Alphonse Bertillon [7].

Thanks to these studies and other researches, it has been possible to establish some anthropometric and phenotypic parameters which characterise the main races. But also the work of Paul Topinard in 1878 contributed to identify and describe the "cephalometric nasal index" [7, 8]. This index is obtained from the percentage ratio between the width and the height of the external nose: The width corresponds to the maximum distance between the lateral rim of the nasal alae while the length is the measure between the subnasal point and the nasofrontal suture. This ratio is calculated by multiplying the width of the nose by 100 and dividing the product by the height. The nasal index allows to categorize narrow or leptorrhine noses (index less than 70) or medium or mesorrhine noses (index between 70 and 85) and wide-broad or platyrrhine noses (index greater than 85). Paul Topinard and Charles Henri Collignon identified three groups of nasal indices which corresponded respectively to the White (Caucasian), Yellow (Asian-Oriental), and Black (African) races [7, 9, 10]. According to some anthropologists and in some countries, in the past this index was one of the elements identifying a hierarchical system, which corresponded to a high status for leptorrhine nasal shapes and to a low status for platyrrhine nasal shake [7].

Nasal index and the shape of the nose are key elements to classify human races. In anthropometry, a leptorrhine nose identifies the category of nasal index which includes relatively tall and narrow noses, which are widespread features among the European Caucasian population and are especially typical of the Mediterranean race and the Dinaric subtype. This last one is a subcategory of the Europid (White-Caucasian) race and, according to Jan Czekanowski, is a mixed biotype consisting of the Nordic race and the Mediterranean race. In the first half of the twentieth century, the Dinaric or Adriatic race indicated the Balkan populations, especially the inhabitants of South-Eastern Europe, showing the dominant phenotypical characteristics such as a prominent strong nose. This nasal feature, also known as "the Roman Nose," was widespread among Italians, Southern French, Spanish, and Portuguese who were classified as Dinaric race. It is a long, prominent, convex, and aquiline nose (leptorrhine) which is also identified with an undefined tip often pointing downwards [7].

According to the classical categorization in Europe, but above all in Italy, four types of conformation of the nasal pyramid are taken as reference: the Greek nose (Venus de Milo), the straight and pronounced Roman nose (Caesar Augustus), the hooked nose (Dante), and the saddle nose (Socrates) [7]. From a more detailed analysis of these main classical physiognomic categories, it is possible to observe a wider morphological and anatomical variability of the nasal biotype in the Mediterranean Basin.

2.3 The Mediterranean Nose

The most common morphological and physiognomic feature of the Mediterranean nose is marked with a dorsal projection of the pyramid; usually the tip has a boxy or bulbous shape depending on skin thickness, with a general presence of rinomegalia and the consequent necessity to satisfy, in the majority of cases, the request for reductive rhynoplasty. Despite the Mediterranean nasal phenotype has some characteristics in common with the Caucasian-derived biotpype, it is surprising to observe how many variants can be found in different ethnic groups and within the same ethnicity.

From an anthropometric perspective, the nasal index and the main structures to be taken as references are the height of the nasion and the nasofrontal angle, the bony dorsum with the nasal bridge, the rhinion and the cartilagineous dorsum, the tip with the conformation and orientation of the alar cartilages, the nasal base, the columella and the shape of the nostrils, the nasolabial angle, and the type and thickness of the skin. These parameters have allowed to classify and identify six main ethnical groups: African, Asian, Mediterannean, Middle Eastern, Northern European, and Latin American (Mestizo). There are significant differences in nasal proportions among the various ethnic groups but there is little evidence that the shape and proportions of the nose have an impact on physiology and pathology.

Nasal variations in the proportions together with the nasal index are the best differentiation parameters with respect to ethnic or racial categories, which are relevant in aestethics and reconstruction surgery. On the contrary, shape and size assume little importance in rhinology research [11, 12]. The most recent anthropometric researches on the shape and size of the nose are due to the studies of Farkas who has identified and discussed the main racial differencies related to the byometric measurement obtained from different populations and within various ethnic groups [13–17].

The Mediterranean nose has a prominent or markedly convex dorsum (Fig. 2.1), compared to the nasion that is considered to be the lowest point of the nasofrontal angle and is filled to varying degrees with subcutaneous soft tissues and cutaneous tissues which are thick at this level.

The nasal bridge, which can be normal or narrow (Fig. 2.2), has a thinner skin covering on the bony dorsum, the rhinion and the cartilaginous dorsum. Usually, the nasal tip has a variable complex structure and an indefinite shape with square and wide alar cartilages at the level of the domes (Fig. 2.3), sometimes malpositioned and vertically oriented in the lateral crura [18].

The tip may also be ptotic due to the weakness of the supporting structures or to the strong depressor nasi septi muscle but, sometimes, it may have a good position with a proper rotation and projection (Fig. 2.4). In some cases, the strong traction of the nasal tip from the depressor muscle of the nasal septum may emphasize the ptosis of the tip and the dorsal convexity (Fig. 2.5).

The nostrils are vertical and have a normal or narrow base, the skin can vary from moderately thick to thin, sometimes it can be greasy and the nasolabial angle can vary from normal to acute. The ideal range of this important angle is comprised between 95 and 105° in women and between 90 and 95 in men.

One of the biggest complaints for some typical Mediterranean patients who present an unpleasant drooping-amorphous tip, a prominent dorsum and a redundancy of soft tissues at the junction of the lateral cartilages, is the length of the nose combined with the subjective perception of a "large and big nose" at the level of the scroll area and the tip (Fig. 2.6). This rinomegalia is due to the strong osteocartilaginous support in the higher two third of the nose and to the weakness of the supporting fibrocartilaginous structures combined with a thicker skin in the lower third [19].

These anatomical, structural and physiognomic parameters are even more marked in some countries of the Mediterranean area, in particular in the Middle Eastern and North African basins, especially concerning the dorsum which shows a wider bridge and convexity that extends, in some cases, up to the nose radix, with a thicker skin [20, 21]. The differences are even more marked than in North European countries where the dorsum is less pronounced or even concave, the nasolabial angle is more obtuse with a more prominent nasal spine and a thinner skin [22].

The skin has a fundamental relevance in some races and, in this regard, this anatomical aspect cannot be ignored when evaluating nasal morphology which represents a distinctive ethnical trait in some populations. Some scientists have studied and classified the skin characteristics and its thickness in the nose is considered to be a relevant risk factor and a fundamental prognostic factor for determining rhinoplasty success

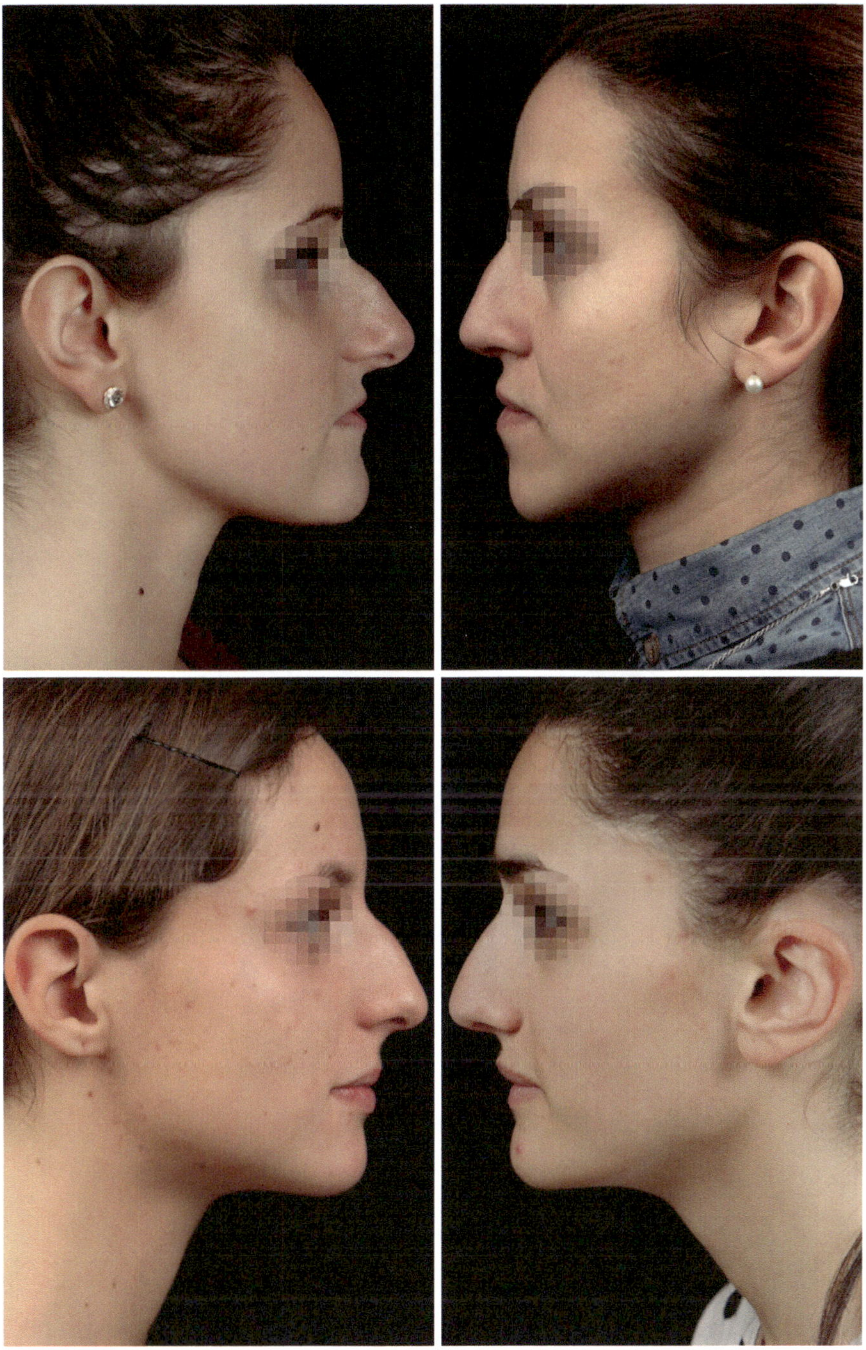

Fig. 2.1 Mediterranean nasal biotypes: prominent nasal dorsum in Italian women

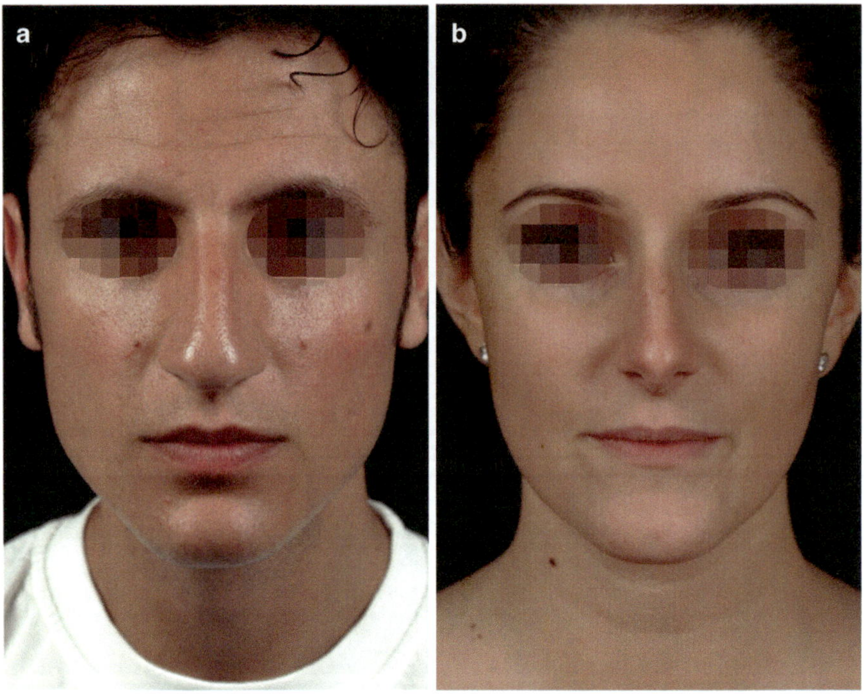

Fig. 2.2 (**a**) Normal nasal bridge. (**b**) Narrow nasal bridge

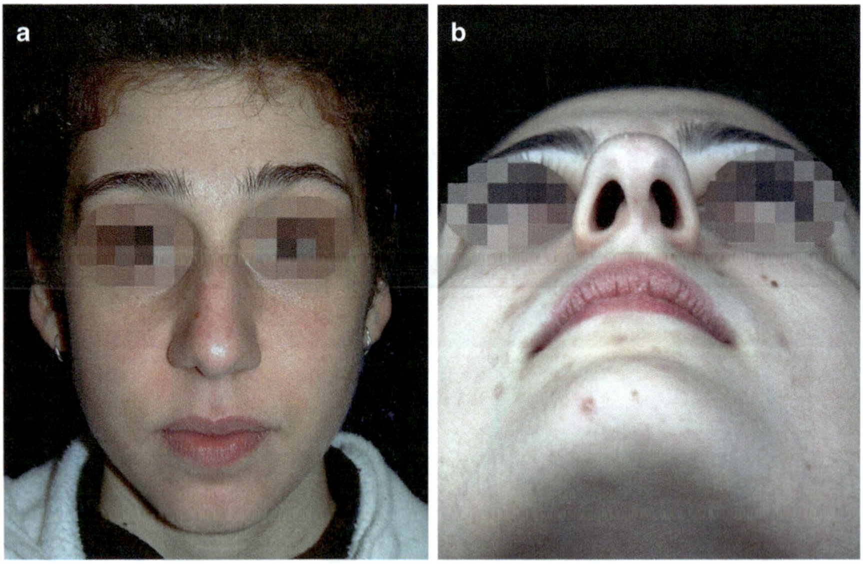

Fig. 2.3 (**a**) Broad and undefined shape of the nasal tip. (**b**) Boxy nasal tip

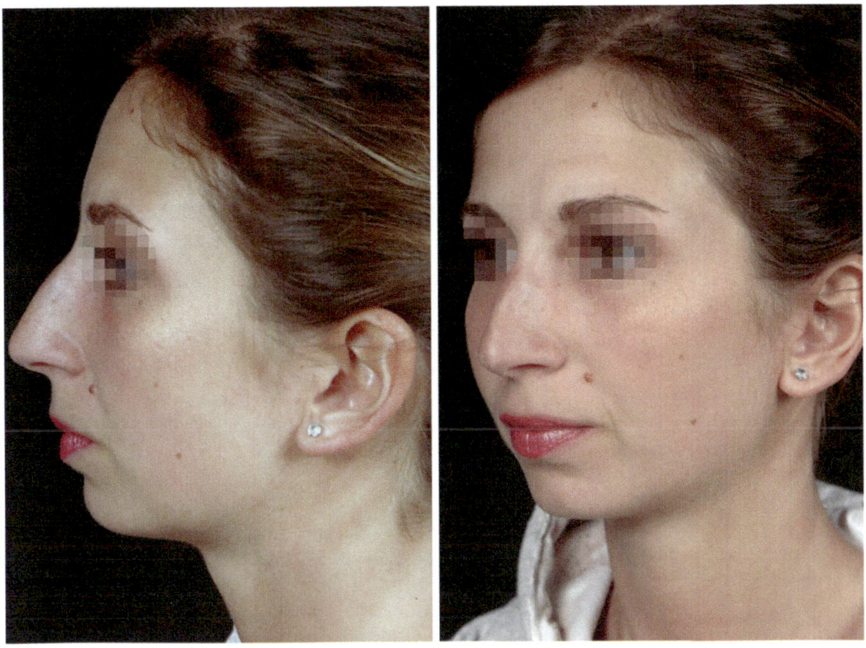

Fig. 2.4 Correct position of the tip with a normal nasolabial angle

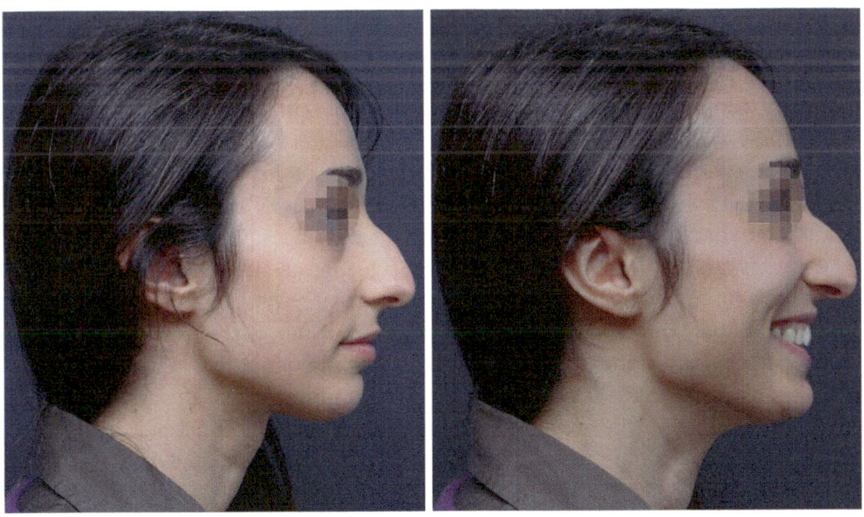

Fig. 2.5 Ptotic nasal tip and convexity of the dorsum in static and dynamic view

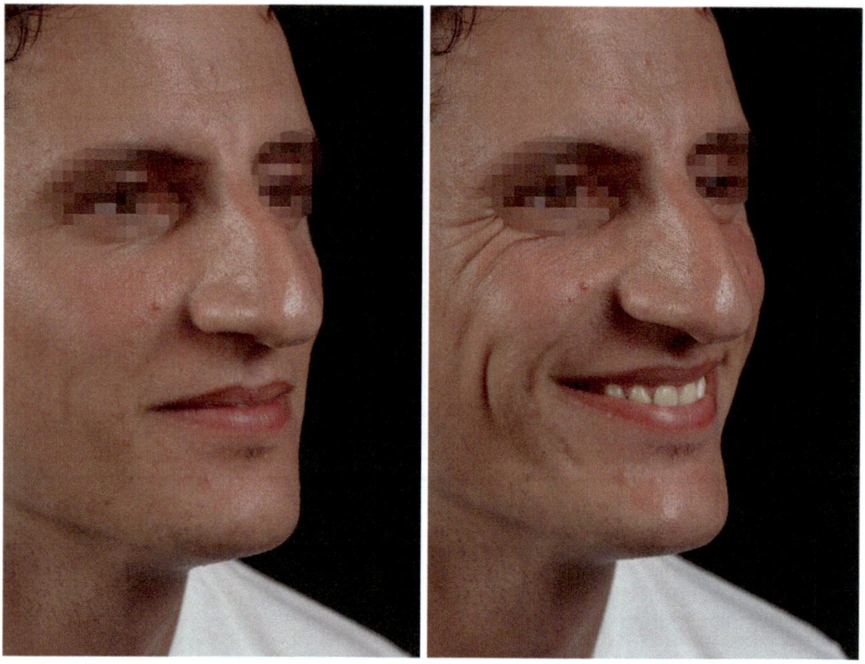

Fig. 2.6 Mediterranean nasal biotypes: rinomegalia with thick skin

[23–26]. Several factors affect the variations in nasal skin thickness such as sex, race, genetics, and ethnicity of the patient. Indeed, the impact of each of them is still unclear. Generally, people who have an extremely thick nasal skin have a more porous overall skin quality, which could affect the nasal appearance after surgery, whereas people who have thinner nasal skin more distinctly show the shape of the underlying cartilages and the nasal framework. Therefore, some minor deformities of the primary or reshaped nasal framework might cause visible and unwanted changes.

Only few studies have examined the impact of nasal skin thickness on the aesthetics results of rhinoplasty. The Mediterannean nose has thick skin at the nasofrontal angle which becomes thinner above the dorsum, thickens again on the tip and becomes thinner above the columella so it is important to evaluate and recognize nasal skin thickness before planning and executing rhinoplasty, thus contributing to the success of the surgery. There are several tools to measure and classify nasal skin thickness but the most widely used ones include some types of calipers (micrometer screw gauge and skinfold), and imaging methods such as standard radiography, ultrasound, and computed tomography (CT) [26]. The skinfold caliper is the most widely used technique for measuring skin thickness due to its accessibility, high feasibility and low cost but its precision has been questioned. On the contrary, CT is the most sensitive and reliable technique because it may depict and measure soft tissues with greater clarity and accuracy [26].

Nasal skin and soft tissues thickness and their objective assessment have a relevant impact on the procedural planning and postoperative outcomes in rhinoplasty surgery. The knowledge of skin thickness variations by demographic group and the single individual, especially in the different subsites, proves to be of great aid to surgeons. These subsites can be evaluated with high-resolution CT images and the ethnic-racial differencies in nasal skin thickness in a single patient may significantly affect the development and planning of the surgical strategies and postoperative outcomes rhinoplasty [25]. Even the type of skin lining of the nose, if it not carefully evaluated, may cause dissatisfaction with respect to the aestethic expectations of the patients. Facial skin is generally classified as dry, normal, and oily. This kind of classification, however, may somewhat result in an arbitrary judgment because the skin type does not correspond to the amount of the secretion of sebum itself. Therefore, this classification has a very limited value and should be re-evaluated applying an objective and standardized analytical instrument capable of quantitative measurement such as a sebumeter, a device which allows to measure sebum levels in any part of the skin [24]. Nasal skin sebum levels may affect periorbital edema and ecchymosis after rhinoplasty; therefore, the ability to predict the effects of the types of nasal skin on these problems may help surgeons to inform the patients in a more correct way [27].

2.4 Ethnic Remarks in Rhinoplasty

There are many reports about rhinoplasty procedures within the medical literature, especially those related to the technique of correction of paradigmatic nasal types which show phenotypical features of Caucasian origin. But, in recent years, the diffusion of plastic and aesthetic surgery has contributed to spread the interest in this procedure even in populations and ethnic groups with highly different and peculiar nasal phenotypical features to the point of coining the definition of the so-called *ethnic rhinoplasty*. In this regard, there is an increasingly frequent demand for personalised rhinoplasty. The ability of the rhinoplasty surgeon must be therefore oriented towards a "tailored rhinoplasty" that takes into account the racial, phenotypic and biometric type of the patient to be treated by applying both an individualized and analytical evaluation and a specific surgical plan adapted to the patient's goals.

Cultural homogenization through the rise of mass media, the improvement of both surgical techniques and the results of rhinoplasty have brought to a more and more widespread diffusion of rhinoplasty among non-Caucasian patients. While in the past the demand for rhinoplasty was especially linked to aesthetic canons and to the typical features of a Caucasian-looking nose, today, despite the implications of globalization, ethnical and cultural differencies are the most important aspects affecting the perception of nasal deformities and, accordingly, the typology of modification demanded. These extra-surgical parameters depend on different aspects such as the patient's background and expectations of the family members, the prevailing cultural models imposed by mass media, the level of racial identification but also on external elements such as the perception of physical attractiveness [28] and the external observers' reaction [29]. When planning a rhinoplasty operation, the nasal aestethics must be considered within the context of race, ethnicity and culture. For nasal types of Caucasian-Mediterranean origin, careful preoperation analysis of nasal and facial features that contributes to having a pleasant nose is based on well-defined and standardized neoclassical canons which are validated by a number of reports within the existing literature. On the contrary, it is not possible to apply these models to non-Caucasian patients since the profound anatomical and morphological differencies do not allow surgeons to adopt universal rhinoplasty procedures among the races; indeed these must be aligned to the ethnic biotype and to the expectations of the individual, thus representing a real challenge for rhinoplasty surgeons in the approach to ethnic rhinoplasty. For this reason, more and more studies on the nose have focused on nasal and facial aestethics models which are essential to approach face plastic surgery and ethnic rhinoplasty.

When analyzing rhinoplasty in ethnic patients, it is necessary to determine their aesthetic goals, which, in many cases, might deviate from the stereotype of the "North European nose." It is, therefore, necessary for rhinoplasty surgeons to satisfy the expectations and wishes of patients by refining the techniques and surgical skills and aligning them to the increasingly and various requests for changes in nasal morphology. A skilled and experienced rhinoplasty surgeon should be able to adapt nose surgery to the physical nuances of the various ethnic subtypes. Furthermore, by virtue of the above-mentioned aspects and following the indications and principles established in rhinoplasty, you can expect a pleasant and harmonious nose without radically altering the ethnicity [30, 31].

The transformation of this rapidly changing world, which appears to be increasingly globalized due to ubiquitous immigration, with increasingly blurred geographical, racial, and economical boundaries, has greatly modified both the conception of ethnic identity and individual perspectives and beauty standards. In this connection, the nasal pyramid which is placed in the center of the face, on the midline, has a crucial importance in the judgment of the individual's attractiveness and plays a significant cosmetic role in the appearance of the whole face as it gives it harmony and balance [16, 17]. Although "contamination" among races and various ethnic groups is unstoppable, this introductory chapter analyzes the main aspects of the Mediterranean nose and the osteocartilaginous anatomical strucures which identify a nasal biotype with neoclassical canons and proportions of beauty.

2.5 Mediterranean Rhinoplasty

In the Mediterranean area, it is possible to observe different nasal phenotypes sharing common structural features: the ethnical groups in the South and South East show stronger nasal structures, especially regarding the dorsal prominence and a more marked skin thickness compared to the smaller nasal hump and the thinnest layer of the skin which identify Northern populations. In some cases, these typical features of the Mediterranean nose may appear unduly accentuated and reflect a real nasal deformity. In the case of primary surgery, it is necessary to consider the patient's demands for change, in compliance with the canons of the Mediterranean ethnic beauty. Usually, when dealing with a reductive rhinoplasty it is necessary to seek for the harmony of the nose with the whole face without altering the unique features of the ethnic biotype.

The surgical approaches must be selected from time to time by applying the most appropriate techniques to correct the various defects according to each individual case trying to preserve, as much as possible, the supporting structures. A skilled and experienced rhinoplasty surgeon should be able to adapt his/her work to the nuances of the various ethnic subtypes. In some cases, the use of cartilage grafts can prove to be very useful in achieving stability over time. From an anatomical and morphological point of view, the shape of the nose and its relations with the whole face greatly differ among races and genders.

Since anthropometric parameters vary with age, sex, and ethnic origin, several authors have attempted to report normative values that can be used as a reference, especially for the Mediterranean nose of Caucasian origin [11, 32, 33]. Anthropometric measurements might help rhinoplasty surgeons to perfom objective and quantitative evaluations of deformities, executing preoperative and postoperative assessments and deciding on proper surgical strategies [11, 34]. These measurements can be obtained from four methods: direct anthropometry (direct measurement), photogrammetry (analysis of photographies), cephalometry (imaging), and three-dimensional anthropometry [14, 32, 35]. Among these methods, digital standardized photographic analysis is considered to be the best, faster, cheaper, and more practical tool to quantify the nasal index and measures [32, 35, 36]. A dorsal hump, a bulbous tip and, in general, a rinomegalia are the most evident deformities of a Mediterranean nose to be corrected, which appear to be more marked in the male gender. The most common request is the reduction of the hump with a straight or slightly concave dorsum to avoid any kind of sagging, especially in men (Fig. 2.7). From an aesthetic point of view, what is mandatory in rhinoplasty

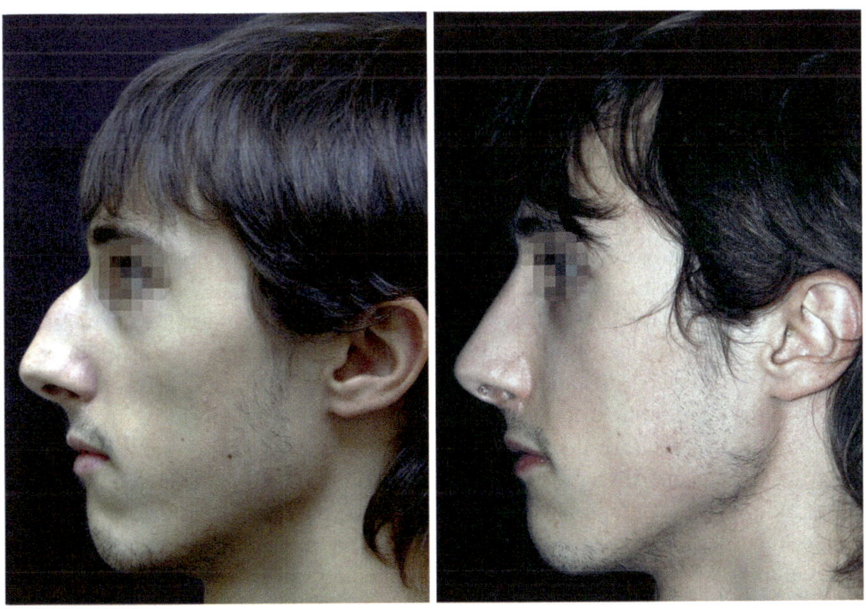

Fig. 2.7 Correction of a dorsal hump with a straight postoperative aspect of the dorsum

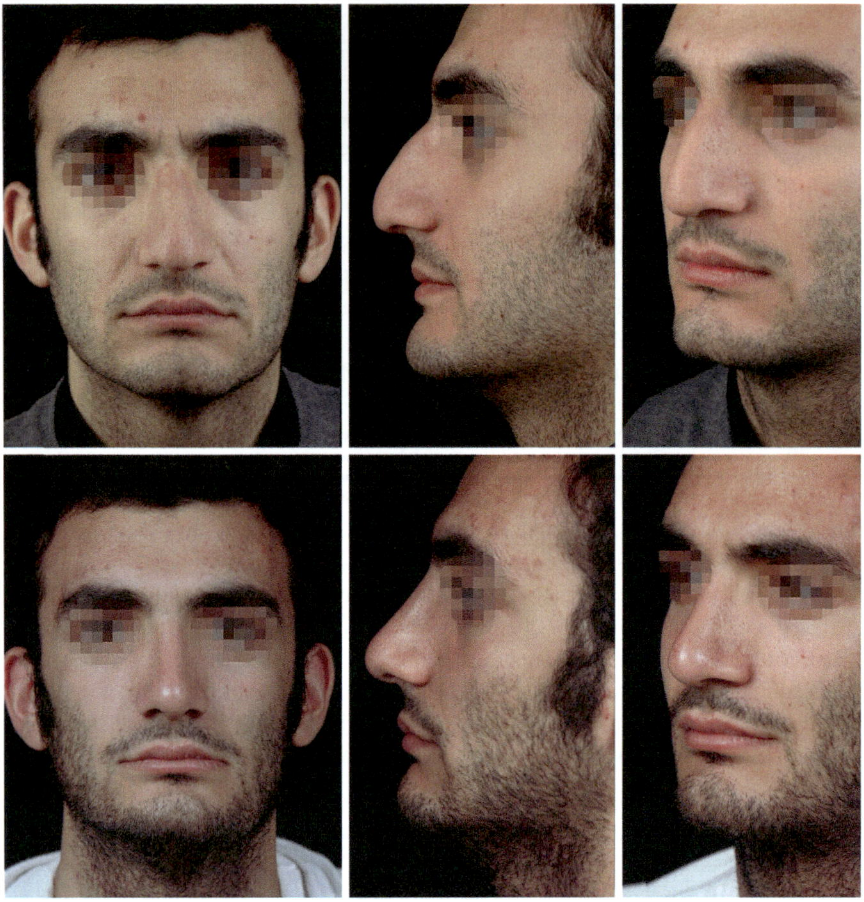

Fig. 2.8 Harmony and balance between the dorsum and the nasal tip in a Mediterranean man

is an improvement of the fullness or the asimmetry in the middle nasal vault [37] and a better definition of the large, amorphous, or ptotic tip [38], seeking to achieve harmony and balance between the dorsum and the tip (Fig. 2.8).

The most used rhinoplasty techniques are the so-called "reductive ones," especially those related to the correction of a dorsal hump. Furthermore, when remodelling the nasal framework it is possible to adopt the most preservative procedures, by also using structural grafts and accurate sutures, especially at the level of the nasal tip, in order to minimize the excision maneuvers. The tip position may also be improved with the above-mentioned strategies in dynamic expressions of the face (Fig. 2.9). A key and strategic element that must be carefully evaluated before planning and performing rhinoplasty, thus contributing to its successfull outcome, is represented by skin thickness, which sometimes can be very thick and sebaceous.

To preserve the ethnic characteristics of a Mediterranean nose, specific skills and accurate surgical maneuvers are necessary to reduce the hump, stabilize the dorsum, especially in the middle vault, with proper support of the tip in order to achieve

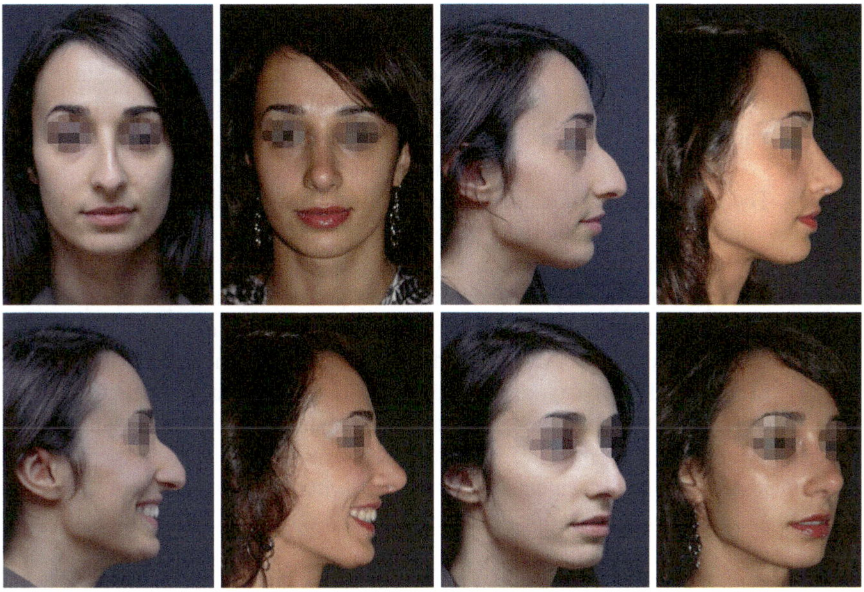

Fig. 2.9 Improvement of a convex dorsum and a ptotic tip in static and dynamic view

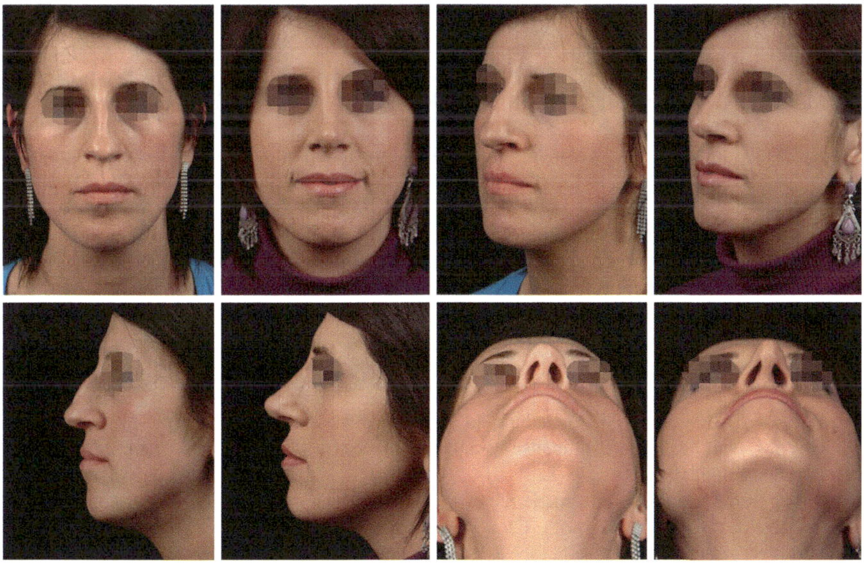

Fig. 2.10 Harmony and balance between the dorsum and the nasal tip in a Mediterranean woman

harmony between the dorsal projection and the correct positioning of the tip (Fig. 2.10) [38, 39]. These procedures are finalized to achieve face harmony while maintaining the characteristics which define ethnic identity. Rhinoplasty is the plastic surgery procedure which is usually performed in the Mediterranean countries. It must take into account the study of nasal morphology so as to provide nasofacial balance and proportions. Beauty is defined by the judgment process of the mind, it is not a feature which can be described or judged in an objective way. Since harmony and simmetry are considered universal elements of beauty, the nasal pyramid plays a visible cosmetic role in the appearance of the whole face because it gives it the sense of proportions, shape, and handsomeness of the neoclassical canons [5, 16, 40]. The appreciation of facial attractiveness, especially the nose, depends on the individual observer. In fact, each observer perceives different features, traits, and shades according to the cultural experience and within the context of ethnic origin but this perception may also be affected by preminent facial phenotypes such as the environment and new models of attractiveness. In most cases, personal identity and facial ethnic features correspond to the requests of the patients for plastic surgery. In fact, in rhinoplasty new models of reference may affect beauty canons, standardizing them to increasingly universal parameters. The ultimate endgoal of rhinoplasty surgery is to improve the shape of the nose, basing it on the patient's desired aestethic appearance and expectations without causing them unwanted changes and functional alterations over time.

References

1. Leong SC, Eccles R. Race and ethnicity in nasal plastic surgery: a need for science. Facial Plast Surg. 2010;26:63–8.
2. Garofano D. The synecdoche of the soul: observations toward a mythography of the nose. Facial Plast Surg. 1999;15:273–83.
3. Mohammed AW, Pathath AW, Al-Kuwaity KW, Ali SI. Rhino physiognomy: a myth or science? J Craniofac Surg. 2018;29:108–11.
4. Farkas LG, Hreczko TA, Kolar JC, Munro IR. Vertical and horizontal proportions of the face in young adult North American Caucasians: revisions of neoclassical canons. Plast Reconstr Surg. 1985;75:328–37.
5. Saad A, Hewett S, Nolte M, Delaunay F, Saad M, Cohen SR. Ethnic rhinoplasty in female patients: the neoclassical canons revisited. Aesthet Plast Surg. 2018;42:565–76.
6. Sullivan R. The identity and work of the ancient Egyptian surgeon. J R Soc Med. 1996;89:467–73.
7. Enciclopedia Italiana Treccani. Naso. Ed. 1949; vol. XXIV:287–291.
8. Williams RI. The nasal index; anthropological and clinical. Ann Otol Rhinol Laryngol. 1956;65:171–89.
9. Romo T III, Abraham MT. The ethnic nose. Facial Plastic Surg. 2003;19:269–78.
10. Ohki M, Naito K, Cole P. Dimensions and resistances of the human nose: racial differences. Laryngoscope. 1991;101:276–8.
11. Leong SC, Eccles R. A systematic review of the nasal index and the significance of the shape and size of the nose in rhinology. Clin Otolaryngol. 2009;34:191–8.
12. Leong SC, Eccles R. The use of race as a demographic variable in clinical research. Rhinology. 2010;48:3–6.
13. Farkas LG. Anthropometry of the head and face. 2nd ed. New York: Raven Press; 1994.
14. Farkas LG, Katic MJ, Forrest CR, Alt KW, Bagic I, Baltadjiev G, et al. International anthropometric study of facial morphology in various ethnic groups/race. J Craniofac Surg. 2005;16:615–46.
15. Farkas LG, Hreczko TA, Deutsch CK. Objective assessment of standard nostril types—a morphometric study. Ann Plast Surg. 1983;11:381–9.

16. Farkas LG, Kolar JC, Munro IR. Geography of the nose: a morphometric study. Aesthetic Plast Surg. 1986;10:191–223.
17. Farkas LG, Kolar JC. Anthropometrics and art in the aesthetics of women's faces. Clin Plast Surg. 1987;14:599–616.
18. Boccieri A. The surgical approach to the Mediterranean nose. Facial Plast Surg. 2010;26:119–30.
19. Palma P, Bignami M, Delù G, De Bernardi F, Castelnuovo P. Rhinoplasty for the Mediterranean nose. Facial Plast Surg. 2002;19:279–94.
20. Daniel RK. Middle eastern rhinoplasty: anatomy, aesthetics, and surgical planning. Facial Plast Surg. 2010;26:110–8.
21. Crognier E. Climate and anthropometric variations in Europe and the Mediterranean area. Ann Hum Biol. 1981;8:99–107.
22. Rowe-Jones J, van Wyk FC. Special considerations in northern European primary aesthetic rhinoplasty. Facial Plast Surg. 2010;26:75–85.
23. Gupta V, Sharma VK. Skin typing: Fitzpatrick grading and others. Clin Dermatol. 2019;37:430–6.
24. Youn SW, Kim SJ, Hwang IA, Park KC. Evaluation of facial skin type by sebum secretion: discrepancies between subjective descriptions and sebum secretion. Skin Res Technol. 2002;8:168–72.
25. Eggerstedt M, Rhee J, Buranosky M, Batra PS, Tajudeen BA, Smith RM, Revenaugh PC. Nasal skin and soft tissue thickness variation among differing races and ethnicities: an objective radiographic analysis. Facial Plast Surg Aesthet Med. 2020;22:188–94.
26. Jomah J, Elsafi RA, Ali KSAE, Abdullah R, Gelidan AG. Plast Reconstr Surg Glob Open. 2019;7:e2450.
27. Erdur ZB, Oktem F, Inci E, Yener HM, Gozen ED, Birben AO, et al. Effect of nasal skin type on skin problems following rhinoplasty. Facial Plast Surg. 2020;36:643–9.
28. Mueser KT, Grau BW, Sussman S, Rosen AJ. You are only as pretty as you feel: facial expression as a determinant of physical attractiveness. J Pers Soc Psychol. 1984;46:469–78.
29. Darrach H, Ishii LE, Liao D, Nellis JC, Bater K, Cobo R, et al. Assessment of the influence of the "other-race effect" on visual attention and perception of attractiveness before and after rhinoplasty. JAMA Facial Plast Surg. 2019;21:96–102.
30. Villanueva NL, Afrooz PN, Carboy JA, Rohrich RJ. Nasal analysis: considerations for ethnic variation. Plast Reconstr Surg. 2019;143:1179–88.
31. Patel PN, Most SP. Concepts of facial aesthetics when considering ethnic rhinoplasty. Otolaryngol Clin North Am. 2020;53:195–208.
32. Santos M, Monteiro D, Coutinho M, e Sousa CA, Ferreira MG. Caucasian Mediterranean patients seeking rhinoplasty—anthropometric measurements and prevalence of major deformities. Clin Otolaryngol. 2019;44:581–7.
33. Jankowska A, Janiszewska-Olszowska J, Jedlinski M, Grocholewicz K. Methods of analysis of the nasal profile: a systematic review with meta-analysis. Biomed Res Int. 2021;2021:6680175.
34. Doddi NM, Eccles R. The role of anthropometric measurements in nasal surgery and research: a systematic review. Clin Otolaryngol. 2010;35:277–83.
35. Tuncel U, Turan A, Kostakoglu N. Digital anthropometric shape analysis of 110 rhinoplasty patients in the Black Sea region in Turkey. J Craniomaxillofac Surg. 2013;41:98–102.
36. Tamir A. Numerical survey of the different shapes of the human nose. J Craniofac Surg. 2011;22:1104–7.
37. Sheen JH. Spreader graft: a method of reconstructing the roof of the middle nasal vault following rhinoplasty. Plast Reconstr Surg. 1984;73:230–9.
38. Toriumi DM. New concepts in nasal tip contouring. Arch Facial Plast Surg. 2006;8:156–85.
39. Crumley RL, Lanser M. Quantitative analisys of nasal tip projection. Laryngoscope. 1988;98:202–8.
40. Zacharopoulos GV, Manios A, De Bree E, Kau CH, Petrousis M, Zacharopoulo I, et al. Neoclassical facial canons in young adults. J Craniofac Surg. 2012;23:1693–8.

3 Mediterranean Noses: The Tension Nose Deformity and Preservation Rhinoplasty

Yves Saban, Masoud Saman, and Abdülkadir Göksel

3.1 Introduction

The term tension nose deformity (hereafter TND) is well familiar for most rhinoplasty surgeons. However, its exact definition may not be clearly understood. The term Tension Nose was first coined by Maurice Cottle [1]. Most popularly, the cause of TND has been attributed to the overgrowth of the septal quadrangular cartilage. However, more recently studies have suggested that the absolute size of the quadrangular cartilage is relatively consistent in various populations [2].

A recent study by Weinstock et al. suggested the external extrusion of the normal sized quadrangular cartilage from its bony encasement as the possible relative enlargement of the septal cartilage in TND. The authors suggest this extrusion to be related to a buckling effect on the cartilage due to limited bony space available [3].

Although Cottle's description of a high and narrow dorsum is commonly seen in the tension nose deformity, what is constantly seen is the overgrowth of the quadrangular cartilage in the sagittal plane [4]. The excessive size, absolute or relative, of the quadrangular cartilage in essence pushes the dorsum high and the lower lateral cartilages forward or downward, thus overprojecting the entire nose or giving an aspect of high, convex, and narrow dorsum associated to an underprojected and slightly droopy tip. It is important to keep in mind that the tip projection is not necessarily related to the length of the nasal tip tripod, but to the underlying overgrown septum at the anterior septal angle that thrusts the tip forward and/or downward. It is interesting to notice that many TND patients are showing a visible anterior septal

Y. Saban (✉)
Facial Plastic Surgery, FPS and Maxillofacial, Nice, France

M. Saman
Saman Rhinoplasty and Facial Plastic Surgery, Manhattan, NY, USA

A. Göksel
ENT Facial Plastic Surgery, Rino Istanbul, Istanbul, Turkey

P. G. Giacomini (ed.), *Mediterranean Rhinoplasty*,
https://doi.org/10.1007/978-3-031-05551-5_3

angle (ASA hereafter) in the supratip area, while the tip looks like pushed downward and lying at a lower level than the ASA. Other frequent findings include a shortening and tethering of the upper lip to the overgrown caudal septum and retrogenia. In this chapter, we aim to discuss the anatomic findings commonly associated with tension nose deformity, as well as surgical considerations related to this deformity.

The evolutionary advantages or reasons for the tension nose deformity are not known. In many animals and insects, an elongated facial appendage, or proboscis, is used for nourishment, enhanced olfaction, showing affection, storing water, and more. In the elephant, the trunk is composed of the nose and the upper lip in which case the advantages of the upper lip muscular interdigitation with the nasal muscles are obvious.

Jankowski in his book "Evo-Devo Origin of the Nose, Anterior Skull Base and Midface" [5] hypothesizes that the redesign of the face because of the bipedism, medialization of the eyes, and retraction of the muzzle has led to an assembly of three organs of quite different nature: the olfactive nose, the respiratory nose, and the paranasal sinuses. The controversial growing forces of these three organs are responsible for the various nasal deformities, acting like tectonic plates. Thus, the quadrangular cartilage acts a major actor of the nasal growth.

Significant debate surrounds the evolutionary reasons for variation in nose morphology across human populations. We must not forget the functions of the nose or nasal appendix: air conditioning and olfaction, while the cosmetic and social aspects can be considered equally important in mammals including humans. In some species, male nasal and sinusal hypertrophy functions as a "sound resonator" for males calling or for territory marking.

Given the function of conditioning of the air passing through the nose prior to reaching the lower airway, adaptations to climate have been cited as the evolutionary reason behind varied nasal shapes as early as 1923 by Arthur Thomson [6]. Best remembered for Thomson's Nose Rule, he suggested ethnic groups inhabiting warm humid climates tend to have short, thicker noses, whereas populations living in cold, arid environments tend to have longer, thinner noses. However, the Mediterranean climate is almost not considered to be rainy nor wet but rather a temperate type. Tension noses are generally considered as so-called "Semitic" noses.

3.2 Anatomical Findings in Tension Nose Deformity and TND Biomechanical Anatomy

Profile view analysis: the anatomical characteristics of TND may be summarized in Figs. 3.1 and 3.2 showing a "typical" TND and the biomechanics.

Convex dorsum lines and dynamic tip ptosis are the main evident deformities; consequently, shortened upper lip, effaced NLA, hanging columella represent the most common associated anatomic deformities.

The enlarged quadrangular nasal septum creates a domino effect on the interplay of several nasal and perinasal structures which should most logically be discussed

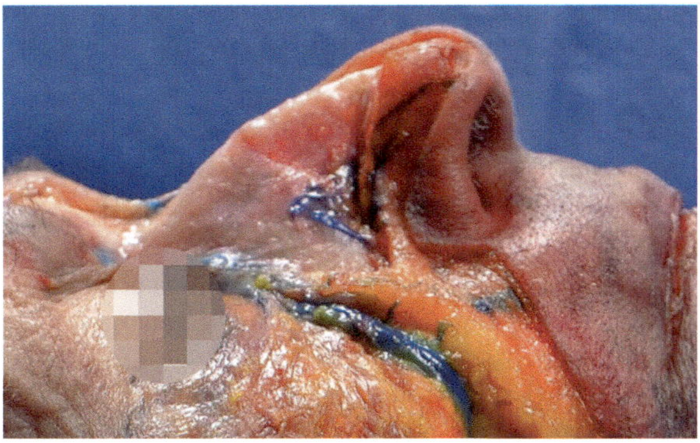

Fig. 3.1 Typical Tension Nose Deformity (TND) Shown on an Anatomic Specimen

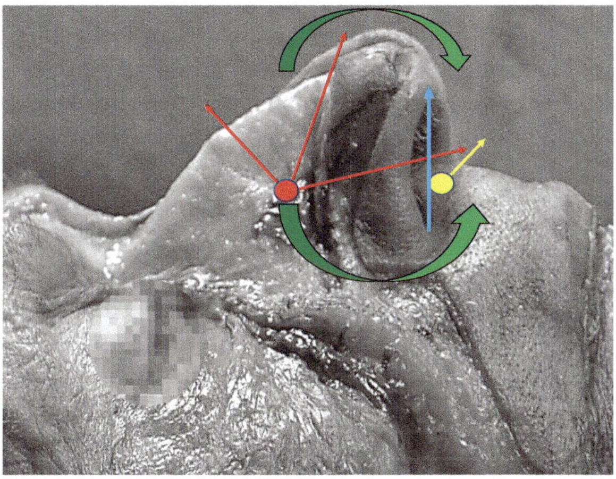

Fig. 3.2 TND Biomechanics: the overgrowth of the quadrangular cartilage provokes (red arrows): (1) DKA and (2) ASA elevation, (3) caudal septal displacement; consequently, some biomechanical effects are induced: (4—green arrow) caudal tip rotation, that may look underprojected, (5—light blue arrow) stretching of the nostrils, (6—yellow arrows) ANS prominence and consequently the nasolabial angle becomes obtuse and, the upper lip looks shorter as it is pulled upward

as a continuum. The forward displacement of the lip-columella junction caused by the overgrowth of the caudal septum together with the anterior nasal spine in tension nose deformity results in blunting of the nasolabial angle and tipping the cranial portion of the philtral columns anteriorly. This in turn may cause tethering of the upper lip to the base of the nose causing a short upper lip and in more severe cases interdigitation of depressor septi nasalis muscle with orbicularis muscles resulting in accentuated dynamic tip ptosis with animation. In addition, the inferior displacement of the medial crura of the lower lateral cartilages due to caudal septal push may result in a hanging columella.

3.3 Preoperative Considerations and Patient's Assessment: The Decision-Making Process in TND

3.3.1 What Are the Critical Questions a Rhinoplasty Surgeon Should Ask to himself While Assessing a Patient Seeking Primary Rhinoplasty? (Table 3.1)

Beyond the ever-so-important psychological evaluation of the patient and their motives for desiring a rhinoplasty, the following four anatomical and aesthetic evaluations are critical in the decision-making process: prior to any decision, the surgeon must ask himself five questions:

(1) Can I preserve the dorsum? Assessment of the Dorsal Aesthetic Lines. (2) Is the tip difficult? Assessment of nasal tip morphology. (3) Is the septum stable? Evaluation for the need for septoplasty and the septal foundation that makes the dorsum stable. (4) How is the breathing? Assessment of the width of the pyriform aperture. (5) How is the global facial harmony? Evaluation for an additional fifth question can be added as regards to some miscellaneous facial procedures such as chin augmentation, upper lip procedures, etc.

3.3.1.1 Question 1: Can I Preserve the Dorsum Lines?

Assessment of the Dorsal Aesthetic Lines: Choosing between three surgical preservation rhinoplasty procedure options (Table 3.2).

A thorough analysis and assessment of the patient's DAL is critical in the decision-making process. In cases where the patient already has pleasing DAL, it would baffle logic to destroy normal anatomy. Thus, in such cases a conservative approach may be warranted. A comprehensive discussion of the nasal dorsum requires conceptual separation of the bony and cartilaginous vaults, as each one may require a separate management. In TND, the entire nasal dorsum should be preserved, i.e. both cartilaginous and bony dorsum, thus allowing for decision-making a choice between a "Full Dorsum Preservation" as preconized by Gola [7] or a "Dorsum Preservation with bony-cartilaginous resurfacing" [8].

In order to select the appropriate surgical procedure, a comprehensive profile analysis must be performed. This analysis must not however be limited to the nasal profile lines, but also with careful attention to the patient's whole face, including the forehead, upper and lower lip, and chin projection.

Table 3.1 Algorithm # 1 in primary rhinoplasty: the decision-making leading questions

The 3 leading questions
1. Can I keep the dorsum intact?
– Yes: Preservation technique
– No: Classic resection or nasal disarticulation
2. Is the tip difficult?
– Yes: Open approach
– No: EndoNasal closed approach
3. Is the septum stable?
– Yes: Classic rhinoplasty paradigm + septoplasty
– No: Cottle's technique or traditional rhinoplasty

Table 3.2 Algorithm # 2 in primary rhinoplasty—decision-making process: correspondences nasal shapes and surgical procedures

Type 1 Straight nose	**En-Bloc Full Dorsal Preservation—No SSTE Elevation**
Type 2 Tension nose	**Dorsal Preservation With Bony-Cartil. Reshaping**
	2a—Reshaping by rasping or rhinosculpture
	2b—Bony cap resection + ULCs "shoulder" shaving
Type 3 Kyphotic nose	**"Cartilage-only Push-down"—"Hybrid Technique"**
Type 4 No Preservation nose	**Resection Following Joseph and/or Structure**

Profile lines analysis is the foundation for biomechanical anatomy understanding in rhinoplasty. The bony radix, the bony-cartilaginous K-Area, and the cartilaginous supradomal segments are the three target areas of this profile analysis applied to preservation rhinoplasty [9]. Radix foundation is comprised of nasal bones covered by thick superficial soft tissues made of fat compartments and procerus muscle [10]. The keystone area may be straight or convex. This area corresponds to the bony-cartilaginous overlapping related to bony cap [11, 12] and the cephalic part of the upper lateral cartilages (ULC). Dorsal Keystone Area (DKA) is extended downward to cranial ULC, covered by a thin skin soft tissue envelope [11]. The supradomal segment, corresponding to the cartilaginous septal W-ASA segment, may be straight or convex, covered by thick skin corresponding to subcutaneous fat and SMAS extensions, and deep Pitanguy ligaments [13, 14].

Considering the thickness, shape, and orientation of nasal bones and cartilaginous DKA, a classification can be proposed, regarding the ability to straighten the nasal profile with dorsal preservation (DP) procedures that are nowadays the gold standard in primary rhinoplasty. However, nasal profile lines are not only related to bony-cartilaginous skeleton: the soft tissue thickness can make the nose look straight, even when the underlying bony-cartilaginous framework is convex. Consequently, the relationship between these three segments directly influences the nasal dorsum profile lines appearance that is anatomy and optic illusion, and therefore the surgical procedure.

3.3.1.2 Question 2: Is the Tip Difficult?

Assessment of the tip; choosing the surgical approach—open transcolumellar, or endonasal closed—depends on tip deformities.

The assessment of tip aesthetics, projection, rotation, and overall shape allows the surgeon to best select the approach that looks most suitable, according to his experience and practice. In many TND noses, the tip already has pleasing aesthetics and may not require complicated, if any, contouring procedures or grafts. In these cases, even the surgeon who prefers open rhinoplasty would be wise to strongly consider the endonasal approach as to prevent unnecessary excessive dissection of the nasal tip.

Tip underprojection is commonly seen in tension nose deformity, even when the tip cartilages are "pulled up" secondary to septal overgrowth and forward and superior position of the anterior septal angle. It is important to remember that the tip cartilages may be normal sized, large, or even deficient and should be assessed in their own right. The underprojected tip in tension nose deformity has surgical implications as reducing the ANS may well result in loss of tip support thereby mandating a need for tip reproduction and support. In cases where the nasal tip is underprojected, after reduction of the quadrangular cartilage especially at the anterior septal angle, foundation support for reprojection must be utilized. Although these maneuvers can be achieved just as optimally using the endonasal approach, many surgeons may prefer the open approach. Such reproduction may be achieved with innovative grafts such as ANSA banner [15], or Teostrut [16], or a columellar strut [17].

3.3.1.3 Question 3: Is the Septum Stable?

Assessment of the septum can modify the decision-making process from a Preservation High-Strip Procedure to a Cottle's Low-Strip Technique, or leading even sometimes to a structural concept.

The common theme of septal cartilage overgrowth often results in a high cartilaginous dorsum. This may or may not be associated with a high bony dorsum. From an evolutionary development point of consideration, one may be accounted for by considering the quadrangular septum and the upper lateral cartilages as one anatomic unit—the septolateral cartilages—as opposed to two separate entities [18].

In all TND cases, the rhinoplasty surgeon must assess the need for septal surgery. Is a septoplasty necessary? TND is generally associated with an inherently straight septum, which may be convex due to the overgrowth, thus not requiring a difficult septoplasty. In these cases, removal of some of the excess cartilage, as one would achieve with removal of a high strip, will allow for the septum to sit straight within the nasal framework without the need for any additional septoplasty.

In cases where the bony septum is deviated, thus distorting the cartilaginous septum, that can be luxated downward most commonly on the left side of the maxillary crest, then a septoplasty following Cottle's "swinging door" procedure may become necessary. Based on the stability of septal framework, the surgeon is able to decide between a typical Cottle's dorsum lowering [8, 19] versus a direct septal reduction. In our hands, the high strip procedure can be easily performed in the majority of cases.

3.3.1.4 Question 4: Is the Pyriform Aperture Narrow?

Assessment of the Pyriform Aperture Size is critical in all cases of rhinoplasty.

Especially in TND, the maxillary bone grows forward and does not expand laterally, leading to a narrow pyriform aperture. We can talk of leptorhinia or even of stenorhinia, the name given to extreme anatomical narrowing. In TND, the dorsal lines look straight and thin, almost narrow. This, in turn, corresponds to the classic "leptorrhine" typology. Moreover, sometimes, the pyriform aperture is so narrow that the nose looks "closed" at the isthmus nasi, a deformity we refer to as "stenorhinia." This assessment is critical as the width of the pyriform aperture is one of the main steps in patient's preoperative assessment [20, 21].

So, is the pyriform aperture narrow? TND is generally associated with leptorrhine morphology and although most tension noses require conservative bony management, in already-narrow pyriform apertures one must be cognizant of avoiding unwanted nasal obstruction due to further narrowing. Anecdotal in our practice, we have noted some patients complaining of nasal obstruction following dorsum preservation procedures related to pyriform aperture narrowing. In these cases, revisionary surgery for aperture widening was performed according to Webster's triangle widening [20]. Objective data analyses of CT measurements and functional/clinical outcomes are underway (Stergiou). Based on our unpublished data [10], it appears nasal obstruction following push-down procedures is mainly observed when dorsum lowering was more than 5 mm. It is therefore our recommendation that in TND, if the dorsum needs to be lowered more than 4–5 mm, a d'emblée bony wedge resection associated to an inferior turbinoplasty should be considered. The name of this procedure is "Let-Down" procedure.

As a complementary analysis, the bony pyramid junction to the facial plane is defining the so-called "nasal parenthesis" [22]. This bony base is generally convex and wide in TND, which in-turn means a bony base reduction is mandatory to achieve a well-balanced postoperative triangular nasal pyramid.

3.3.1.5 Question 5: How Is the Facial Global Harmony?

How are the nostrils, upper lip, and chin? Are any complementary maneuvers indicated to improve the facial appearance?

In TND, nostrils are thin and elongated while the nasal base looks nicely triangular. One must keep in mind that nasal dorsum deprojection may further deproject the tip as tip support may be lost secondary to ASA lowering. Consequently, a widening of the nostril base and associated rounding effect of the nostrils' apertures may be apparent. These deformities may be unwanted, hence requiring additional surgical procedures to reproject tip and give it support. Of note, most of Mediterranean TND patients show normal skin thickness, a favorable anatomy for creating aesthetic tip remodeling and definition.

Additionally, patients presenting for rhinoplasty usually expect a precise and bespoke analysis solely of their noses. Often, they are surprised if other facial disharmonies are discussed outright. However, as mentioned, a complete profile analysis is crucial in achieving a balanced final result. In our experience, the "not-only-the-nose" concerns are best analyzed at the end of the patient's profile assessment while performing (and at the end of) the computer simulation. Simply commenting: "let's see together if some additional changes may improve the aesthetic result" may be helpful in attracting their attention to other deformities present. In our experience, conversely, if such a comment is made at the beginning of the visit, the patient may lose trust and become resistant for a full analysis: "I am here for my nose, and I don't have any issues with my chin!"

However, patients with Tension Nose Deformity are often noted to have retruded chins. This retrogenia may result from an optic illusion related to the anterior overgrowth of the nose. However, in our experience (clinical case here after—patient photos) most of our TND patients require a genioplasty that is performed either intraoperatively, or in the postoperative period through filler injections. The question is how and when to suggest this procedure to the patient visiting for nose surgery and who has never noticed any chin concern. Surgeons must be aware of rhinoplasty patient's psychology.

3.3.2 What Are the most Common Primary Rhinoplasty Procedures Preserving the Natural Dorsum Aesthetic Lines as the First-Choice Procedures According to the Patient's Anatomy and to the Best Benefit-Risk Ratio, in 2021? [8]

Across the structural-preservation continuum, one can describe and collectively group the following narrow range of rhinoplasty procedures that share the same philosophy (Tables 3.3 and 3.4).

1. Primary rhinoplasty Type 1: Full dorsum preservation without soft tissues elevation.
2. Primary rhinoplasty Type 2: Dorsum preservation with bony cartilaginous resurfacing.
3. Primary rhinoplasty Type 3: Partial dorsum preservation: cartilaginous vault only preservation or bony dorsum only preservation (Göksel in press).

Table 3.3 Classification of preservation rhinoplasty procedure based on high strip septal excision and bony cartilaginous vaults disarticulation

Rhinoplasty procedures from high strip	
1. *Without dorsal disarticulation*	
• Goodale	(1898)
• Gola	(1989)
• Saban	(2006)
• Kovacevic	(2019)
2. *With cartilaginous vault disarticulation*	
a. Partial LKA disarticulation	
• Göksel	(2017)
• Ishida LC	(2020)
b. Total dorsal disarticulation	
• Saban *(Sparing roof technique)*	(2012–2013)
• Ferreira *(Spare roof technique)*	(2016)

Table 3.4 Classification of preservation rhinoplasty procedure based on Cottle's technique and bony cartilaginous vaults disarticulation

Septo-rhinoplasty procedures from Cottle's
Without dorsal disarticulation
Cottle's Original (1956)
Dewes's SPAR (2000)
Finocchi's SPQR (2019)
Neves' TETRIS (2019)
Most's Intermediate Flap (2020)
With total cartilaginous disarticulation
• Ishida J

Table 3.4 (continued)

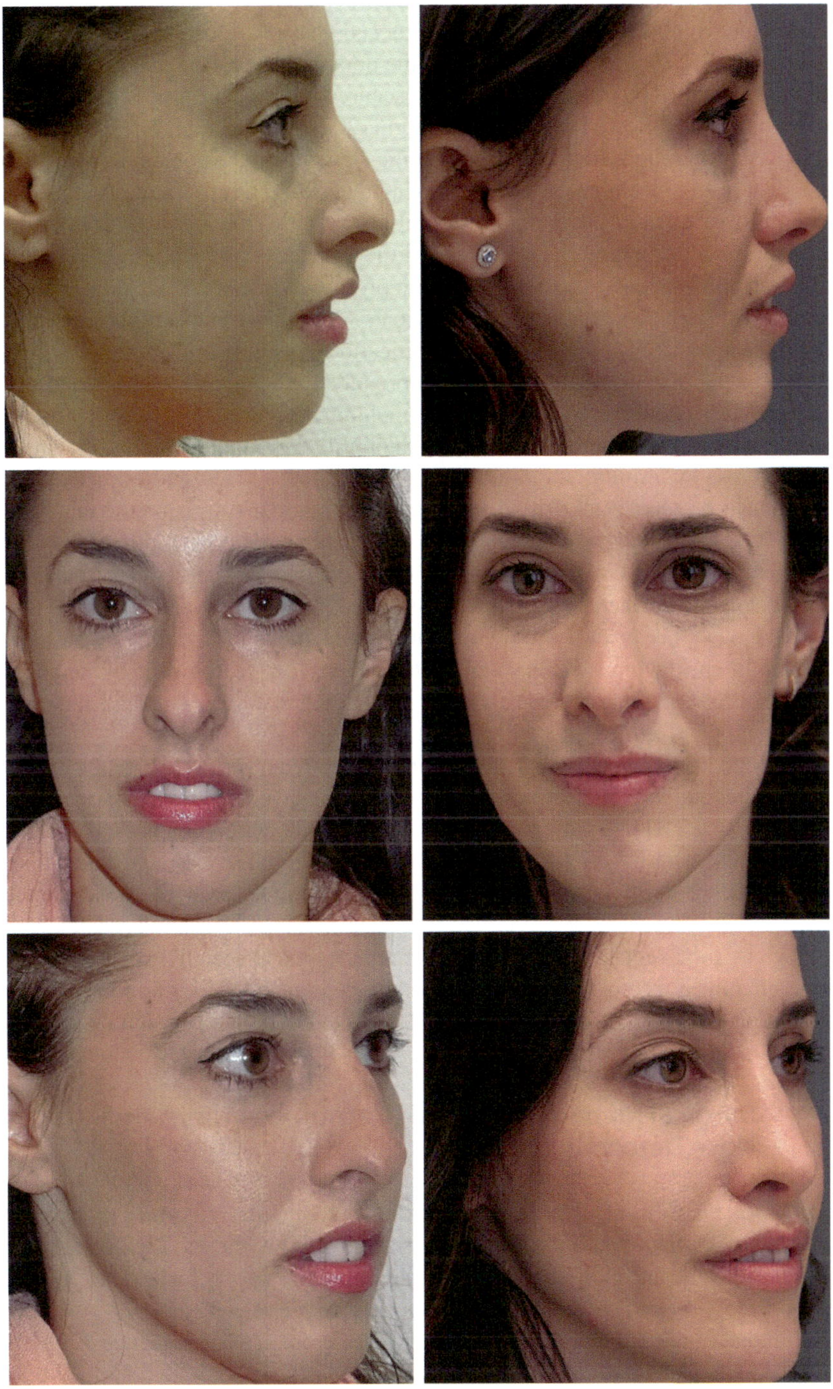

4. Primary rhinoplasty traditional procedures: Dorsum resection following Joseph or/and structural reconstruction.

Structure rhinoplasty for management of TND has previously been discussed in great depth [23]. These include reducing the dorsal septal cartilage height and caudal septal length. The frame L strut is then secured with various grafts. In 2021, it is our opinion—as followed recently by Toriumi (2021)—no place is left for structural rhinoplasty techniques for addressing specific elements of the dorsum in TND. With the recent resurgence of interest in preserving the natural nasal structures in primary rhinoplasty, a plethora of literature describing various techniques in Preservation Rhinoplasty (PR) has emerged. However, little guidance has been provided in technique selection related to various anatomic profiles. Saban's 2021 guidelines [21], based on retrospective analysis of 352 patients who underwent septorhinoplasty by the senior author (YS), introduces a classification system based upon the patient's dorsum profile lines (DPL) and the appropriately applicable PR technique. In this guideline, varied distinct nasal profiles, including TND were discussed. In this chapter, we will focus on Preservation Rhinoplasty technique guidelines related to Tension Nose Deformity.

We have previously classified Preservation Rhinoplasty procedures into three types: Type 1 PR: Full preservation of dorsum without any skin soft tissue envelope dissection, so-called Gola's technique; Type 2 PR: Dorsal preservation with bony cartilaginous resurfacing, so-called Saban's Technique; and Type 3 PR: Cartilaginous-Only preservation with bony-cartilaginous disarticulation and push-down of the cartilaginous vault, so-called Ishida's technique, followed by Jankowski as nasal disarticulation procedure. One must add that in case of deviated and unstable septum, the Cottle's procedure should be considered.

Although an elaborate discussion of details of varied nasal profiles and technique types are beyond the scope of this chapter (Table 3.2), we will emphasize the details pertinent to the TND. In patients with straight noses, in whom the surgical objective is to reduce dorsal height while maintaining shape, nasal valves, and dorsal lines, Type 1 PR, i.e., full preservation of the dorsum, appears to be most suitable. However, the surgeon must be vigilant in recognition of the tension nose deformity as they can look remarkably similar to straight noses, especially in cases of high radix, effectively camouflaging the dorsal hump. In the aforementioned guideline, application of Type 1 PR technique to TND resulted in higher revision rates.

3.4 Surgical Management and Procedures in Tension Nose Deformity

It is important to remember that there is no one singularly correct or universal approach or technique in rhinoplasty that is suitable for all noses. Technique choice is highly dependent upon the patient's anatomy and expectations, as well as the surgeon's facility and capability in his or her technique of choice.

With that in mind, it is our aim to herein present our typical sequence of the surgical steps in TND, namely, Preservation Rhinoplasty type 2 with resurfacing and tip remodeling.

Once the operative plan is reviewed, the patient's nose and septum are injected with local anesthetic. The patient's entire face is then prepared with antiseptic solution of choice and the patient is draped sterilely with the whole face visible.

3.4.1 The Dorsum: Type 2 Preservation Rhinoplasty with K-Area Resurfacing [24]

Type 2 PR is indicated generally in typical TND patients and in patients showing small bony humps, S-shaped nasal bones [25] who have pleasing aesthetic dorsal lines. The sequence of surgical steps is of upmost importance to avoid any issues (Figs. 3.3, 3.4, 3.5, and 3.6).

1. Approach: the endonasal septal vertical approach without any lateral intercartilaginous incisions will be preferred. The elevation of skin soft tissue envelope is performed either the sub-SMAS or subperichondrial/subperiosteal plane.
2. Dorsum step: once accessed, the nasal bones are resurfaced by either rasping or superficial ostectomy performed without any DKA disarticulation. If ULC vault looks squared shape, the cartilaginous shoulders will be shaved with a scalpel. Bony

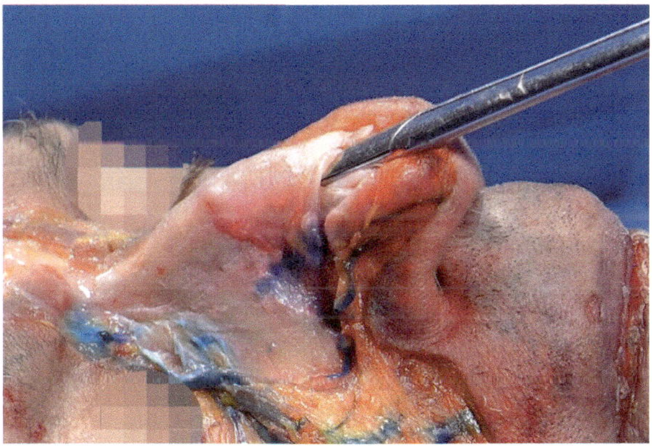

Fig. 3.3 Anatomic Dissection. Septal Stage: High Septal Cross-Section is Starting at the W-Point

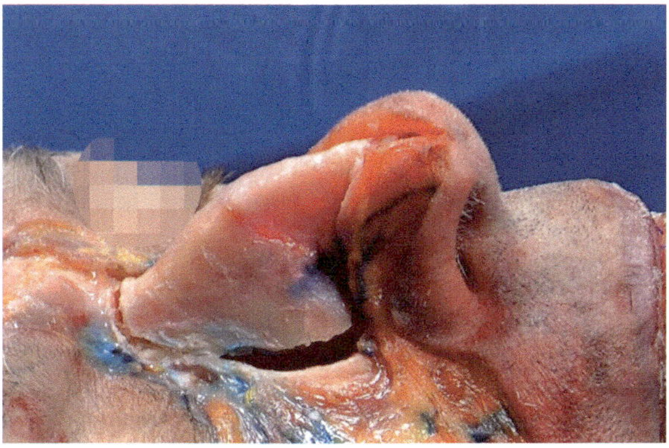

Fig. 3.4 Anatomic Dissection; Osteotomies and Maxillary Bony Wedge Resection (Let-Down Procedure Separate Completely the Bony Nasal Pyramid from its Facial Attachments

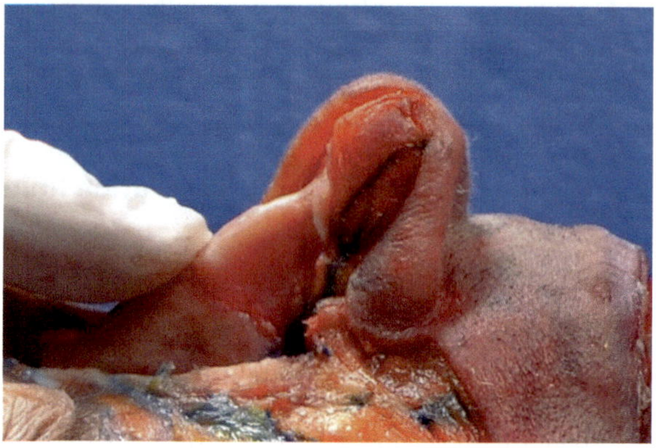

Fig. 3.5 Anatomic Dissection; the Push-Down Procedure is Reducing the Dorsum Height and Flattening the Dorsum Lines

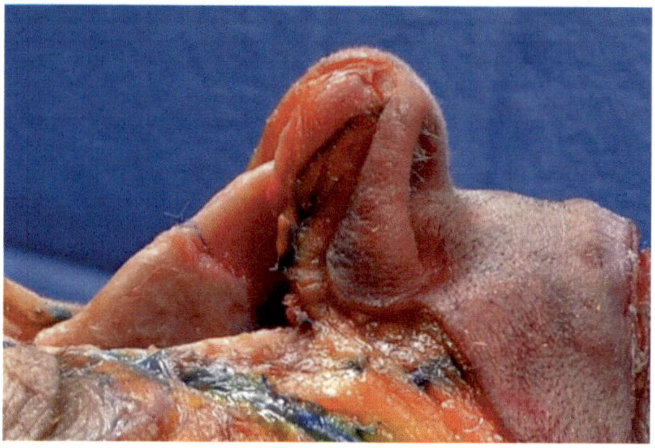

Fig. 3.6 Anatomic Dissection; Stabilization by Cerclage Sutures is Securing the Long-Lasting Result

hump resurfacing not only decreases the bony height, but also displaces the keystone osseocartilaginous pivot point cephalically an effect we previously termed "Rhinion Shift" [21], allowing for hinging the cartilage at a higher point, thereby reducing the hump and flattening the dorsum, effects that are often desired in TND.

3. Septal step: after superior septal tunnels, 1 cm height, done in the subperichondrial/subperiosteal plane, a high septal strip incision is then made as previously described. Next, the septum will be lowered by incremental strip excisions which in turn provides space for dorsum lowering, accordingly to the intraoperative need for. Careful cleaning of the subdorsal septum remnants is critical to avoid the "coat-hanger effect" [24] that would block the dorsum straightening maneuvers.
4. Bony pyramid step: osteotomies are performed next with complete lateral (or let-down where indicated), transverse and radix osteotomies. At this point, importantly to remind that the mobilization must never been done prior to the septoplasty that must be the first step, the bony cartilaginous pyramid mobilization is performed in standard fashion.
5. Profile harmonization: We, then, allow a few minutes to pass and observe the dorsum convexity. If the dorsum appears to spring back, causing recurrence of

the hump, we perform release of lateral K-area as well as the pyriform ligaments to reduce any spring effect tension on the dorsum, procedure named "ballerina maneuver" by Göksel [26].

6. Stabilization step: at the end of these bony-cartilaginous pyramid stages, stabilization must be ensured by specific sutures. These sutures may be done using a cerclage technique either through the endonasal approach or percutaneously.

3.4.1.1 Discussion

Inadequate resurfacing, dorsally and in some cases along the lateral keystone area (LKA) [26] may result in need for revisionary surgery in tension nose deformity. In the interest of a comprehensive discussion, one could discuss Cottle's variation SPQR procedure [19] in TND when a septoplasty must be associated as the first surgical stage. Then, considering the cartilaginous vault, a few patients show ULC "shoulders" that give an aspect of square cartilaginous dorsum; in these cases, resurfacing consisting of obliquely shaving the cartilaginous ULC angles to smooth the DAL must be considered. We recommend the endonasal approach allowing for preserving the nasal ligaments, thus facilitating and shortening the healing process in the postoperative period.

3.4.2 The Tip and the Concept of "Structure-Preservation Rhinoplasty"

Tip surgery will depend on the patient's anatomy and aesthetic goals and may require extended marginal approach, lower lateral cartilage cephalic reduction or folding manipulations, lateral crural re-orientation according to tip sutures and if necessary, either Cakir tip-plasty with lateral crus steal and columellar strut. In TND, nasal tip, even when pulled upward, is generally underprojected. Therefore, tip projection or, at least, tip support is required. Maneuvers for tip support and reprojection, such as Neves' ANSA Banner [15] or Dogan's Teostrut domal suspension graft [16] may be utilized in these cases.

In rare cases, the nasal tip in TND is overprojected secondary to the relative or absolute large septal size. The lower later cartilages may be overgrown, adequate, or deficient. As such, after reducing the dorsum, following the "deprojection-reprojection" concept described by Johnson et al. [27], the tip cartilages should be assessed in their own right. The expert rhinoplasty surgeon will have an armamentarium of suture techniques, structural grafting, and lower lateral cartilage overlay techniques at their disposal.

3.4.3 Miscellaneous Maneuvers

Representing the last surgical steps, some harmonization of the nose may be necessary. In TND, nasal base is usually well triangular and aesthetically pleasing, often not requiring any manipulation. However, if nasal dorsum deprojection is provoking nasal tip lowering, a biomechanical widening of the nasal base and subsequent nostrils flaring may occur. Thus, an alar base reduction may be needed. The surgeon must be aware of this possible iatrogenic deformity and the patient must be counseled preoperatively about possible need for alar base reduction.

Mobile tip management. In many cases, resection of the depressor septi nasalis muscle may be required.

Deepening the naso-labial angle. Reduction of nasal spine must be weighted very carefully at the end of the procedure and as judged by the surgeon. Most often, there is no requirement for such procedure.

Upper lip replacement. Adjunctive profileplasty procedures, such as upper lip frenulum Z-cheiloplasty is almost always necessary "to free" the upper lip.

In TND cases associated with microgenia, chin augmentation by means of either surgical genioplasty, or chin implant placement, or fat grafting, or nonsurgical injections may be indicated. In selected cases when abundant bony-cartilaginous material is left at the end of the septorhinoplasty, an autologous transfer may be performed through a limited chin endobuccal vertical subperiosteal approach. This procedure offers excellent aesthetic results and neither any postoperative issues, nor complaints of the patients who appreciate this additional procedure, generally done without any additional fees, in our hands.

3.5 Clinical Case

This 22 year old young nice lady, is visiting for a nose-job. No history of trauma nor nasal pathology except some breathing concerns. No psychological issues. Computer simulation and full explanations were done and got her agreement. Informed consent and authorization for recording movie of her surgery; written agreement for publication of the photos.

She is presenting a typical tension nose deformity: nice convex dorsal lines, slightly underprojected tip, straight septum, narrow pyriform aperture causing breathing issues, thin tent nostrils, retracted upper lip, and microgenia. Consequently, she required an endonasal preservation procedure, pyriform aperture widening, not difficult tip surgery, and no specific septoplasty. Miscellaneous procedures on nostrils, upper lip, and chin.

She underwent an endonasal Preservation Rhinoplasty Type 2: hump resurfacing, 9 mm septum high-strip excision, 6 mm Let-Down Operation procedure to improve airway and avoid any breathing issues after push-down. Caudal septum 2 mm edge reduction. Tip exclusive marginal approach, dome sutures and cranial LLC reduction. Upper lip cheilo-Z-plasty. Nostrils alar base reduction. Chin augmentation through endoral vertical subperiosteal approach and autologous nasal bony-cartilaginous transfer.

The results are shown after 6 years post-op follow-up. She did not need any revision (Clinical Case 3.1).

3.6 Conclusion

Tension Nose Deformity is a common finding in Mediterranean noses. The first and most important factor in management of the Tension Nose Deformity is identification and correct diagnosis. Many of the common findings in the typical tension nose have been described in this chapter. However, the management should be guided by specific findings.

Herein, we have presented the modification required for successful TND management using dorsal preservation techniques that are becoming the current gold standard procedures. Management of the tip should be performed after the dorsum has been managed and in accordance with patient's specific anatomy and aesthetic goals and desires, and as always, in a customized and bespoke manner for the individual patient.

Complementary maneuvers such as nostrils plasty, upperlip Z-cheiloplasty, and chin augmentation must be customized and utilized for the specific anatomy at hand.

References

1. The Cottle nasal syndromes. Rhinology: the collected writing of Maurice H. Cottle. The American Rhinologic Society; 1987. p. 189–90.
2. Pernia NER, Galvez JAC, Victoria FA. The dimensions of the nasal septal cartilage: a preliminary study in adult Filipino Malay cadavers. Philipp J Otolaryngol Head Neck Surg. 2011;26(2):10–2.
3. Weinstock MS, Stupak HD. Bony/cartilaginous mismatch: a radiologic investigation into the cause of tension nose deformity. Plast Reconstr Surg. 2018;141(2):312–21.
4. Johnson CM, Godin MS. The tension nose. Plast Reconstr Surg. 1996;97(1):246.
5. Jankowski R. The Evo-Devo origin of the nose, anterior skull base and midface; 2013.
6. Thomson A, Buxton LHD. Man's nasal index in relation to certain climatic conditions. J R Anthropol Inst Great Britain Ireland. 1923;53:92–122.
7. Gola R. Conservative rhinoplasty. Ann Chir Plast Esthet. 1994;38(3):239–52.
8. Saban Y. Preservation septoplasty and rhinoplasty in deviated noses. In: Çakir B, Saban Y, Daniel RK, Palhazi P, editors. Preservation rhinoplasty. 1st ed. Turkey: Septum Ed; 2018. p. 295–315.
9. Daniel RK. The preservation rhinoplasty: a new rhinoplasty revolution. Aesthet Surg J. 2018;38(2):228–9.
10. Saban Y, Daniel RK, Polselli R, Trapasso M, Palhazi P. Dorsal preservation: the push down technique reassessed. Aesthet Surg J. 2018;38(2):117–31.
11. Palhazi P, Daniel RK, Kosins AM. The osseocartilaginous vault of the nose: anatomy and surgical observations. Aesthet Surg J. 2015;35(3):242–51.
12. Daniel RK, Palhazi P. Rhinoplasty: an anatomical and clinical atlas. New York: Springer; 2018.
13. Saban Y, Andretto Amodeo C, Hammou JC, Polselli R. An anatomical study of the nasal superficial musculoaponeurotic system: surgical applications in rhinoplasty. Arch Facial Plast Surg. 2008;10(2):109–15.
14. Saban Y, Polselli R. Atlas d'Anatomie Chirurgicale de la Face et du Cou. Florence: SEE Ed; 2009. (Book in French and Italian).
15. Neves JC, Tagle DA. Lateral crura; control in nasal tip plasty: cephalic oblique domal suture, 7X suture and ANSA banner. Ann Plast Reconstr Surg. 2020;4(3):1059.
16. Dogan T. Teorhinoplasty book.

17. Cakir B. In: Çakir B, Saban Y, Daniel RK, Palhazi P, editors. Preservation rhinoplasty. 1st ed. Turkey: Septum Ed; 2018.
18. Varoquier M, Rumeau C, Vuissoz PA, Perez M, Hossu G, Jankowski R. Do the upper lateral nasal cartilages exist? The concept of septolateral cartilages. Eur Ann Otorhinolaryngol Head Neck Dis. 2021;138(2):77–81.
19. Finocchi V. SPQR technique. Preservation rhinoplasty meeting. Rome, Italy; 2019.
20. Saban Y, Polselli R. Pyriform aperture and rhinoplasty. In: Saban Y, Braccini F, Polselli R, Micheli-Pellegrini V. Rhinoplasties; The monographs of CCA group n°32. Paris; 2002.
21. Saban Y, de Salvador S. Guidelines for dorsum preservation in primary rhinoplasty. Facial Plast Surg. 2021;37(1):53–64.
22. Jankowski R. Le nez en tension. In Septoplastie et Rhinoplastie par Désarticulation. France; Issy-les-Moulineaux: Elsevier Masson; 2016 (Book in French). pp 261–266.
23. Toriumi D. EAFPS 43rd annual meeting. Joseph lecture. Live webinars. 2020. https://eafps.org/video/members-only. Accessed 25 Dec 2020
24. Saban Y. Step by step closed rhinoplasty with dorsum preservation. In: Saban Y, Çakir B, Daniel RK, Palhazi P, editors. Preservation rhinoplasty. 2nd ed. Kazim; 2019. pp. 251–265.
25. Lazovic GD, Daniel RK, Janosevic LB, Kosanovic RM, Colic MM, Kosins AM. Rhinoplasty: the nasal bones—anatomy and analysis. Aesthet Surg J. 2015;35(3):255–63.
26. Goksel A, Saban Y. Open piezo preservation rhinoplasty: a case report of the new rhinoplasty approach. Facial Plast Surg. 2019;35(1):113–8.
27. Johnson CM, Godin MS. The tension nose: open structure rhinoplasty approach. Plast Reconstr Surg. 1995;95(1):43–51.

4 Morphological and Diagnostic Tools in Rhinoseptoplasty: Italian Experience

Stelio Antonio Mocella, Rosario La Rosa, Riccardo Nocini, Mariapia Guerrieri, and Giorgio Giacomini

4.1 Introduction

Rhinoplasty is one of the most common facial plastic surgery procedures performed in the Western world, Mediterranean area included. The nose being one of the facial landmarks that define ethnic identity, surgeons need to pay particular attention to the expectations of patients requiring both functional and aesthetic nasal surgery, since the outcome must be both functionally and aesthetically satisfying, still maintaining a natural look that does not alter the ethnic identity of the patient. Otherwise, the risk of unsatisfaction and the need of a re-intervention is very high. To this purpose, in order to avoid surgery failure, it is advisable to perform a thorough preoperative diagnostic work-up, informing the patient on the exact possible final result.

S. A. Mocella (✉)
Centro di medicina Day Clinic di Verona, Verona, Italy

R. La Rosa
Casa di cura Villalba, Bologna, Italy

R. Nocini
Department of Otorhinolaryngology, University of Verona, Verona, Italy

M. Guerrieri
Department of Otorhinolaryngology, University of Rome "Tor Vergata", Rome, Italy

G. Giacomini
Department of Plastic Surgery, University of Rome "La Sapienza", Rome, Italy

P. G. Giacomini (ed.), *Mediterranean Rhinoplasty*,
https://doi.org/10.1007/978-3-031-05551-5_4

4.2 Preoperative Evaluation: Imaging Techniques

A careful preoperative diagnostic work-up is fundamental when planning both aesthetic and functional nasal surgery. Functional rhinological tests like acoustic rhinometry and rhinomanometry, together with subjective questionnaires investigating the grade of nasal obstruction are valid tools to assess nasal dysfunction (see Chap. 5).

Patients seeking for functional nasal surgery often wish, at the same time, to improve the aesthetic of their nose. In these cases, preoperative nasal evaluation must consider both functional and anatomical aspects.

At this regard, evaluating patients asking for aesthetic nasal surgery with Computed Tomography (CT scan), which is widely used in the diagnostic work-up of paranasal sinuses pathologies, is nowadays up for debate [1].

Modern high resolution CT scan allows to obtain a three-dimensional reconstruction of facial tissues, from the bone to muscles and skin.

In our opinion, nowadays CT scan offers the chance to study nasal anatomy more accurately, giving the rhinologist a precise idea of the sites that need surgical correction, in order to preserve or improve nasal airflow during rhinoplasty. Furthermore, the morphological evaluation of nasal structures through CT scan can also be a precious tool when planning aesthetic correction of the nose, as it allows to identify preoperatively the structures that need particular attention in order to reach the best result.

The standard high-resolution CT scan used for the previously mentioned reason can be even modified with a workstation so as to obtain high resolution images while the new Cone Bean CT technique can be used for preoperative diagnostic plans and postoperative control as it offers the advantage of a relatively low exposition to radiations and a lower cost of the machine which is now very popular in many medical offices.

In some of our previous works on MRI in Rhinoplasty, we have stressed the importance of such a method to carry out the assessment of the morphology of the nose and of cartilages, especially in cases of secondary rhinoplasty [2]. With the help of radiologists, it is possible to accurately detect the bone structures and the different portions of nasal cavities and of cartilaginous structures, especially with the use of surface coils.

On the base of tomographic dataset of nose and paranasal sinuses, it is possible to obtain the so-called diANA (Digital Analysis of Nasal Airflow) a computational fluid dynamics study, that might allow surgeons to better choose and select the indications for surgery [3].

During rhinoplasty, it is absolutely mandatory to correct the fluid dynamics of airstream inside the nose, with the aim to have the whole cavity reduced at the end of the procedure, so that the patient could have a different sensation and perception of the inset airstream.

In 2007, we presented the exact volume of nasal and paranasal cavities detected on CT scan data integrated with workstation procedures; it is possible to evaluate

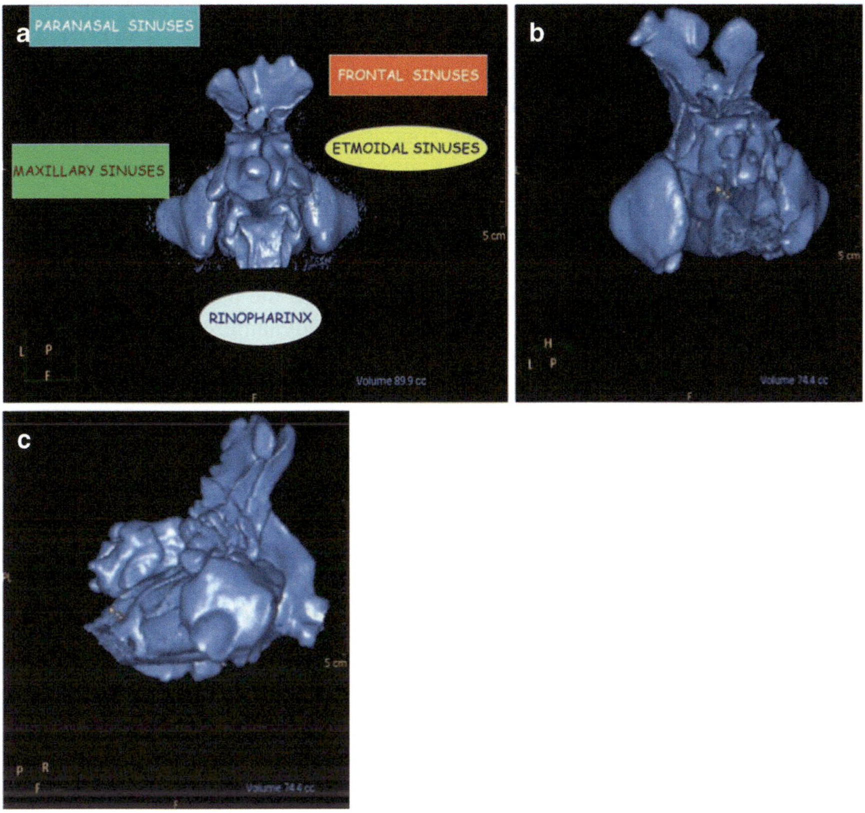

Fig. 4.1 (**a**) Volumetric reconstruction with CT three-dimensional configuration of nasal cavities; in the picture, the posterior part of nasal cavity laterally the maxillary sinuses and above the frontal and ethmoidal sinuses are visible. In this case, the preoperative volume is 74.4 cc with a ¾ view (**b**) and a lateral view (**c**)

precisely the volume of nasal cavities in different position of the obtained series of axial and sagittal scans [4] (Fig. 4.1).

After a first experience in 2014 [5], in 2015 Quadrio et al., from the Department of Aerospace Sciences and Technologies, suggested that the study of fluid dynamics could be applied to CT sections of nasal cavities so to obtain a virtual functional representation of nasal passage and also to perform virtual surgery in order to locate the exact structures to modify and to foresee the outcome [6]. In recent literature, an Italian contribution on fluid dynamics of the internal nose has been given by the school of engineering and otolaryngology of Milan, with the work of Covello et al. (2018), which pointed out the significant advances in Computational Fluid Dynamics (CFD) techniques for the study of the nasal airflow improving the general imaging and providing a quantitative analysis tool with a high unprecedented analytic power [7].

Another important contribution has been provided by the Italian Rhinology school and in particular by the second author of this article (La Rosa 2020). On the bases of his experiences with the collaboration of aerodynamics and fluid dynamics engineering, he observed that many patients have normal nasal resistances despite important septal deviations and, on the contrary, patients with normal endoscopic appearance may have difficult nasal ventilation [8, 9].

This is really important especially during rhinoplasty, as the patient's objective is the correction of both morphology and function of the nose.

Another important concept introduced in modern practical rhinosurgical activity is that it is important not only to correct and increase the nasal fluxes but also to realize structural modifications to restore the fluid dynamics and the receptorial activity in order to obtain a satisfied sensation of flux. According to some authors (Eccles 2000; Willet 1996), it is the temperature of the inspired air that could stimulate the activation of trigeminal receptors which are localized in the derma of nasal vestibule [10].

Despite the observation of Hoshino (1988) and Tsubone (1989) that have proven in animal experiments the presence of thermal receptors in the mucosa [11, 12], they are not histologically proven in the human mucosa but there is evidence of a very rich free not corpuscolated terminations.

Another important concept is the geometry of nasal cavities for the analysis of internal aerodynamics. With CT scan, we can get radial sections of the head, obtained using the hyoid bone as central point as shown in the Fig. 4.2.

These sections can be used to obtain the so-called *circular equivalence* (Fig. 4.3a), which represents the relationship between equivalent diameter and the CT sections of origin; an elliptic model with a representation of elongated section can also be obtained (Fig. 4.3b).

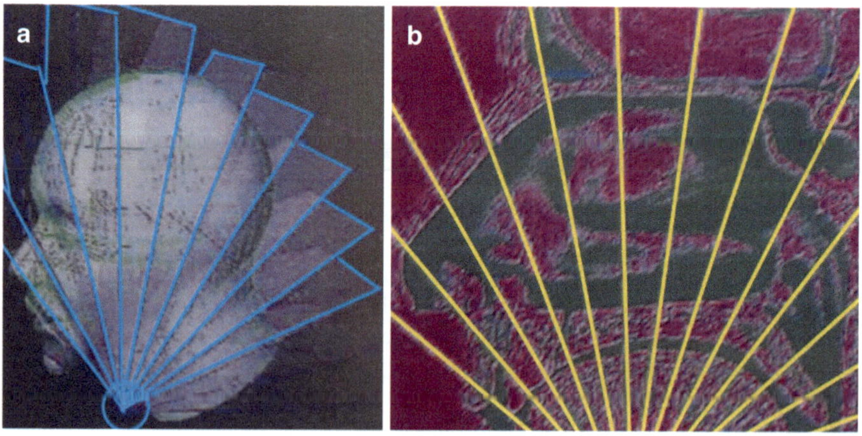

Fig. 4.2 (**a**) Radial sections on three-dimensional image. (**b**) Nasal sagittal section with evidence of radial sections used in studies fluid dynamics

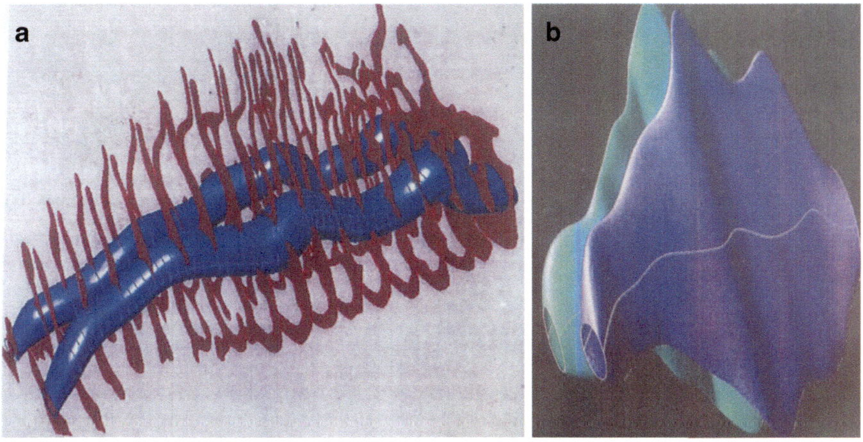

Fig. 4.3 (**a**) Circular Equivalence, relationship between equivalent diameter and the CT sections of origin. (**b**) Elliptical model in internal three-dimensional representation of the nasal cavities

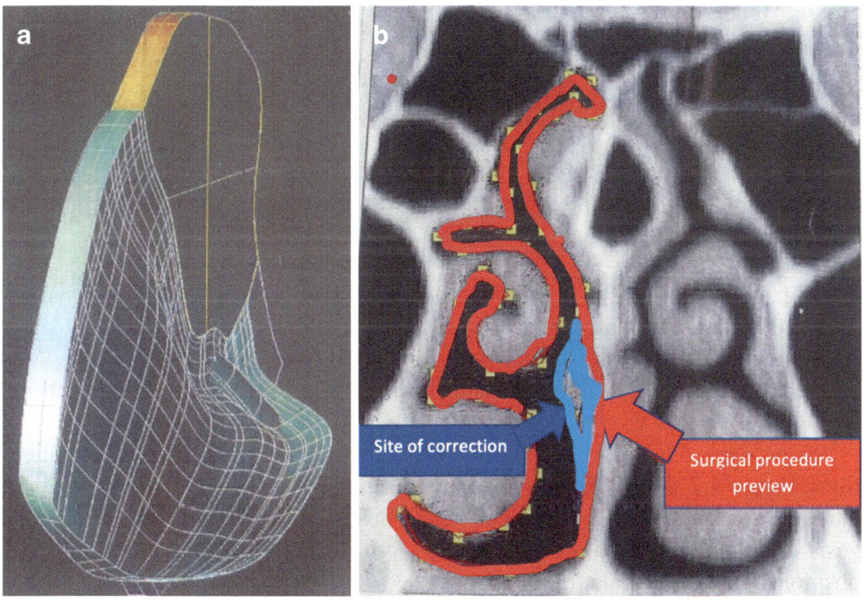

Fig. 4.4 (**a**) Study with four-sided grid for representation of the flow in a case of severe septal deviation. (**b**) Simulation of septoplasty on CT section

At the same time, Computational Fluid Dynamic (CFD) can be used to analyse the internal fluid dynamic of the nose using a programme of simulation called SNIFF (Simulation for Nasal Internal Flow Forecast).

Based on the use of these techniques, the second author has developed new concepts in the simulation of septal surgery (Fig. 4.4) and in the correction of Empty Nose Syndrome (Fig. 4.5) [9].

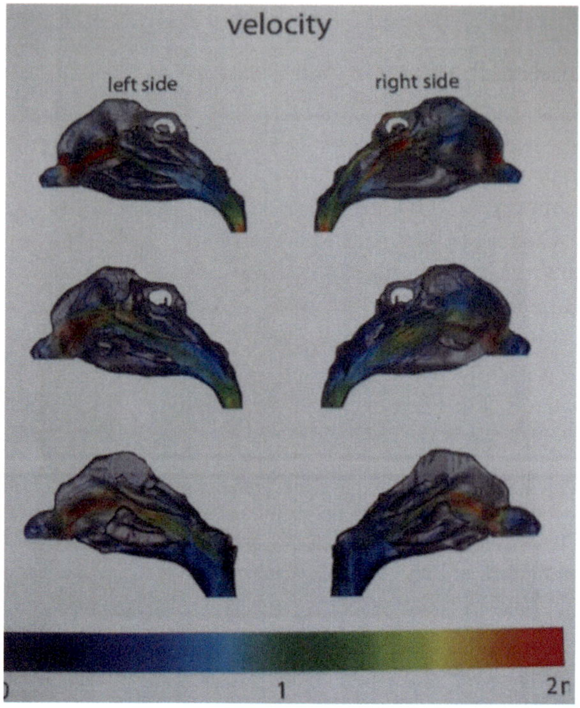

Fig. 4.5 CFD: coloured representation of the velocity of air molecules in the two nasal cavities, in a patient with empty-nose syndrome

4.3 Clinical Cases

When planning surgery, it is important to obtain elaborate CT images to make a correct diagnosis especially in case of secondary rhinoplasty, where we do not know what has been done previously and which materials have been used.

Case 1 presents a patient of balcanic origins who affirmed to have some material inside his nose after a surgical procedure (Fig. 4.6).

We performed a CT scan analysis with elaborations and workstation modifications. Figure 4.7 shows the normal axial CT scan (a) and an elaborated CT scan at the same level, with a strange presence of air inside the septum area (b), which suggests an infection due to aerobic bacteria, probably due to heterogenic material positioned into the septal area.

During surgery, we removed the material showed in the picture (Fig. 4.8a). Hence the auricular cartilage was harvested, modified and positioned between the two perichondral septal layers during an open rhinoplasty (Fig. 4.8b, c).

In the images obtained with cone bean CT scan, 1 month after surgery, we could see the auricular cartilage positioned in the septal site and two silicone sheets in each nasal side (Fig. 4.9).

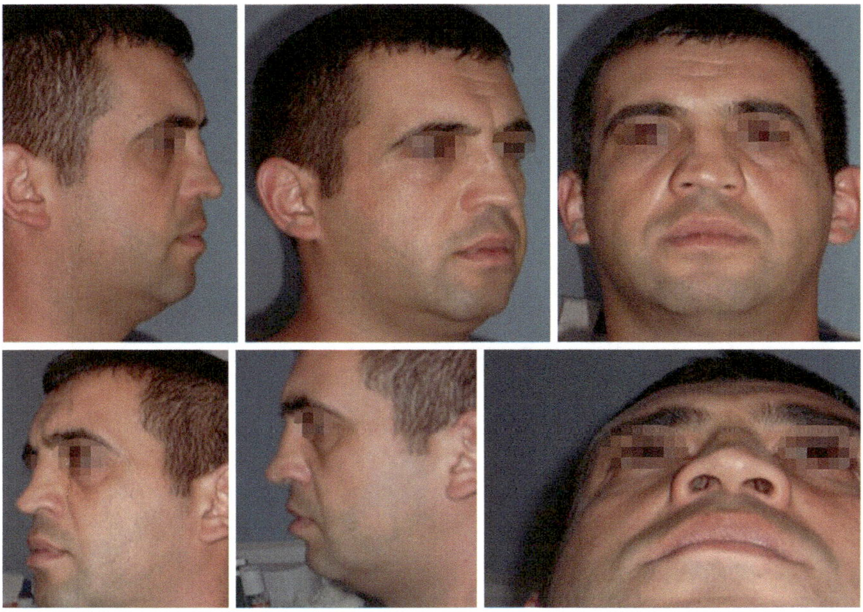

Fig. 4.6 Preoperative view

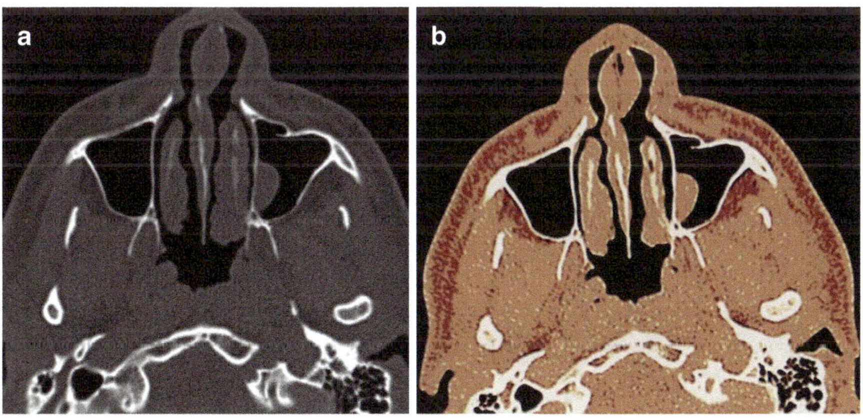

Fig. 4.7 (**a**) Axial CT section. (**b**) Elaborated CT section at the same area shows air inside the nasal septum, due to the infection of foreign material

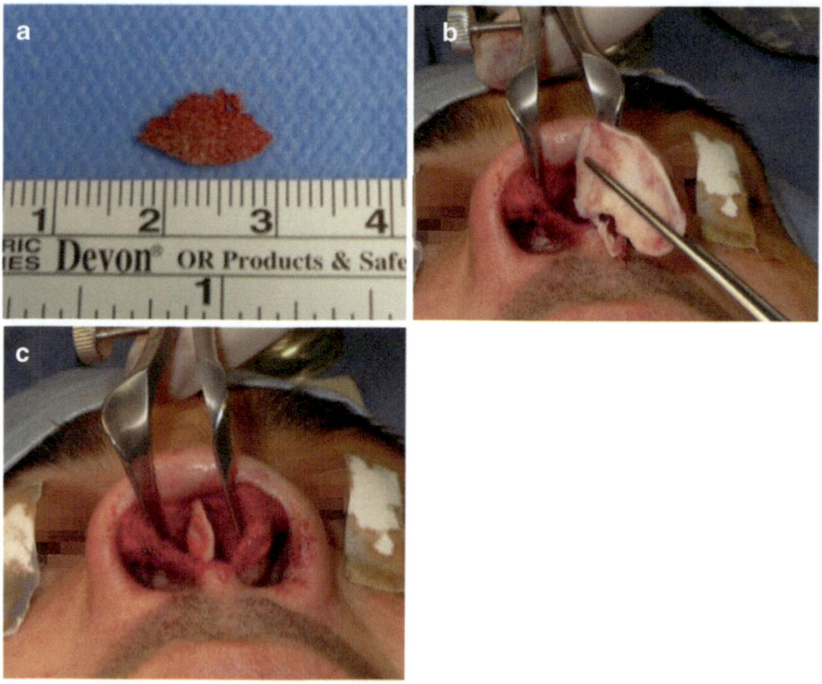

Fig. 4.8 (**a**) Foreign material removed from the patient's nose. (**b**, **c**) A graft of auricular cartilage is positioned between the two perichondral septal layers

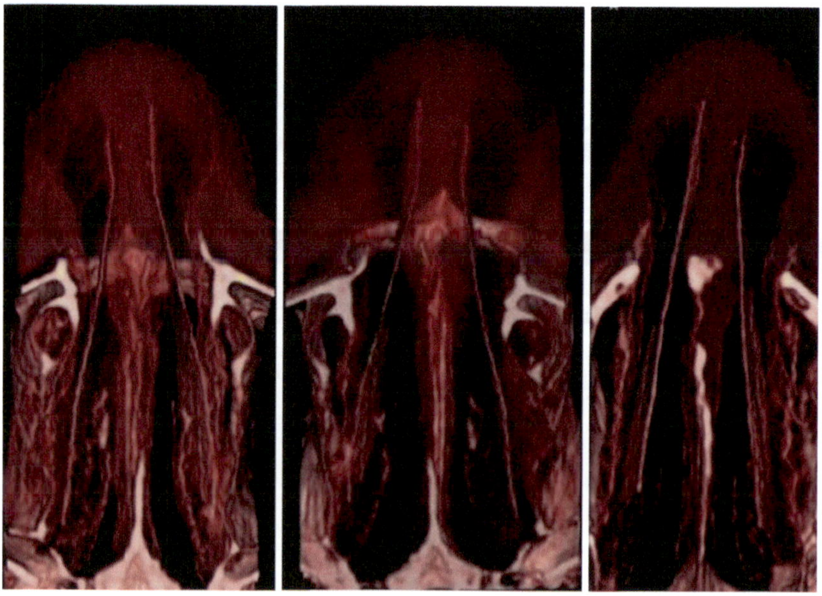

Fig. 4.9 Cone bean CT scan with elaboration: it is possible to visualize the auricular reconstruction of the septum and the silicone sheets in each nasal cavity

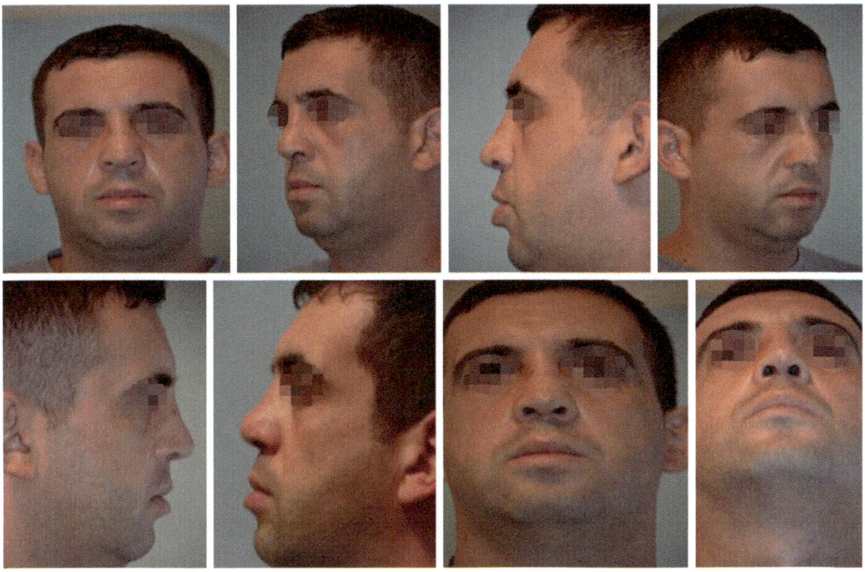

Fig. 4.10 Postoperative result

These sheets were removed in a next surgery. Figure 4.10 shows the complete result obtained 6 months after surgery.

Case 2 presents another complex septal deformity and contemporary bulbous large tip. An open rhinoplasty was performed (Figs. 4.11, 4.12, 4.13, 4.14, 4.15, and 4.16).

Case 3 shows a case of post-traumatic nasal deformity (Figs. 4.17, 4.18, and 4.19).

Case 4 shows a case of tip surgery where 3D CT scan reconstruction was used during preoperative planning (Figs. 4.20 and 4.21).

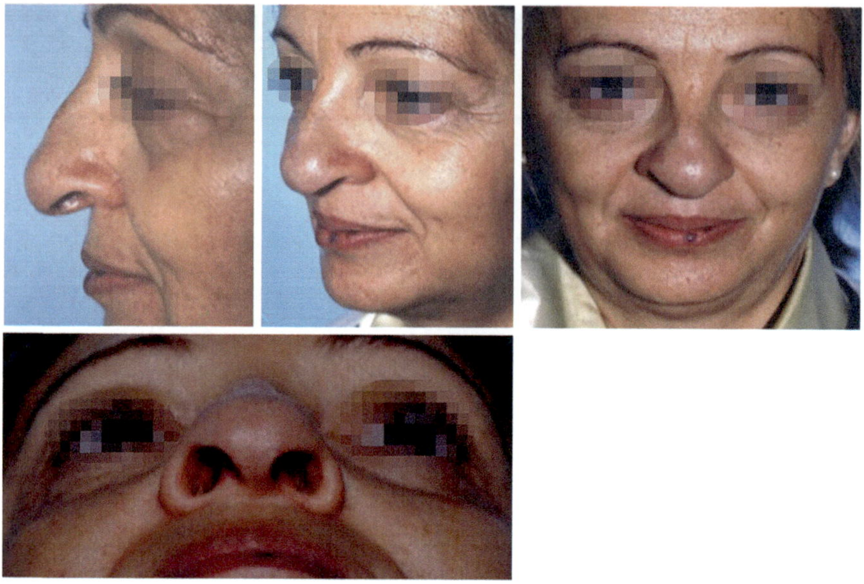

Fig. 4.11 Pre-operative view of a female patient with a post-traumatic morphology nose

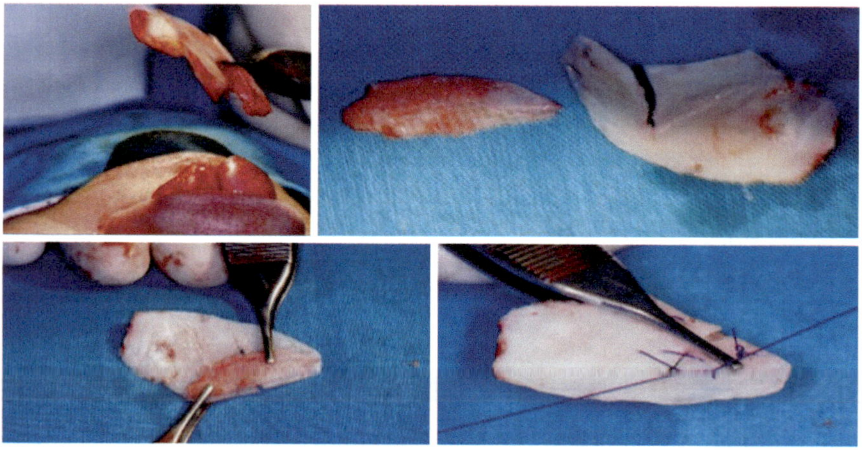

Fig. 4.12 Septal reconstruction with employment of hump to stabilize the new septum

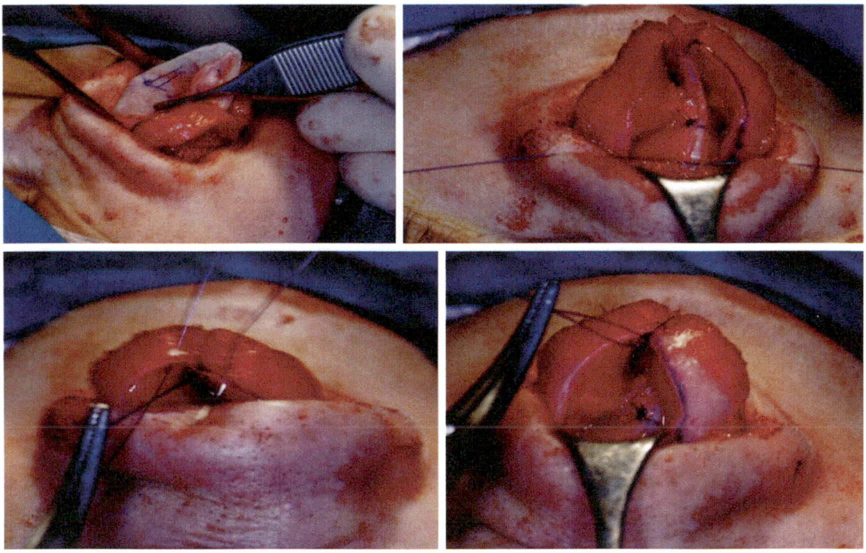

Fig. 4.13 Septal repositioning during the open approach and tip remodelling with interdomal sutures

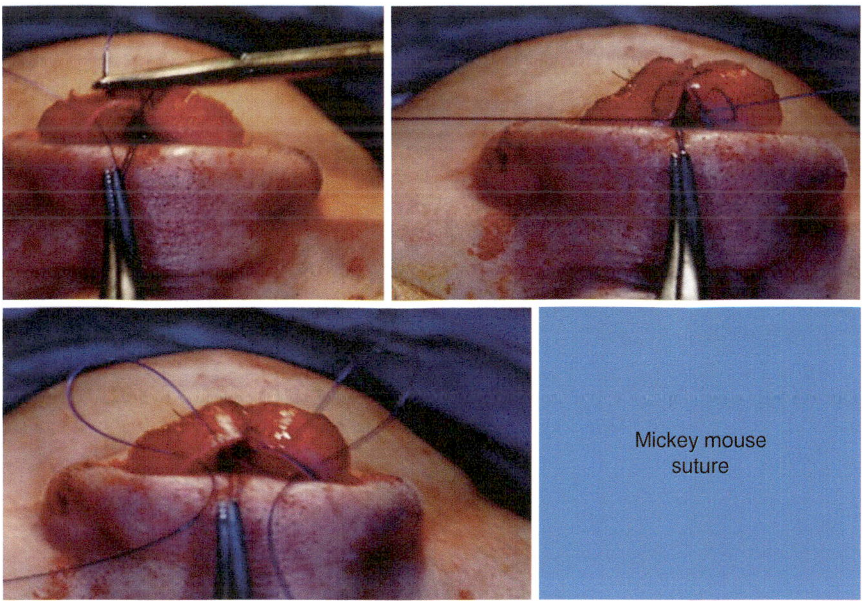

Fig. 4.14 Tip "Mickey mouse" sutures

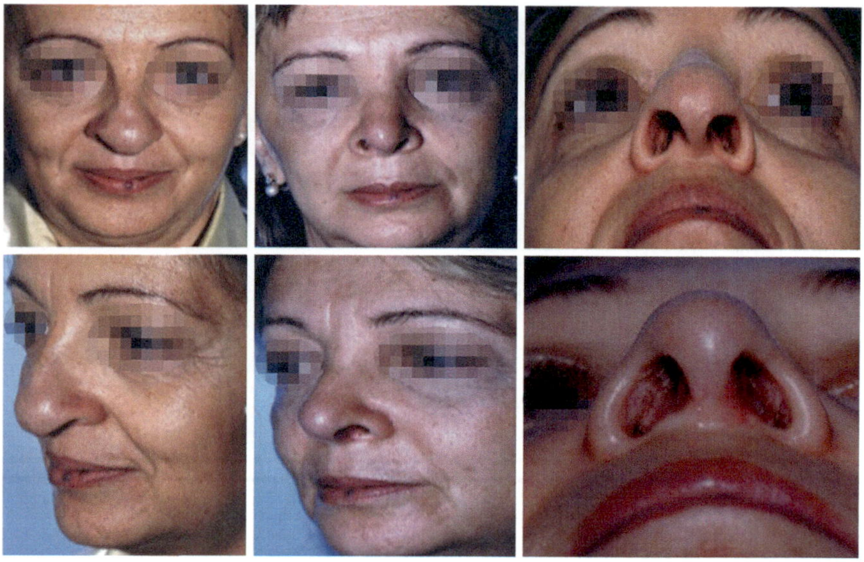

Fig. 4.15 Pre and postoperative views in particular basal views of the tip

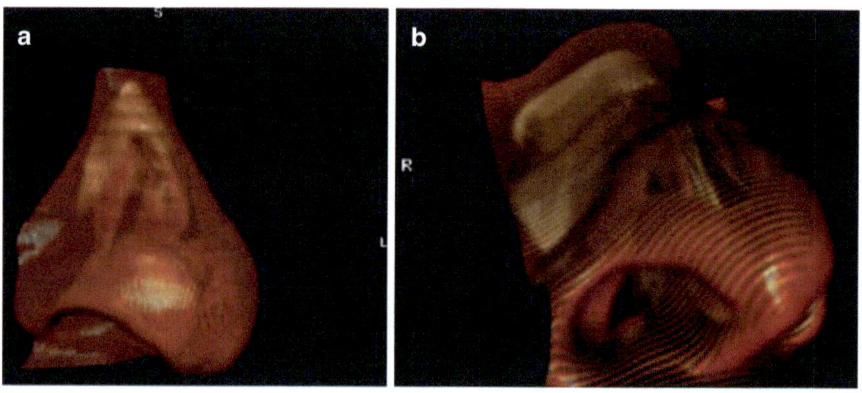

Fig. 4.16 High-definition CT scan reconstructions with evidence of tip modifications and tissue under the surface, pre (**a**—left) and postoperative (**b**—right) images

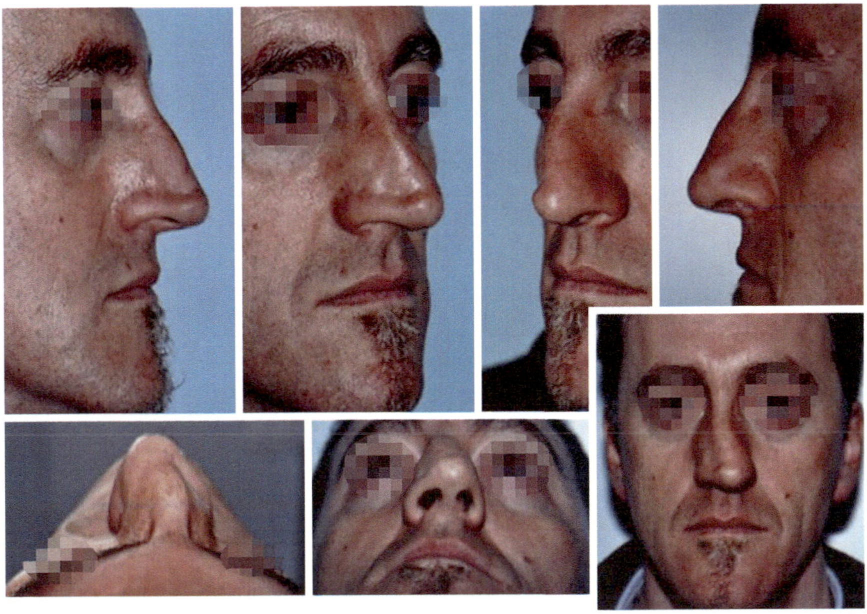

Fig. 4.17 Different projections of man with a post-traumatic nasal deformity

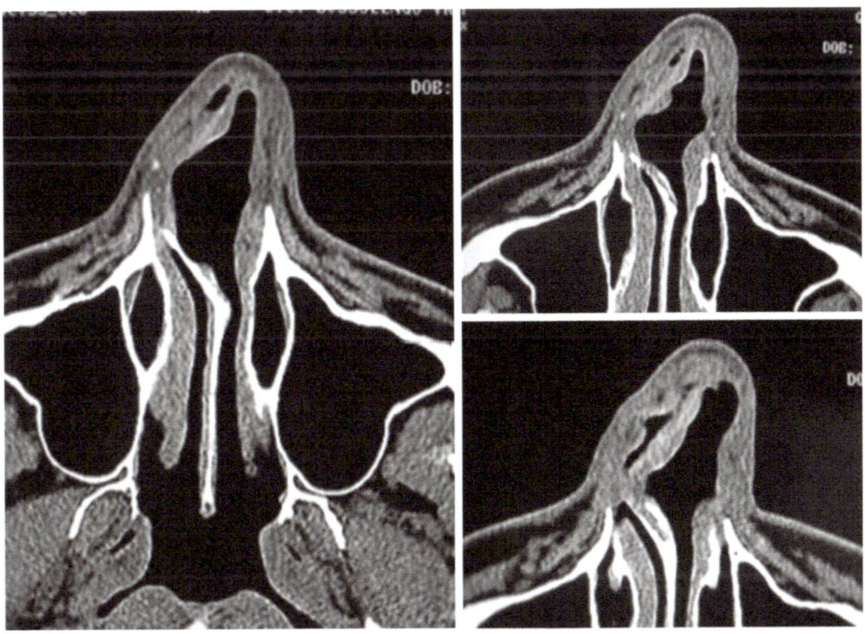

Fig. 4.18 CT axial scans of the previous case with evidence of the septal deformity and latero-deviation of the pyramid

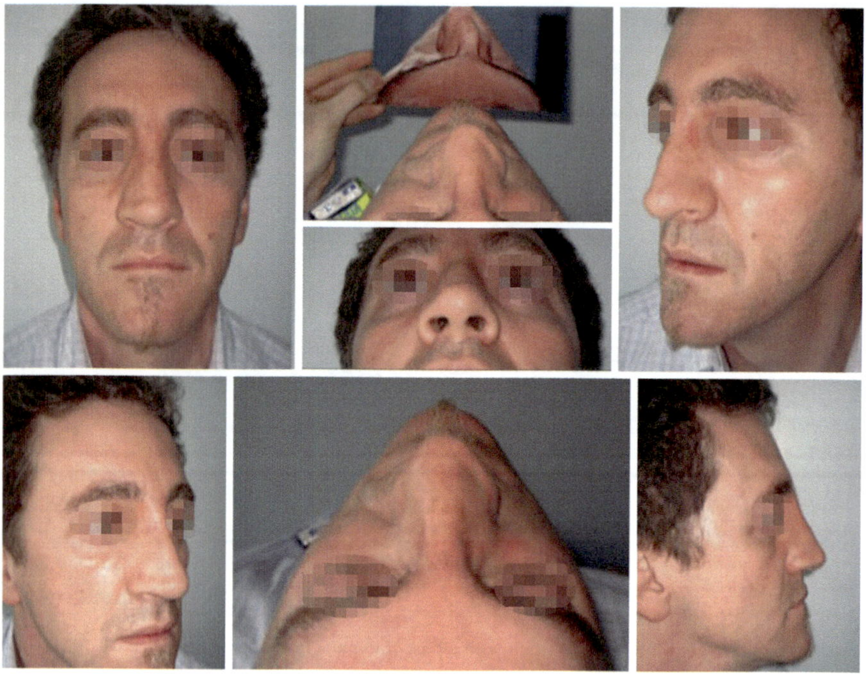

Fig. 4.19 Postoperative pictures of the previous man case with evidence of the result in particular at the helicopter view

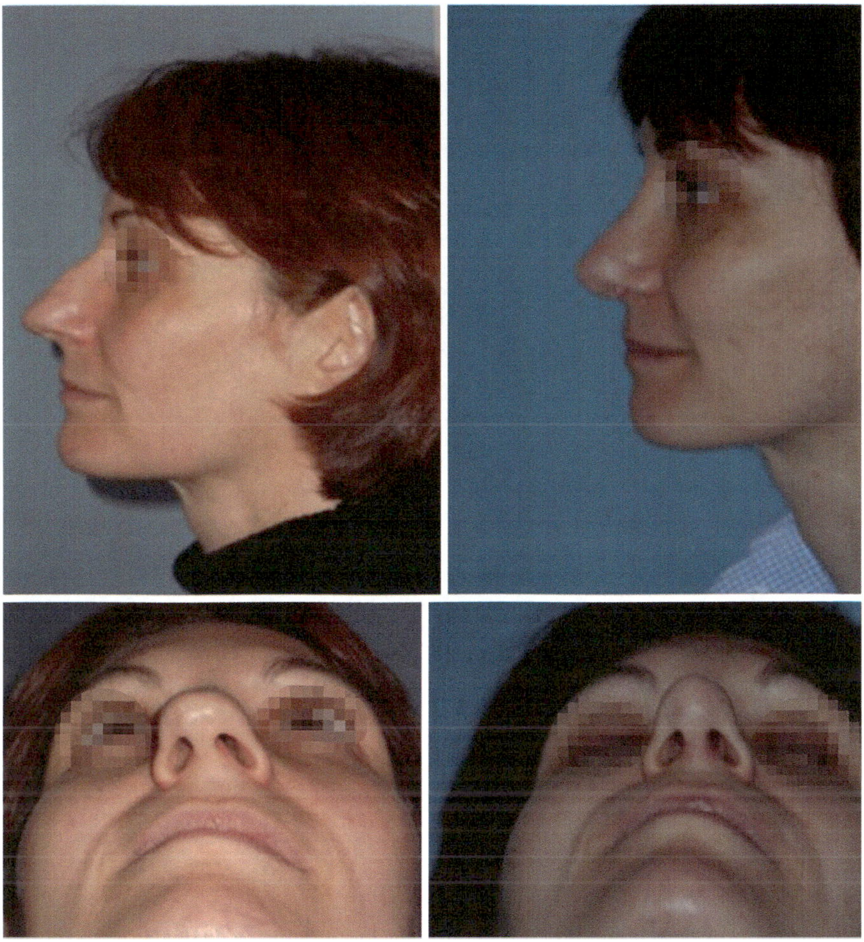

Fig. 4.20 Pre and postoperative view of a patient who underwent rhinoseptoplasty with tip surgery

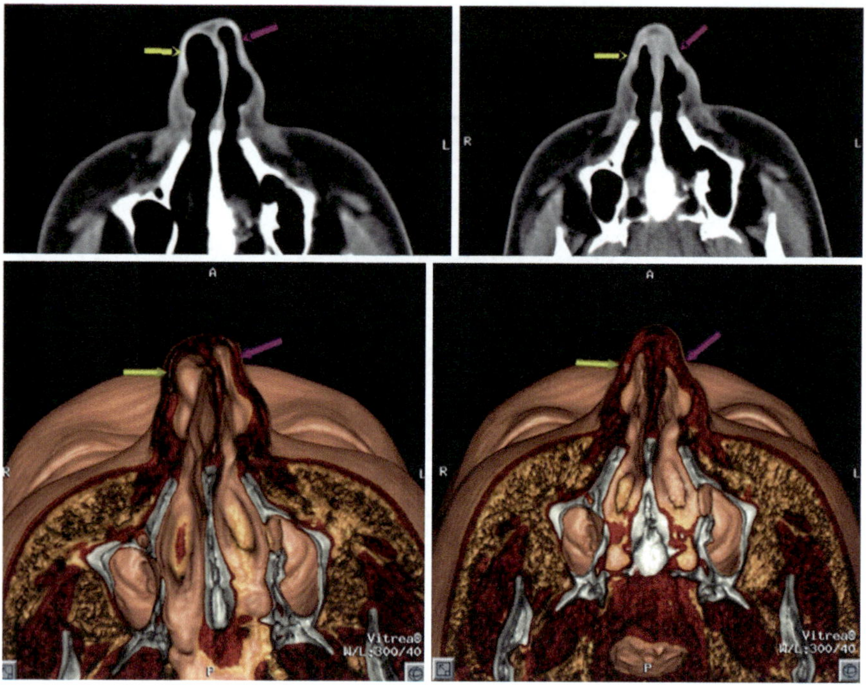

Fig. 4.21 Nasal tip view obtained with 3D CT Reconstructions elaborated—pre and postoperative scans with evidence of the result obtained after 6 months, in particular the reorientation of the tip

4.4 Conclusions

Rhinoseptoplasty is a complex procedure and pre-operative analysis of both function and aesthetic of the nose is fundamental.

At this regard, the surgeon has to collect as many information as possible in order to avoid postoperative complications but also, and more importantly, to reach the most satisfying result for the patient.

For this reason, the authors suggest considering the use of CT scan data when planning aesthetic surgery. We have in fact demonstrated that through the elaboration of CT scans and images, especially considering the data derived from aerodynamic studies, it is possible to assess pre-operative true functional site of obstruction and to evaluate virtual surgical outcomes, in order to predict real post- operative results both in their aesthetic and functional aspects. "Cone bean" CT scan is really important, especially in the post-operative period. Further studies will be necessary to expand our knowledge of the complex physiology of nasal cavities, in order to improve nasal surgery, both functional and aesthetic, and to obtain more satisfying results.

References

1. Hildebrandt T, Bruening JJ, Schmidt NL, et al. The healthy nasal cavity—characteristics of morphology and related airflow based on a statistical shape model viewed from a surgeon's perspective. Facial Plast Surg. 2019;35(1):9–13. https://doi.org/10.1055/s-0039-1677721.
2. Mocella S, Bianchi N, Cerini R, Beltramello A. Magnetic resonance imaging in primary and secondary septorhinoplasty. Facial Plast Surg. 1996;12(4):321–32. https://doi.org/10.1055/s-2008-1064503.
3. Hildebrandt T, Brüning J, Lamecker H, et al. Digital analysis of nasal airflow facilitating decision support in rhinosurgery. Facial Plast Surg. 2019;35(1):3–8. https://doi.org/10.1055/s-0039-1677720.
4. Mocella S, Biasiutti C. Nasal cavities and paranasal sinuses volumes detected with high resolution CT data. 2007.
5. Quadrio M, Pipolo C, Corti S, et al. Review of computational fluid dynamics in the assessment of nasal air flow and analysis of its limitations. Eur Arch Otorhinolaryngol. 2014;271(9):2349–54. https://doi.org/10.1007/s00405-013-2742-3.
6. Quadrio M. Fluid dynamics of the nasal cavity: how to, what for. 34.
7. Covello V, Pipolo C, Saibene A, Felisati G, Quadrio M. Numerical simulation of thermal water delivery in the human nasal cavity. Comput Biol Med. 2018;100:62–73. https://doi.org/10.1016/j.compbiomed.2018.06.029.
8. La Rosa R. Le basi della moderna aerodinamica nasale per la chirurgia funzionale. Basi Della Mod Aerodinamica Nasale Chir Funz. 2020.
9. La Rosa R. Empty nose syndrome. Moderne tecnologie per la diagnosi ed il trattamento chirurgico—Monografia; 2021.
10. Eccles R, Griffiths DH, Newton CG, Tolley NS. The effects of menthol isomers on nasal sensation of airflow. Clin Otolaryngol Allied Sci. 1988;13(1):25–9. https://doi.org/10.1111/j.1365-2273.1988.tb00277.x.
11. Hoshino T. In vitro electrophysiologic studies on nasal airway receptors of the rabbit. Ann Otol Rhinol Laryngol. 1988;97(3 Pt 1):294–7. https://doi.org/10.1177/000348948809700317.
12. Tsubone H. Nasal "flow" receptors of the rat. Respir Physiol. 1989;75(1):51–64. https://doi.org/10.1016/0034-5687(89)90086-8.

Functional Diagnostic Tools in Rhinoplasty: Italian Experience

5

Francesco Maria Passali, Eleonora Ciaschi, Laura Loccisano, and Stefano Di Girolamo

5.1 Introduction

Rhinoplasty is a plastic surgery procedure aimed to correct and reconstruct the nose. There are two types of rhinoplasty surgeries: functional rhinoplasty, used to improve the shape and function of the nose, and cosmetic rhinoplasty, the goal of which is to improve its appearance. To distinguish, in the "functional rhinoplasty", patients look for improvements in nasal breathing and olfaction, without radically changing the aesthetic of the nose. In most cases, functional improvements may be achieved without significantly altering the shape of the nose, such as when a septoplasty or certain types of nasal vestibular stenosis (valve) repair are performed.

The success of a cosmetic rhinoplasty is very important for patients, as the operation fundamentally changes a part of their appearance that has bothered them for years. However, rhinoplasty has relatively low satisfaction rates compared to other cosmetic procedures, causing high revision operation rates (about %15) and hence more physical and financial discomfort for the patient; nasal airway obstruction was found to be the most common indication for secondary surgery [1].

One of the reasons for the low satisfaction rate is failing to set the patient's expectations right before operation, due to the lack of the right use of communication and diagnostic tools. The perception of the patient and the surgeon might be different for the results of the operation. It is of utmost importance to reach a mutually agreeable set of expectations during the pre-surgery consultation utilizing the tools available for pre-surgery planning [2].

It is well known that breathing through the nose is the only physiological form of breathing, as it is proved by the anatomical, functional, and psycho-behavioural alterations induced by breathing through the mouth. However, this natural and

F. M. Passali (✉) · E. Ciaschi · L. Loccisano · S. Di Girolamo
Department of Otorhinolaryngology, University of Rome "Tor Vergata", Rome, Italy
e-mail: passali@med.uniroma2.it

P. G. Giacomini (ed.), *Mediterranean Rhinoplasty*,
https://doi.org/10.1007/978-3-031-05551-5_5

apparently simple way of breathing implies the existence of fine mechanisms and functions of cleaning and heating of the air breathed in, with which the nasal mucosa is endowed. It is, indeed, the role of the nose to change the physical characteristics (temperature and humidity) of the air, making them suitable for the gas exchange in the lungs and providing in addition a barrier from pollution, allergens, viruses and bacteria.

The nose is a distinct landmark in facial aesthetics, being it the focal point of the face with a complex three-dimensional structure. The morphological integrity of the osteo-cartilaginous structures, as well as of the mucosa and epithelium that cover them, is an indispensable prerequisite to carry out a physiological nasal breathing and for the ventilation of the paranasal cavities. Reductive rhinoplasty reduces nasal size and may compromise nasal airway width; thus, the ideal rhinoplasty includes preservation or improvement of the respiratory function.

To measure nasal function objectively is a constant challenge for plastic surgeons, otolaryngologists, speech pathologists, physiologists and allergists. The patient's perception is important but does not define the degree of obstruction or the degree of improvement after a certain treatment.

Nasal breathing takes place under conditions of resistance over 50% higher than that of the oropharyngeal tract. In the course of breathing in, the inspired volume of air, which crosses the nasal valve at the speed of 2–3 m/s, is distributed in three main streams: the main one passes through the middle meatus, another accounting for 5–10% with an almost vertical route reaches the olfactory bulb, and the third one laps the nasal floor. Moreover, to this laminar flow crossing the three meati, microturbulences are added, especially behind the nasal valve. Microturbulences are required in order to guarantee an adequate flow's merging and to increase the contact between the air and the mucosa. This phenomenon is aimed to improve heating and humidification, as well as the cleaning process of the inspired air [3].

The internal nasal valve cross-section is delimited by the head of the inferior turbinate, the nasal septum and the upper lateral cartilage. The external nasal valve is bordered by the alar lobule, medial crus of the lower lateral cartilage, caudal septum, alar rim and nasal sill [4]. The nasal valves are responsible for one-third of total nasal resistances [5], they respond to mechanical stresses and are modulated by voluntary muscles. Two thirds of nasal resistances are due to the turbinates valve [6], i.e. the neurovascular control cavernous tissue of the turbinates [7]. This is why it is more correct to speak about the "nasal valve area" (Fig. 5.1) or "flow-limiting segment" [8] where cartilages, muscles, mucosa, and epithelium contribute to prepare and provide the air for the lower respiratory apparatus and for the pulmonary gas exchanges.

Thanks to the *nasal valve area*, the airflow through the nasal cavities follows the Poiseuille's law with a laminar flow and microturbulences around the unevenness of the nasal fossae walls. This way, the contact of the air with the mucosa is increased, reaching the ideal air temperature and humidity, and promoting the cleansing from pollution, allergens, viruses and bacteria made by the ciliated epithelium.

The important role of the internal nasal valve in nasal airflow has been widely discussed in literature [9]. Iatrogenic internal nasal valve obstruction is frequently

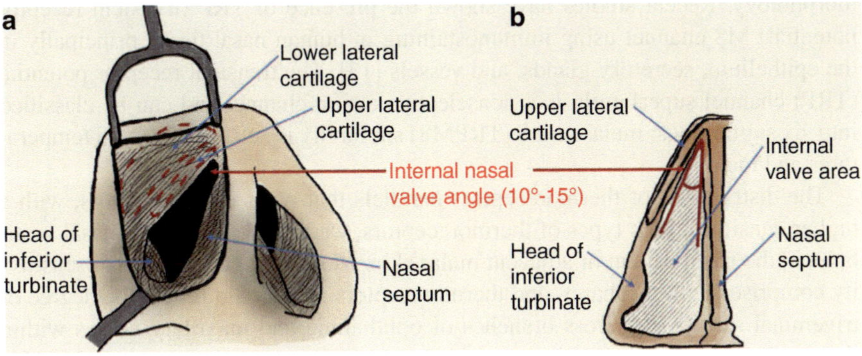

Fig. 5.1 Schematic view of the "nasal valve area". (**a**) The internal nasal valve area is delimited by the head of the inferior turbinate, the nasal septum and the upper lateral cartilage. (**b**) The internal nasal valve angle mesures usually 10–15°

secondary to collapse of the mid-vault after composite dorsal hump reduction or vestibular stenosis [10]. Moreover, if an iatrogenic cause of obstruction is identified, such as internal nasal valve collapse or synechiae, the rhinoplasty revision treatment will be required but should be delayed for at least 1 year to allow complete resolution of edema and maturation of scar tissue.

Studies have demonstrated that air flowing from the nostrils to the nasopharynx increases to 95% humidity and nearly 30 °C [11]. In fact, the air conditioning is guaranteed by the presence of the cavernous tissue and the arterious-venous shunts of the turbinates' microcirculation. The breathing of cold air enhances, in a reflex way, the opening of the arterious-venous shunts, increasing the heat exchanges at the air–mucus interface, while, on the other hand, breathing in hot air leads to the constriction of afferent arterioles.

The degree of repletion of the cavernous spaces, moreover, is modulated by the conditions of environmental humidity: if the air is dry, the water transudes from the turgid sinusoids toward the mucosa surface as a result of osmotic phenomena.

Previous studies have focused on the involvement of tactile receptors and mechanoreceptors in the sensation of nasal airflow. The major distribution of mechanoreceptors has been proved to be on the nasal vestibule, which is therefore the predominant sensitive nasal area. Indeed, the nasal vestibule represents the start of the respiratory system and histologically resembles skin lined by stratified squamous epithelium. The high concentration of mechanoreceptors and thermoreceptors in the anterior nasal valve/vestibule region may reflect an optimized confluence of trigeminal sensitivity to allow the detection and modulation of inspiratory air [4].

Worth of mention, among all these complex functions and the neurovegetative reflexes controlling them, is the presence of cold thermoreceptors involved in nasal patency sensation.

The idea of cold thermoreceptors in the nasal mucosa was proposed several years ago by Eccles [12], who reported that menthol topic administration produces the illusion of decongestion and improves nasal airflow without actually altering nasal morphology. Recent studies have shown the presence of TRP (transient receptor potential) M8 channel using immunostaining in human nasal tissue principally in the epithelium, secretory glands, and vessels [13]. The transient receptor potential (TRP) channel superfamily is a nonselective cation channel and can be classified into six subfamilies; melastatin 8 (TRPM8) subfamily is activated by cold temperatures and menthol.

The distribution of thermoreceptors parallels that of mechanoreceptors, with a higher density of both types of thermoreceptors, warm and cold, in the nasal vestibule, in the nasal cavum or adjacent malar skin. Moreover, general somatosensitivity comprises both mechano- and thermoreceptors and should reflect the degree of trigeminal sensitivity across branches of ophthalmic and maxillary nerves within the nasal cavity.

The dynamic cooling, though, is not just a function of the static air temperature or humidity in the environment; it also depends on the interaction between an individual's nasal airway structures (cartilages and mucosa) and the inspired air flow. Sensation of the nasal cavity mucosa is supplied by branches of the maxillary and ophthalmic divisions of the trigeminal nerve [4].

The preoperative consultation for rhinoplasty serves as an opportunity to obtain the patient's nasal history, to examine the nasal airway and perform nasofacial analysis. In this chapter, we will discuss about the functional diagnostic tools in rhinoplasty.

5.2 Assessment of Nasal Airflow

A good preoperative nasal breathing is not a guarantee of same postoperative breathing. The main idea behind volumetric rhinoplasty is as follows: If the size of the nose is reduced, the internal elements should be adjusted even if the patient has no impairments in nasal breathing for an adequate nasal airway width. Minimal septal deviations, concha bullosa, weak lateral cartilages or any other potential breathing problem not reported before the rhinoplasty may cause nasal obstruction [14].

This phenomenon is quite common and, if considered in itself, it limits the outcomes of functional surgery: After a reduction rhinoplasty, a decrease in the internal volume may be expected. According to Sheen et al. [15], this situation can be seen in about 75% of patients, nonetheless only about 10% of subjects develop nasal obstruction.

This complex array of variables may vary as a consequence of the surgical procedure. Thus, it is important to assess nasal airflow both before and after the rhinoplasty.

The patient should be examined for collapse of the external nasal valves on deep inspiration, and a Cottle test should be performed to evaluate patency of the internal nasal valves. Internal nasal examination is aided with the use of a nasal speculum. Narrowing or collapse of the internal valves with inspiration should be reported as well as inferior turbinate hypertrophy, which is typical in patients with septal deviation.

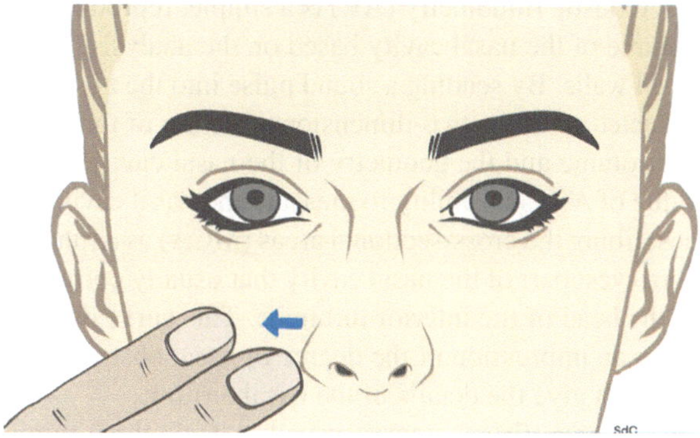

Fig. 5.2 Cottle manoeuver

The Cottle manoeuver (Fig. 5.2) is performed by gently pulling laterally on the cheek directly adjacent to the nose to open the nasal valve on the side of the nose being evaluated [16].

Septal deformities such as deviation, tilt, spurs and perforations must be identified. The shape and the availability of the septal cartilage has to be assessed, as this is the main source of autogenous graft material. The presence of nasal polyps or tumours may require further investigations and specific treatment [10].

Most measurements developed for nasal function have focused on evaluating nasal obstruction. They can be divided into two categories: **patient-reported (subjective)** and **objective** measurements.

5.2.1 Objective Methods

Traditionally, nasal ventilation is **objectively** measured using rhinomanometry or acoustic rhinometry.

Rhinomanometry is a dynamic test of nasal function that calculates nasal airway resistance (NAR) by measuring transnasal pressure and airflow in the nasal passage during respiration [17].

The following three kinds of rhinomanometry are used:

- The most commonly used method is *active anterior rhinomanometry (AAR)*, in which the patient actively breathes through one nasal cavity while the transnasal pressure, or difference in pressure from the naris to the nasopharynx, is measured with a pressure probe placed at the contralateral nostril.
- *Passive anterior rhinomanometry* the pressure is also measured for each nasal cavity separately, but at a given airflow.
- *Active posterior rhinomanometry* measures choanal pressure with a sensor placed at the back of the nasal cavity via the mouth [18].

In AAR, two parameters are recorded: *flow* and *pressure gradient* from the nostril to the rhinopharynx.

Acoustic rhinometry (AR) is a simple, reproducible technique for measuring the volume of the nasal cavity based on the analysis of sound waves reflected from the nasal walls. By sending a sound pulse into the nose and recording and analysing the reflected sound, a two-dimensional picture of the nasal cavity is made, from which the volume and the geometry of the nasal cavity can be deduced [19]. The clinical value of AR is its ability to measure the nasal cavity dimensions in terms of a curve describing the cross-sectional areas (MCA) as a function of distance, identifying the narrowest part of the nasal cavity that usually corresponds to the nasal valve area or to the head of the inferior turbinate. This curve describes nasal airway patency and gives an impression of the degree of nasal obstruction [20], but on the other hand it does not give the details of the nasal airflow.

The area-distance curve usually shows three minimum notches or deflections, which represent the narrowest parts in the nasal cavity. Two of these notches are situated in the most anterior part of nasal cavity (up to 3 cm from the nares), representing the nasal valve and the head of the inferior turbinate [21].

All types of rhinomanometry are supposed to determine a relationship between pressure and flow. In other words, this method can reveal how much pressure decay in the nasal cavity is needed to bring about the amount of flow that meets the demands of adequate nasal physiology and the needs for respiration and gas exchange.

Since 1984, the permanent Standardization Committee on Rhinomanometry [22] published the following statements to perform rhinomanometry on uniformity: concerning pressure gradient measure, the basic method is the adhesive tape technique which gives an airtight seal with a minimal distortion of the nostril and is easy to perform.

To assess the flow, a facial mask is usually employed: the advantages are minimum-to-no nasal valve deformation and little chance of leakage at the level of the nostril. However, any kind of mask that does not result in deformation of the nose and does not allow leaks is acceptable. The mask should be transparent so that deformation of the nostril or kinking of the pressure tube can be noted and eliminated. Calibration of equipment is needed, the recording should always be performed during quite breathing, and the patient should be in a sitting position and have a rest and adaptation time to the environment temperature. The $x - y$ recording is considered the best because it shows very well the relationship between pressure gradient and flow. The resistance is preferably expressed at the fixed pressure of 150 Pa, and the flow is expressed in cm^3/s [3].

With rhinomanometry, the dynamic changes of airway resistance during respiration are continuously assessed. To obtain a single outcome value, the nasal airflow at a transnasal pressure difference of 150 Pa is frequently reported. This pressure difference reflects conditions at low physical efforts, provides information on nasal resistance when mixed laminar and turbulent flow prevails and can be achieved also by patients with poor respiratory strength. Mucosal decongestion with α-imidazoles may help to differentiate mucosal congestion from skeletal abnormalities. Mean flow increases ranging between 20 and 40% after mucosal decongestion have been reported [18].

However, despite the efforts of the *International Standardization Committee*, the introduction of the computerized analysis of the results, the studies of different authors devoted to solving methodological problems and the realization of technical devices, after more than 35 years since its first appearance into the clinical practice, AAR still represents a topic of discussion and a subject for critical reviews [22].

At this regard, for example, the problem of standardization does not end with the reference variables (flow measured in cm^3/s at a fixed pressure of 150 Pa) but includes many aspects that have a decisive influence on the results. Among them, the method of application of the receptors does not represent a triviality, on the contrary, it constitutes an element of extreme importance for the reliability of the collected data: this delicate phase, key to the entire test, is subjected exclusively to the examiner expertise. Consequently, his/her degree of experience and attention represent a variable that can influence the validity of the exam in a positive or negative sense [3].

Another method to measure nasal airflow is the peak nasal inspiratory flow (PNIF). This method assesses the highest airflow through both nostrils during the maximum forced nasal inspiration, but does not measure the transnasal pressure difference and does not reflect the dynamic changes of nasal resistance during breathing, neither represents physiological conditions because normal oronasal breathing starts at much lower tidal volumes compared to the maximum nasal inspiration.

PNIF measures the forced maximal inspiratory airflow through the nose. A portable Youlten peak flow meter is used to assess maximal inspiratory flow; the patient is asked to do about three satisfactory maximal inspirations each time at basal condition and in sitting position, with at least 30 s interval between each inspiration. After this, only the highest of the three values recorded is considered [23].

Peak nasal inspiratory flow is a reliable, cheap and simple method to assess nasal airflow with an acceptable correlation with anterior active rhinomanometry both in healthy and obstructed noses [24].

Recently, the use of four-phase rhinomanometry (4PR) has been recommended to assess nasal obstruction. Nasal airway resistance is calculated using hundreds of resistances continuously recorded during the whole breathing cycle [22]. In 4PR, the most important parameters are the *effective resistance* of the entire breath (Reff) and its *logarithmic value* (logReff). Four-phase rhinomanometry (4PR) is advantageous because a result can be obtained for all patients, as it is not necessary to reach a designated pressure on the pressure–flow curve [25]. Two different studies compared 4PR and PNIF in the study of rhinological patients finding the two instruments to be comparable in results, with PNIF correlating better than 4PR with the nasal symptoms. Both studies concluded that PNIF, being inexpensive, fast, portable, simple and reliable, has practical advantages over 4PR and should be available in daily practice for the assessment of nasal obstruction [26, 27].

The biggest problem, however, is the frequent detection of a discrepancy between the subjective sensation of the degree of nasal obstruction/patency, the objective parameter recorded with rhinomanometry, and the endoscopic picture. The patient's perception is important but does not define the degree of obstruction or the degree of improvement after a certain treatment.

However, the fact that the patient's subjective complaints of nasal obstruction cannot be verified objectively does not mean they are not real and valid symptoms originating from a physical abnormality.

This problem has been pondered over for decades [28]. Several studies have demonstrated that applying substances such as camphor, eucalyptus, L-menthol, vanilla or lignocaine to the nasal or even palatal mucosa can cause a marked sensation of increased nasal airflow without any change in nasal resistance as measured by rhinomanometry. Conversely, infiltration or topical application of local anaesthetics in the nasal vestibule or damage of trigeminal sensory nerve endings may cause a sensation of decreased nasal patency, again without any measurable effect on nasal resistance.

Accordingly to Bermuller et al. [23] approximately 25% of symptomatic patients with functionally relevant nasal structural deformity remained undetected with both AAR and PNIF. Both methods are considered helpful to support the diagnosis of functionally relevant nasal structural deformities, but a negative test outcome does not exclude functionally relevant nasal stenosis. About that patient-centred questionnaire may represent a more practical and informative option to discern outcomes for the rhinoplasty patient. These data are critical in guiding surgical counselling for patients [29].

5.2.2 Subjective Methods

Beyond all the aforementioned objective evaluation methods used to assess nasal obstruction, it would be important to highlight the importance of the subjective evaluation methods as in rhinoplasty the patient perception must be taken under consideration. The aesthetic goals following rhinoplasty are largely dependent on the patient's concerns and expectations. For patients who present without nasal airway impairment, respecting and preserving the key structures is a fundamental requisite. Moreover, patients require careful attention in pre-surgical consultations, and clear communication should be prioritized to ensure that the surgeon understands the patient's expectation. At this regard, patient-reported questionnaires are increasingly becoming a tool to better assess the patient's appeasement and the nasal functional condition.

Subjective analysis of nasal patency is generally based on patient-reported outcome measures (PROMs) with visual analogue scales and/or questionnaires. In relatively recent publications few questionnaires used by plastic surgeon for rhinoplasty were used to assess both the cosmetic or psychosocial aspects, and pre/postoperative functional evaluations [30].

These validated questionnaires were the *Standardized Cosmesis and Health Nasal Outcomes Survey* (SCHNOS) and the "*nasal obstruction symptom evaluation test*" (NOSE), which have the specific goal of evaluating nasal symptoms including subjective obstruction [29].

The **Nasal Obstruction Symptom Evaluation** (NOSE) is a five-item, disease-specific patient-reported outcome measure of nasal obstruction [31]. Elements are scored from 0 to 4, or "Not a problem" to "Severe problem". Total point is summed and multiplied by 5 to allow a minimum score of 0 and a maximum score of 100. Higher results correlate with severity of nasal obstruction. In literature NOSE is described as the most common subjective questionnaire used for rhinoplasty [29] and a total score of 30 is established as the cut off to differentiate between a normal nasal airflow and nasal obstruction. Moubayed et al. developed a classification in which patients are categorized in **mild** (range, 5–25), **moderate** (range, 30–50), **severe** (range, 55–75), or **extreme** (range, 80–100) nasal obstruction [32].

The **Standardized Cosmesis and Health Nasal Outcomes Survey** (SCHNOS) is a 10-item, disease-specific patient-reported outcome measure for functional and cosmetic rhinoplasty: The elements from 1 to 4 are about the nasal obstruction; the item from 4 to 10 evaluate patient perception of the nasal aesthetic. Elements are scored from 0 to 5, or "No problem" to "Extreme problem," for a maximum score of 50; the maximum score is 100 [32].

5.3 Our Experience

In our experience, the most used diagnostic tool in rhinoplasty is the standardized photography, characterized by the frontal projection, lateral, oblique and basal ones. Moreover, an additional photo during smiling is taken because it may reveal nasal tip ptosis, static or dynamic, with a shortening of the upper lip or a transverse crease in the mid-philtral area [10]. This procedure is mandatory for every patient in the pre-surgical stage, as it is a crucial component of the medical record for preoperative planning and evaluation of postoperative results.

The use of diagnostic imaging techniques such as CT scan is required for the analysis of nasal patency, especially the internal nasal valve area. Moreover, imaging techniques are also needed in order to obtain more anatomical details of the structural causes of nasal obstruction for a better pre-surgical functional planning.

Besides morphological tools, we also administer NOSE questionnaire, a scale for the symptomatic measurement of nasal obstruction both in presurgical evaluation and in postoperative follow up. Subjective methods such as NOSE were found to be a promising and reliable tool to assess symptomatic improvement of nasal obstruction, especially after functional rhinoplasty [33].

To a lesser degree for the preoperatory planning of functional rhinoplasty, we analyse the nasal breathing using rhinomanometry and acoustic rhinometry. The main advantage of those objective measurements is the possibility to show any asymmetry in the nasal passage during the exam. Besides in patients that undergo functional rhinoplasty for severe nasal obstruction, it would be advisable to repeat AR and RMM after surgery to objectify the post operatory results.

5.4 Conclusions

Accurate preoperative evaluation of the nasal airway, along with the clarification of both the patient's expectations and the surgeon's goals, is the key to cosmetic and functional good result. Considering both subjective instruments of nasal obstruction evaluation (such as the *Nasal Obstruction Symptom Evaluation Scale*—NOSE and *Standardized Cosmesis and Health Nasal Outcomes Survey*—SCHNOS) and objective parameters such as rhinomanometry or acoustic rhinometry, patient history, and objective examination, it can be generally stated that: when anatomic anomalies on one or both sides are present, the symptom of nasal obstruction is constant, and the inspection assesses the kind and location of the stenosis. In the preoperative planning for rhinoplasty, nasal history should be investigated as well as a thorough examination of the nasal airway should be performed, together with nasofacial analysis. Also, intraoperatively, adequate anatomical exposure of the nasal deformity, preservation and restoration of the normal anatomy, correction of the deformity and restoration or preservation of the nasal airway are required. These steps added to a thorough evaluation of patient's expectations is the key that leads to successful outcomes following rhinoplasty.

References

1. Thomson C, Mendelsohn M. Reducing the incidence of revision rhinoplasty. J Otolaryngol. 2007;36(2):130–4. https://doi.org/10.2310/7070.2007.0012.
2. Saleh HA, Beegun I, Apaydin F. Outcomes in rhinoplasty. Facial Plast Surg. 2019;35(1):47–52. https://doi.org/10.1055/s-0039-1677829.
3. Passali F, Ottaviano G, Passali G, Girolamo S. The role of rhinomanometry and nasal airflow evaluation in the diagnosis of atrophic rhinitis. 2020. pp. 77–87. https://doi.org/10.1007/978-3-030-51705-2_7.
4. Shen J, Hur K, Li C, Zhao K, Leopold DA, Wrobel BB. Determinants and evaluation of nasal airflow perception. Facial Plast Surg. 2017;33(4):372–7. https://doi.org/10.1055/s-0037-1603788.
5. van Dishoeck HAE. Elektrogramm der Nasenflügelmuskeln und Nasenwiderstandskurve. Acta Otolaryngol. 25(4):285–95. https://www.tandfonline.com/doi/abs/10.3109/00016483709127966. Accessed 15 Apr 2021.
6. Haight JS, Cole P. The site and function of the nasal valve. Laryngoscope. 1983;93(1):49–55. https://doi.org/10.1288/00005537-198301000-00009.
7. Kern EB. Surgical approaches to abnormalities of the nasal valve. Rhinology. 1978;16(3):165–89.
8. Bloching MB. Disorders of the nasal valve area. GMS Curr Top Otorhinolaryngol Head Neck Surg. 2007;6:Doc07.
9. Howard BK, Rohrich RJ. Understanding the nasal airway: principles and practice. Plast Reconstr Surg. 2002;109(3):1128–46; quiz 1145–1146. https://doi.org/10.1097/00006534-200203000-00054.
10. Rohrich RJ, Ahmad J. Rhinoplasty. Plast Reconstr Surg. 2011;128(2):49e–73e. https://doi.org/10.1097/PRS.0b013e31821e7191.
11. Sommer F, Kroger R, Lindemann J. Numerical simulation of humidification and heating during inspiration within an adult nose. Rhinology. 2012;50(2):157–64. https://doi.org/10.4193/Rhino11.231.

12. Eccles R, Jones AS. The effect of menthol on nasal resistance to air flow. J Laryngol Otol. 1983;97(8):705–9. https://doi.org/10.1017/s002221510009486x.
13. Liu S-C, Lu H-H, Fan H-C, et al. The identification of the TRPM8 channel on primary culture of human nasal epithelial cells and its response to cooling. Medicine (Baltimore). 2017;96(31):e7640. https://doi.org/10.1097/MD.0000000000007640.
14. Kamburoglu HO, Bitik O, Vargel İ. Airflow considerations and the effect of Webster's triangle in reduction rhinoplasty. Aesthetic Plast Surg. 2021;45(5):2244–54. https://doi.org/10.1007/s00266-021-02168-9.
15. Sheen JH. Spreader graft: a method of reconstructing the roof of the middle nasal vault following rhinoplasty. Plast Reconstr Surg. 1984;73(2):230–9.
16. Das A, Spiegel JH. Evaluation of validity and specificity of the Cottle maneuver in diagnosis of nasal valve collapse. Plast Reconstr Surg. 2020;146(2):277–80. https://doi.org/10.1097/PRS.0000000000006978.
17. Zhao K, Frye RE. Nasal patency and the aerodynamics of nasal airflow in relation to olfactory function. In: Handbook of olfaction and gustation. Hoboken: Wiley; 2015. p. 353–74. https://doi.org/10.1002/9781118971758.ch16.
18. André RF, Vuyk HD, Ahmed A, Graamans K, Nolst Trenité GJ. Correlation between subjective and objective evaluation of the nasal airway. A systematic review of the highest level of evidence. Clin Otolaryngol. 2009;34(6):518–25. https://doi.org/10.1111/j.1749-4486.2009.02042.x.
19. Grymer LF, Hilberg O, Pedersen OF, Rasmussen TR. Acoustic rhinometry: values from adults with subjective normal nasal patency. Rhinology. 1991;29(1):35–47.
20. Ottaviano G, Fokkens WJ. Measurements of nasal airflow and patency: a critical review with emphasis on the use of peak nasal inspiratory flow in daily practice. Allergy. 2016;71(2):162–74. https://doi.org/10.1111/all.12778.
21. Nigro CEN, de Aguiar Nigro JF, Voegels RL, Mion O, Mello Junior JF. Acoustic rhinometry: anatomic correlation of the first two notches found in the nasal echogram. Braz J Otorhinolaryngol. 2005;71(2):149–54. https://doi.org/10.1016/s1808-8694(15)31303-3.
22. Vogt K, Bachmann-Harildstad G, Lintermann A, Nechyporenko A, Peters F, Wernecke KD. The new agreement of the international RIGA consensus conference on nasal airway function tests. Rhinology. 2018;56(2):133–43. https://doi.org/10.4193/Rhin17.084.
23. Bermüller C, Kirsche H, Rettinger G, Riechelmann H. Diagnostic accuracy of peak nasal inspiratory flow and rhinomanometry in functional rhinosurgery. Laryngoscope. 2008;118(4):605–10. https://doi.org/10.1097/MLG.0b013e318161e56b.
24. Døsen LK, Kvinnesland K, TarAngen M, Shiryaeva O, Gay C, Haye R. Unilateral and bilateral PNIF in quality control of nasal septal surgery. Int J Otolaryngol. 2018;2018:7846843. https://doi.org/10.1155/2018/7846843.
25. Vogt K, Zhang L. Airway assessment by four-phase rhinomanometry in septal surgery. Curr Opin Otolaryngol Head Neck Surg. 2012;20(1):33–9. https://doi.org/10.1097/MOO.0b013e32834e6306.
26. van Egmond MMHT, van Heerbeek N, Ter Haar ELM, Rovers MM. Clinimetric properties of the Glasgow health status inventory, Glasgow benefit inventory, peak nasal inspiratory flow, and 4-phase Rhinomanometry in adults with nasal obstruction. Rhinology. 2017;55(2):126–34. https://doi.org/10.4193/Rhin16.296.
27. Ottaviano G, Scadding GK, Iacono V, Scarpa B, Martini A, Lund VJ. Peak nasal inspiratory flow and peak expiratory flow. Upright and sitting values in an adult population. Rhinology. 2016;54(2):160–3. https://doi.org/10.4193/Rhin15.180.
28. Burrow A, Eccles R, Jones AS. The effects of camphor, eucalyptus and menthol vapour on nasal resistance to airflow and nasal sensation. Acta Otolaryngol. 1983;96(1–2):157–61. https://doi.org/10.3109/00016488309132886.
29. Okland TS, Kandathil C, Sanan A, Rudy S, Most SP. Analysis of nasal obstruction patterns following reductive rhinoplasty. Aesthet Plast Surg. 2020;44(1):122–8. https://doi.org/10.1007/s00266-019-01484-5.

30. Barone M, Cogliandro A, Di Stefano N, Tambone V, Persichetti P. A systematic review of patient-reported outcome measures after rhinoplasty. Eur Arch Otorhinolaryngol. 2017;274(4):1807–11. https://doi.org/10.1007/s00405-016-4359-9.
31. Stewart MG, Witsell DL, Smith TL, Weaver EM, Yueh B, Hannley MT. Development and validation of the nasal obstruction symptom evaluation (NOSE) scale. Otolaryngol Head Neck Surg. 2004;130(2):157–63. https://doi.org/10.1016/j.otohns.2003.09.016.
32. Moubayed SP, Ioannidis JPA, Saltychev M, Most SP. The 10-item Standardized Cosmesis and Health Nasal Outcomes Survey (SCHNOS) for functional and cosmetic rhinoplasty. JAMA Facial Plast Surg. 2018;20(1):37–42. https://pubmed.ncbi.nlm.nih.gov/28880988/. Accessed April 14, 2021.
33. Shafik AG, Alkady HA, Tawfik GM, Mohamed AM, Rabie TM, Huy NT. Computed tomography evaluation of internal nasal valve angle and area and its correlation with NOSE scale for symptomatic improvement in rhinoplasty. Braz J Otorhinolaryngol. 2020;86(3):343–50. https://doi.org/10.1016/j.bjorl.2019.08.009.

Northern Mediterranean Nose Correction: Italian Experience—Closed Approach

6

Pier Giorgio Giacomini, Giorgio Giacomini,
and Mariapia Guerrieri

6.1 History of the Procedure

After a first attempt of saddle nose correction published by Roe in 1887 [1], the modern rhinoplasty has been categorized in Germany by Joseph, who presented his revolutionary concepts at the Medical Society of Berlin in 1898. He is considered the father of modern rhinoplasty; his ideas rapidly spread worldwide and the endonasal rhinoplasty has since then been refined and performed up today by several facial plastic surgeons. Among these, in the USA, Aufrict, Safian, Fomon, Cottle and Goldman shared their experience organizing courses of rhinoplasty in order to train new surgeons, as many others did all over the world. In Italy, for example, during the second half of the last century, surgeons such as Valerio Micheli-Pellegrini, Giorgio Sulsenti and Lionello Ponti popularized the teachings of Maurice Cottle from Chicago and Irving Goldman from New York. Their contribution to the education of countless early modern rhinoplasty surgeons has led to the actual trends in closed rhinoplasty in Mediterranean geographical area. Among many others, we can cite nowadays names as Foda in Egypt, Apaydin in Turkey, Costantinidis in Greece, Faki in Lebanon, Sousa Vieira in Portugal, Morero in Spain, Saban in France, Tasca and Scattolin in Italy, Pipic in Croatia and Austria. The debate between endonasal and open approach in nasal surgery has been carried out in the last two decades and has actually greatly subsided in favour of an integrated vision of the matter: different approaches for different problems. Lately, a re-evaluation of Cottle principles has led European-Mediterranean surgeons such as Ives Saban, Baris Chakir and

P. G. Giacomini (✉) · M. Guerrieri
Department of Otorhinolaryngology, University of Rome "Tor Vergata", Rome, Italy
e-mail: piergiorgio.giacomini@uniroma2.it

G. Giacomini
Department of Plastic Surgery, University of Rome "La Sapienza", Rome, Italy

P. G. Giacomini (ed.), *Mediterranean Rhinoplasty*,
https://doi.org/10.1007/978-3-031-05551-5_6

Peter Palhazi to develop the concept of "preservation rhinoplasty" applied to the endonasal approach. The art and science of rhinoplasty in Europe are constantly updated and shared by many distinguished and dedicated surgeons through associations devoted to scholar and clinical activities such as the European Academy of Facial Plastic Surgery (EAFPS), the same target is pursued locally by single national associations: specifically in Italy the Association of Facial Aesthetic and Functional Surgery (AICEFF). Their activity of constant sharing and spreading of rhinoplasty knowledge is of paramount importance to improve patient and surgeon benefit and satisfaction.

From the patient's point of view, the ideal aesthetic proportions may vary depending on gender, age and race or geographical area. During the years, artists, behavioural scientists, and physicians have been trying to elaborate a canon of ideal beauty for nose proportions, which could apply for all kind of ethnicities (symmetry, frontal view straightness, nasal-facial harmony, orbito-nasal smooth lines) or just for selected cases such as white patients (smooth dorsal profile, nasal sidewall shadowing, tip rotation, definition and projection, supratip break, etc.) or Asian and African (increased width of the nasal base, flat nasal bridge, etc.).

Current trend is anyway to acknowledge the specific ethnic features of the nose and to tailor its correction on the patient's needs and expectations, preserving his/her ethnic identity. At this regard, Palma et al. have analysed several kind of Italian noses in order to classify them according to the most frequent defects (strong prominent nose, drooping nose, northern nose, heavy nose), in order to suggest the best way to deal with each case [2].

6.2 Endonasal Rhinoplasty

6.2.1 Indications

Any rhinoplasty surgeon can approach the nasal pyramid re-shaping either by endonasal or external (trans-columellar) route, the patient's features will lead to different rhinoplasty indications according to the surgeon's experience and personal preference [3].

Dealing with endonasal rhinoplasty some tips can be underlined [4]:

- Decreased need for surgical dissection
- Decreased potential for nasal tip support reduction
- Reduced post-operative edema
- Corresponding decrease of the potential overall scarring or iatrogenic insult to the nose
- Ability to make exact changes in situ
- Via intra-operative tactile palpation, a more immediate and predictable ability to feel the changes produced on the nose
- Ability to make targeted improvements without opening the nose apart
- Shorter operative times

- Theoretical reduction in morbidity, especially in older patients
- Elimination of any risk (however minimal) for developing a visible external columellar scar
- Reduced post-operative edema
- Quicker return to a normal appearance

6.2.2 Endonasal Techniques

In primary rhinoplasty, the endonasal approach to the tip may be carried out via either a **non-delivery** or **delivery** technique (Figs. 6.1 and 6.2). Different incisions are therefore performed according to the planned technique: trans-cartilaginous or inter-cartilaginous incisions reserved for the former, alar marginal and inter-cartilaginous incisions for the latter. The different complexity of tip correction required in different cases will lead to non-delivery for simpler cases (Figs. 6.3, 6.4, 6.5, and 6.6) and delivery for more complex (Fig. 6.7) alar cartilages re-shaping

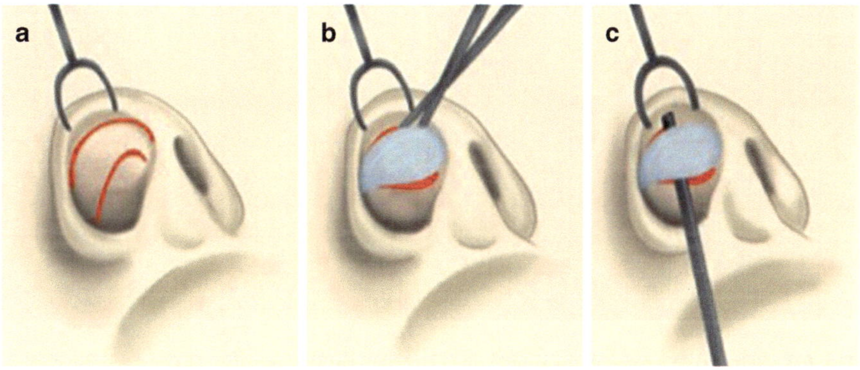

Fig. 6.1 Delivery approach. (**a**) Two incisions on the nasal valve, (**b**, **c**) exposure of the alar cartilage

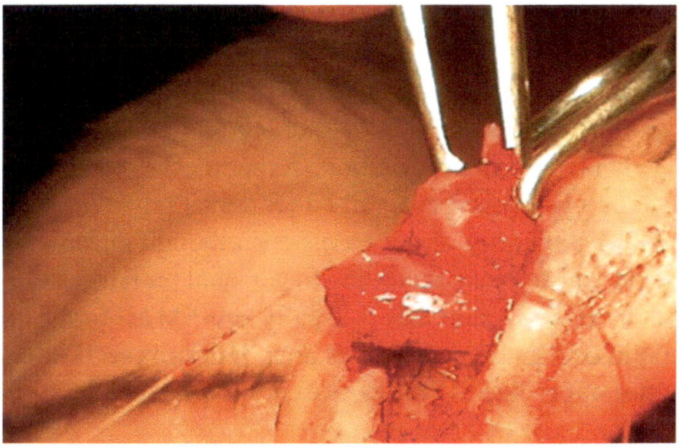

Fig. 6.2 Delivery technique, intraoperative view

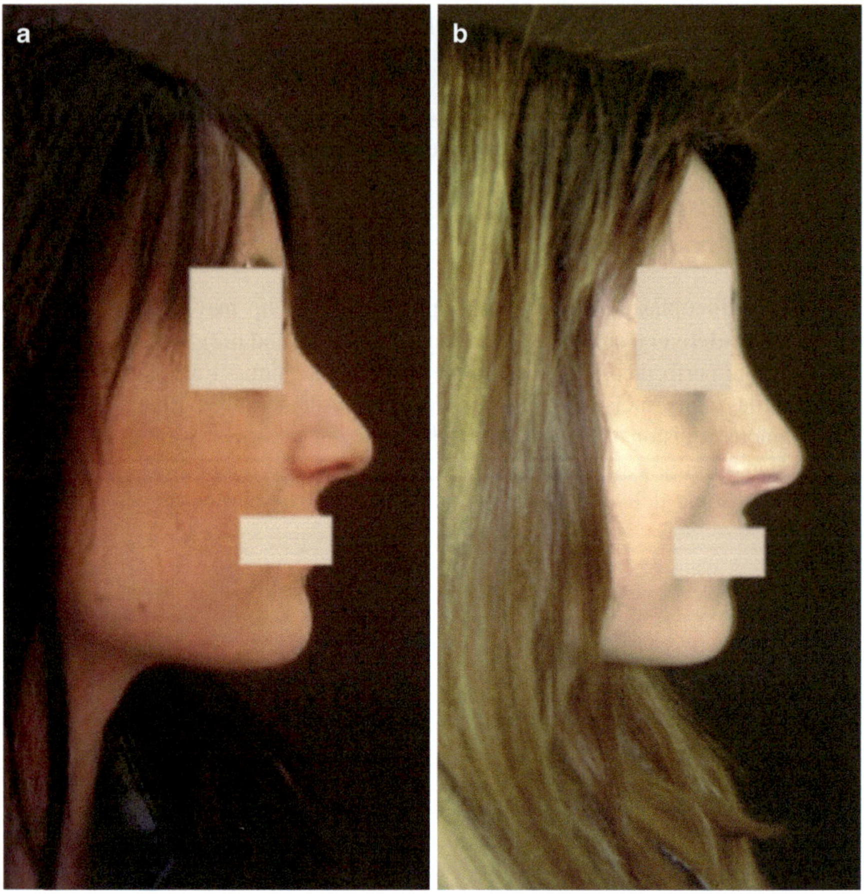

Fig. 6.3 Retrograde approach for simple tip correction. (**a**) Preoperative, (**b**) postoperative

when extensive resection and/or grafting is felt necessary as well as reorientation by multiple stitching. The same incisions are the route to approach the nasal dorsum either in sub-SMAS or sub-pericondral-periosteal plane of dissection. In our experience, a non-delivery technique is suited for tip correction roughly in 50% of our patients since non-interruptive alar re-shaping by minor cephalic resection and reorientation with limited stitching allows correction of slight tip bulbosity with/without light under rotation, sometimes with the adjunct of different grafts. Tip surgery is planned generally after dorsal hump resection (Fig. 6.8) that is needed in the vast majority of our cases, even though different timing is followed usually by different surgeons according to personal preferences. The same is felt for the correct plane of dissection that is usually sub-SMAS in the cartilaginous dorsum and sub-periosteal in the nasal bones area. **Hump resection** either “en-block” or piecemeal after upper lateral cartilages-septum de-connection (as preferred) is carried out in

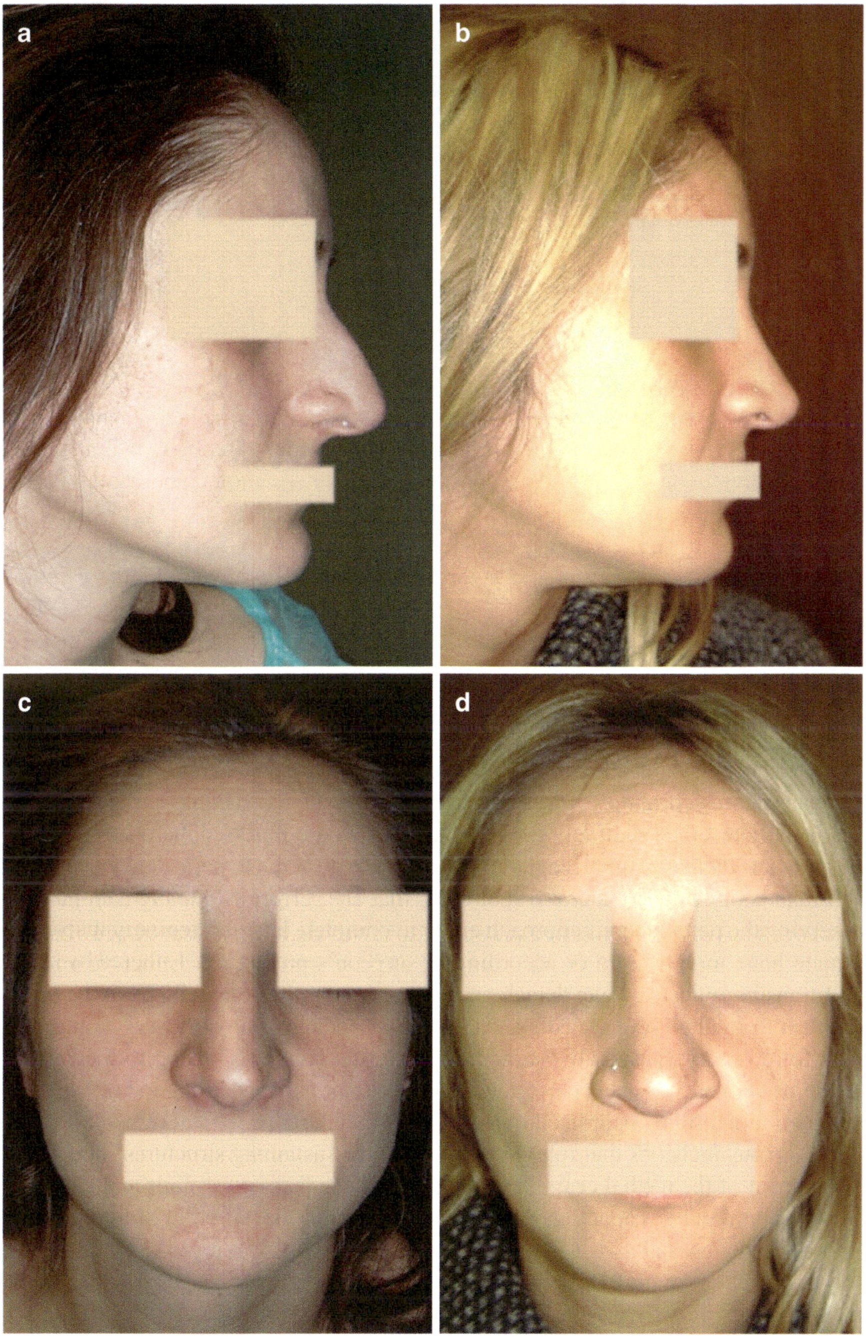

Fig. 6.4 Minimal tip correction combined with significant hump resection. (**a**, **c**, **e**) Preoperative, (**b**, **d**, **f**) postoperative

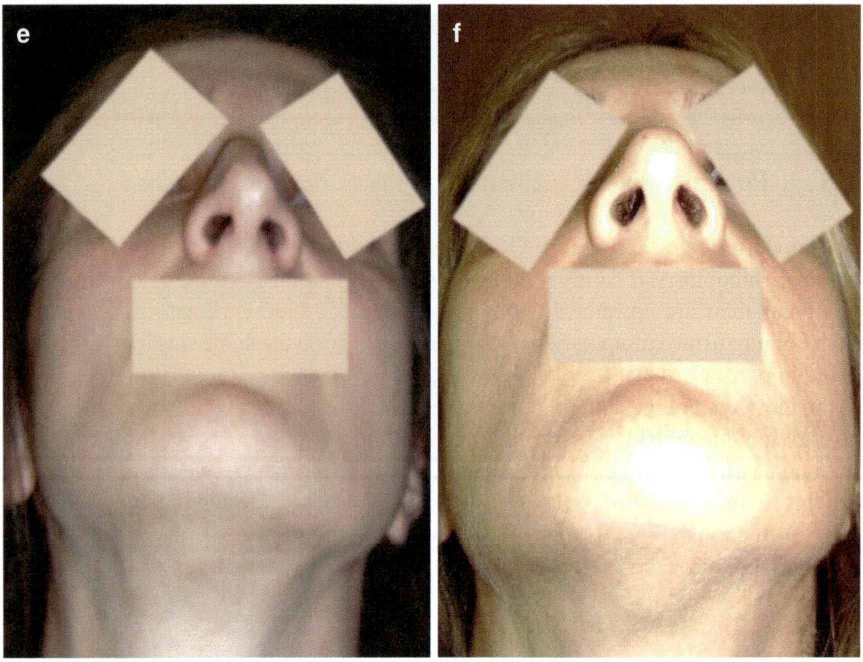

Fig. 6.4 (continued)

extra-mucosal fashion almost always. Similarly, low-to low lateral osteotomies plus in-fracture are felt almost uniformly useful while medial-paramedial osteotomies are usually reserved routinely for twisted noses where fibrous adherences between nasal bones counteracting free mobilization are expected. No periosteal elevation is felt mandatory prior to lateral osteotomies that are performed mostly endonasally, reserving the percutaneous approach either to complete lateral osteotomy with inadequate bone mobilization or according to surgeon's preference. Either an emi- or full-transfixion incision can detach partially or totally the columella from the **nasal septum** to re-align it, proceeding with a sub-pericondral sub-periosteal flap elevation followed by conservative condrotomies/osteotomies according to the "swing door" principle [5]. This is performed in 90% of our patients with good results. **Tip projection** is often jeopardized during these procedures: e.g. total transfix + intercartilaginous incisions that release most of the tip-sustaining structures such as the attachment of the medial crural footplates to the caudal membranous and cartilaginous septum and the attachment of the lower lateral (alar) cartilages to the upper lateral cartilages, and its preservation must be pursued. At this regard, re-connecting the nasal septum with the medial crura of lower lateral cartilages by a "tongue in

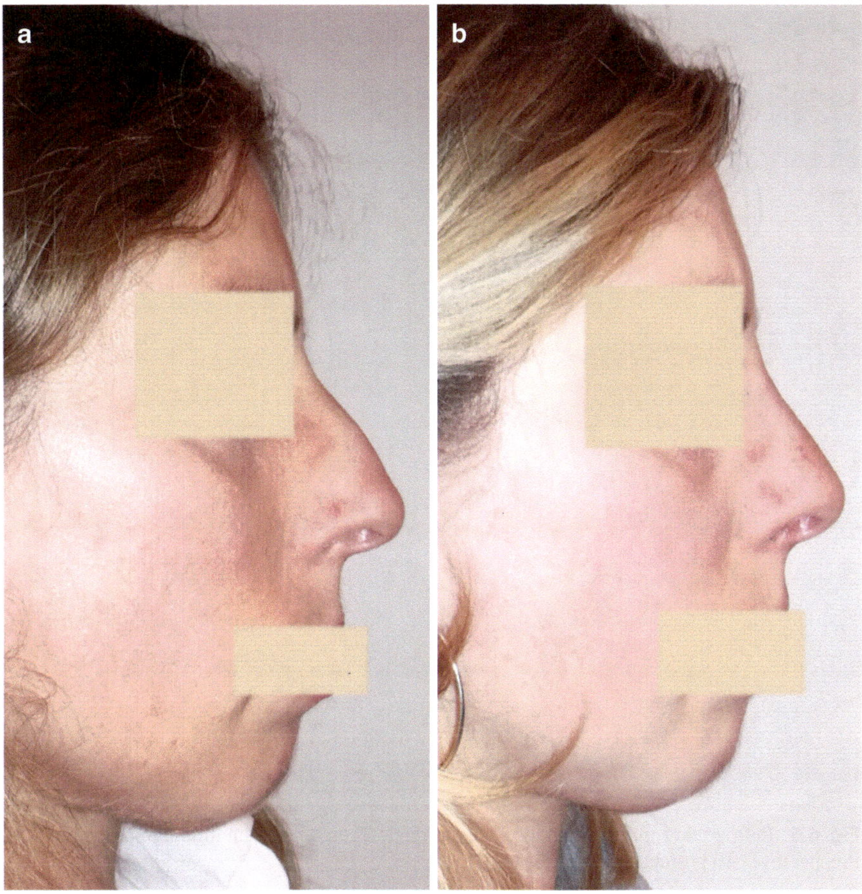

Fig. 6.5 Minimal tip correction combined with mild hump correction. (**a**) Preoperative, (**b**) postoperative

groove" suture or reinforcement of the crura by a columellar strut graft are felt worth to be carried out. Avoiding over resection of cartilaginous structures of the nose remains crucial.

The main cue in our rhinoplasty technique is preservation, reorientation, and reshaping of cartilages. Cartilage resection is limited to a reasonable minimum. Such a policy is mandatory both in thin-skinned patients, to avoid postoperative visible irregularities, and in thick-skinned subjects to avoid unpredictable scar retractions due to lack of structural support from weakened cartilage framework. The former type of skin is seldom observed in our cases, which more frequently show heavy tip skin.

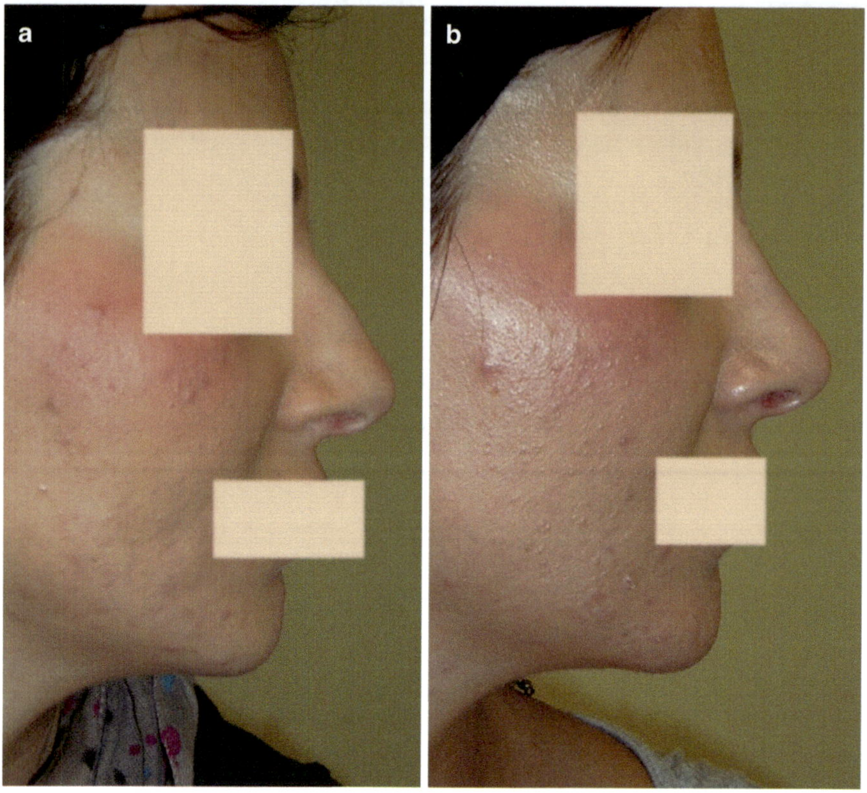

Fig. 6.6 Retrograde approach for simple tip correction combined with mild hump resection. (**a**) Preoperative, (**b**) postoperative

6.2.3 Saddle Nose and Valve Collapse

Dorsal convexities are very frequent in our cases, their conservative and "step by step" correction is usually pursued to avoid over resection. At the moment, a saddle nose aspect is felt unpleasant by the vast majority of patients and not desirable. Therefore, progressive lowering of the dorsum is pursued using initially scalpel and osteotome, followed by rasping to further lower and smooth the dorsum. Care is always taken to lower the anterior septal angle under the domal height to prevent a "polly beak" (Fig. 6.9). Regarding the so-called supratip break, it is not mandatory in our patient's desires; therefore, it is not a priority in our targeted results. A dreaded unwanted result is the inferomedial displacement of the upper lateral cartilages leading to nasal valve collapse and subsequent nasal obstruction and possibly different degrees of "inverted V" (Figs. 6.10 and 6.11) deformity due to scar retraction. The incidence of narrow and tension noses with significant hump cartilaginous component is not negligible in Mediterranean area patients, and these are in danger for postoperative unstable upper lateral cartilages and valve collapse. The

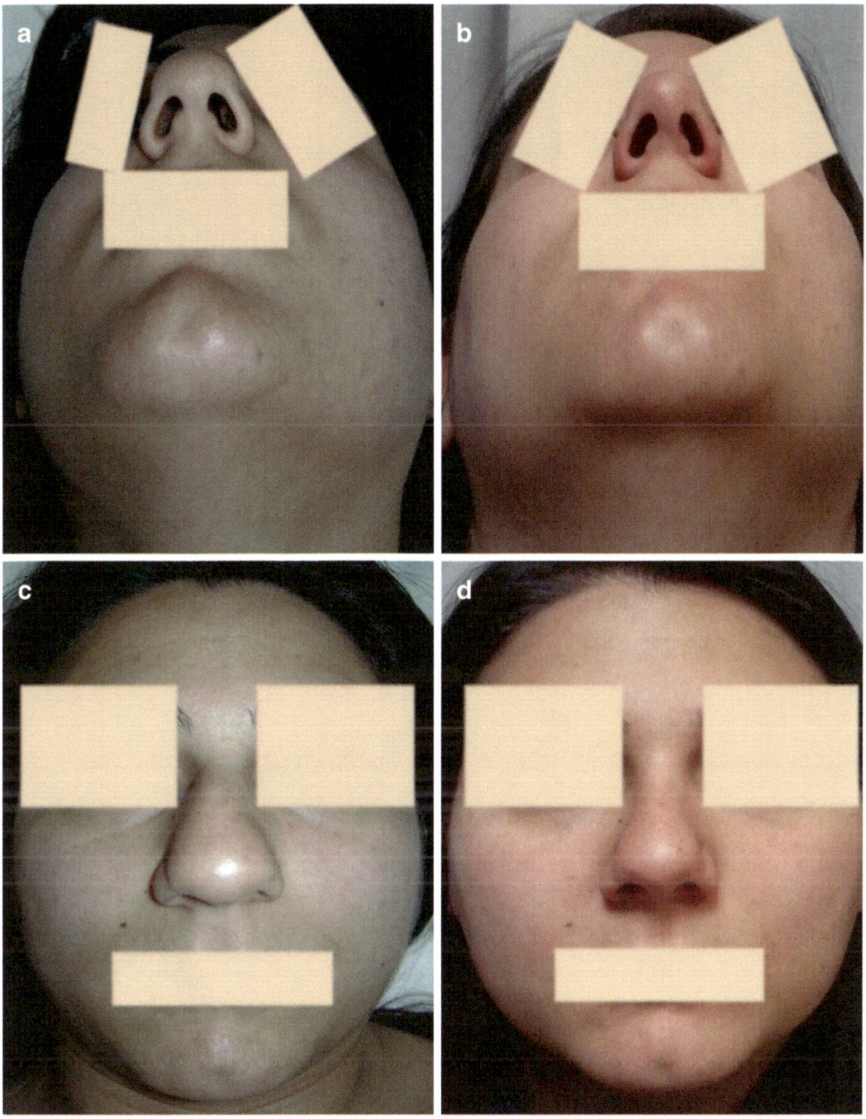

Fig. 6.7 Delivery approach for bulbous tip correction. (**a**, **c**, **e**) Preoperative, (**b**, **d**, **f**) postoperative

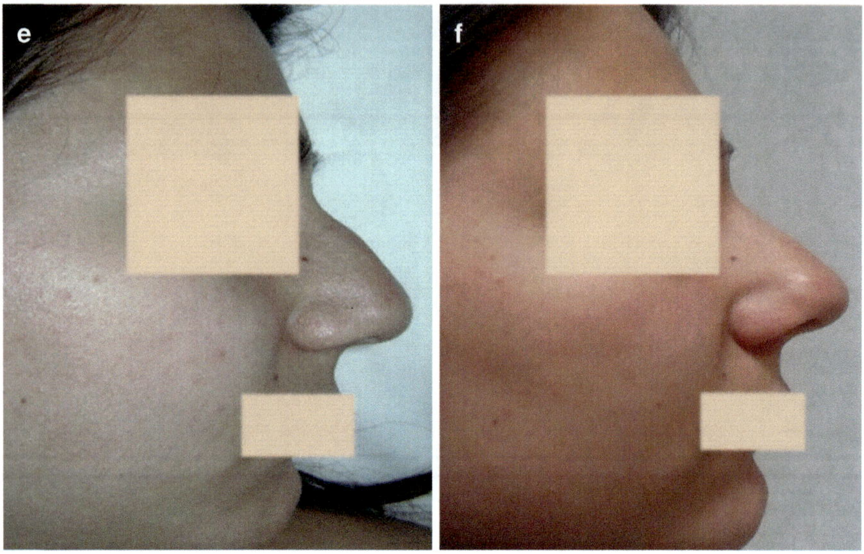

Fig. 6.7 (continued)

Fig. 6.8 En-block Hump resection

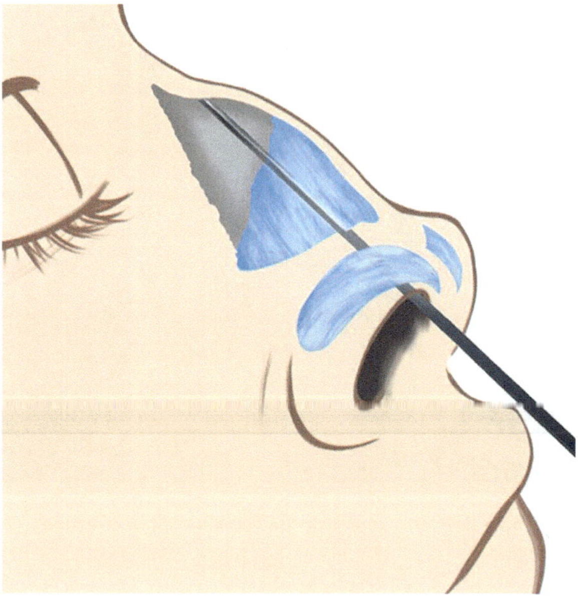

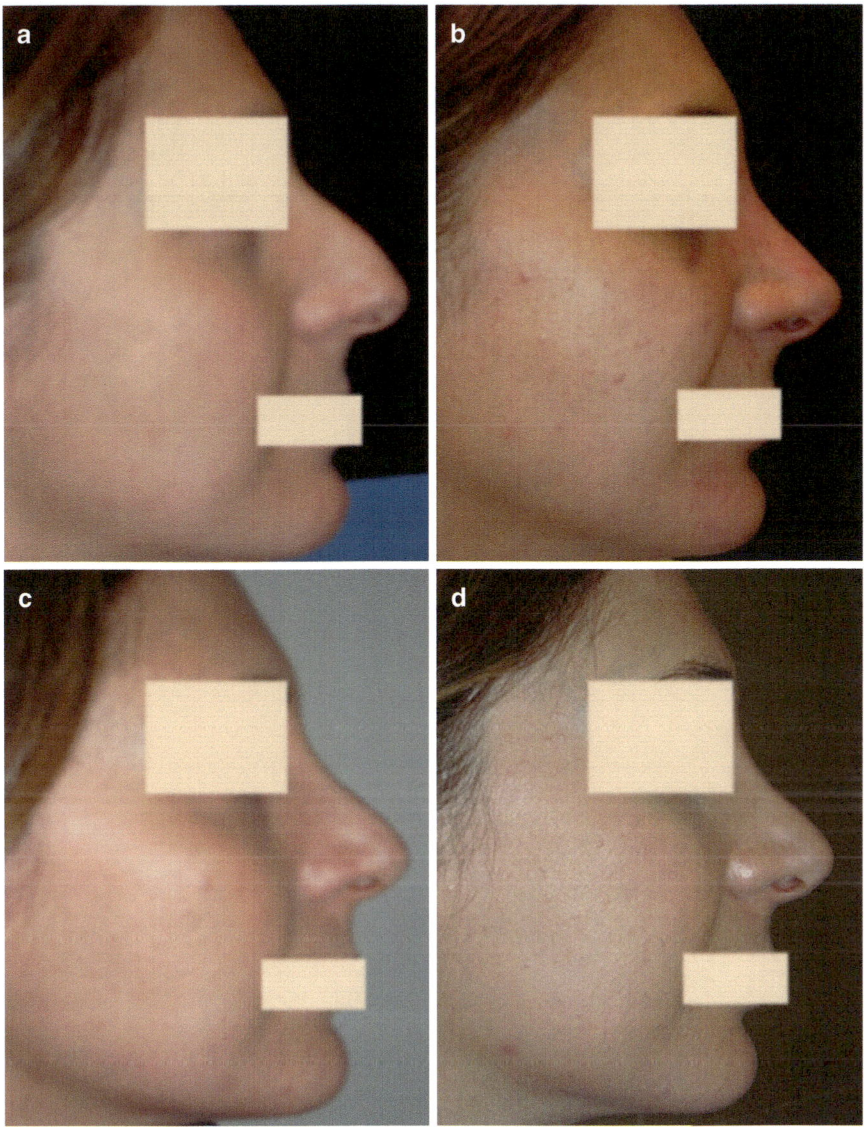

Fig. 6.9 Polly beak development over time and correction by steroid injection. (**a**) Preoperative; (**b**) postoperative early results, (**c**) postoperative late results with polly beak, (**d**) correction by steroid injection

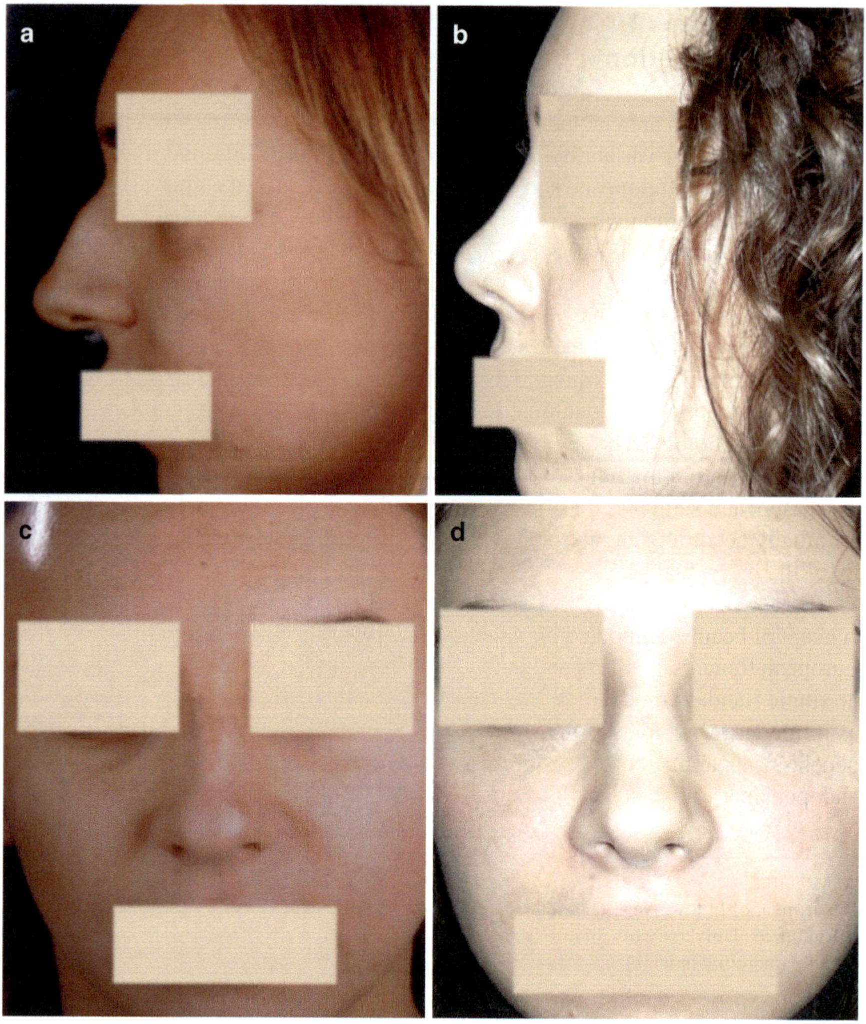

Fig. 6.10 Late Inverted-V deformity development. (**a**, **c**) Preoperative, (**b**, **d**) postoperative (**d**—Inverted V deformity due to short nasal bones)

positioning of spreader grafts (Figs. 6.12 and 6.13) is advisable in such case. Properly placed spreader grafts serve to preserve or increase middle vault width, expand the cross-sectional area of the internal nasal valve, and decrease the risk of inferomedial collapse of the upper lateral cartilages [6].

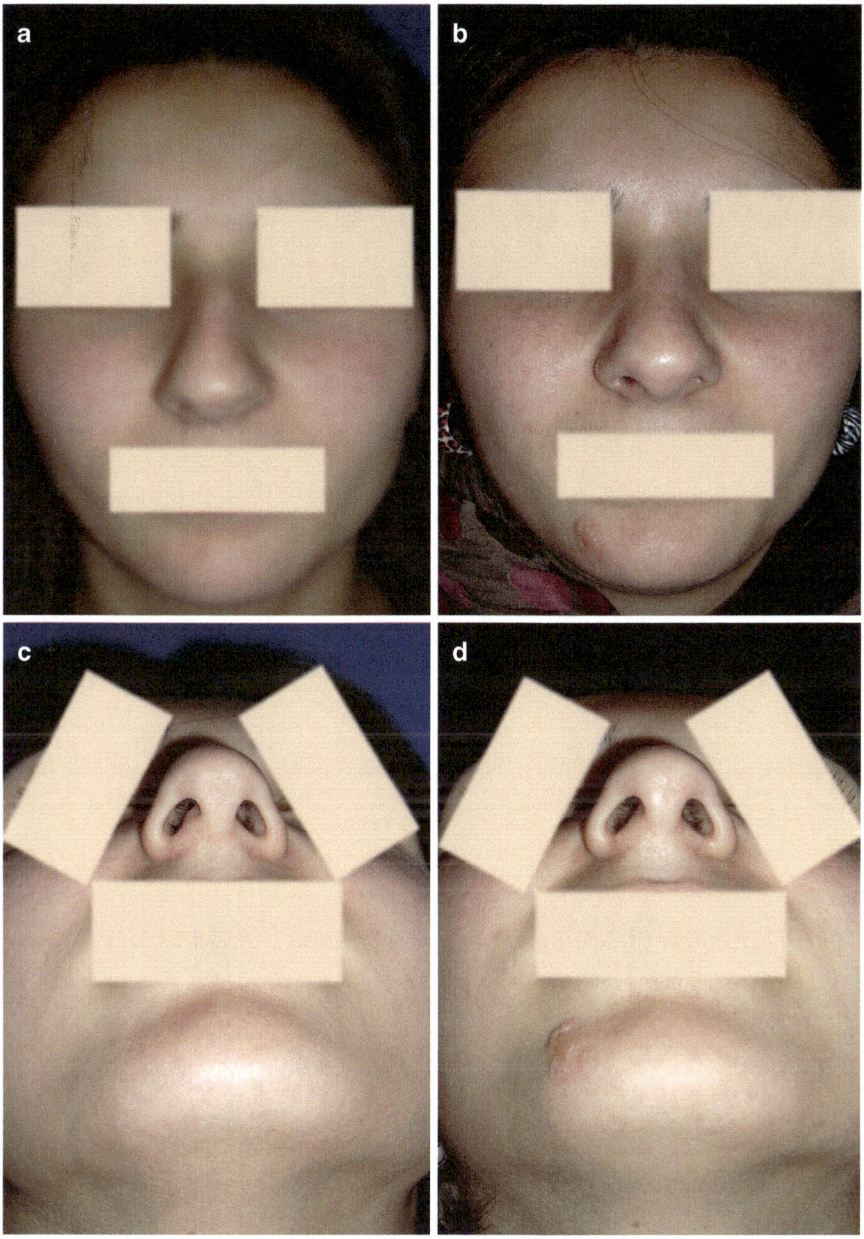

Fig. 6.11 Late development of inverted V deformity due to short nasal bones. (**a**, **c**, **e**) Preoperative; (**b**, **d**, **f**) postoperative (**b**: inverted d deformity)

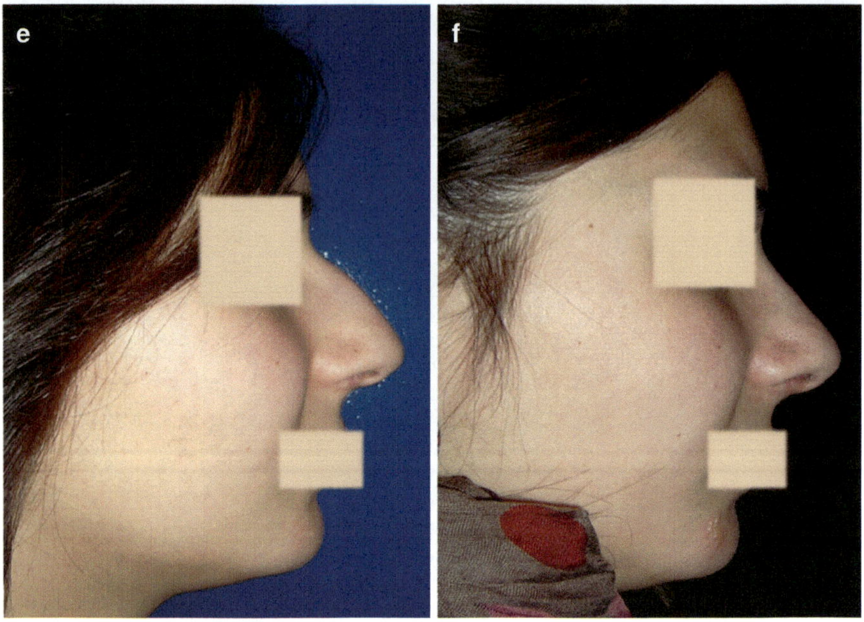

Fig. 6.11 (continued)

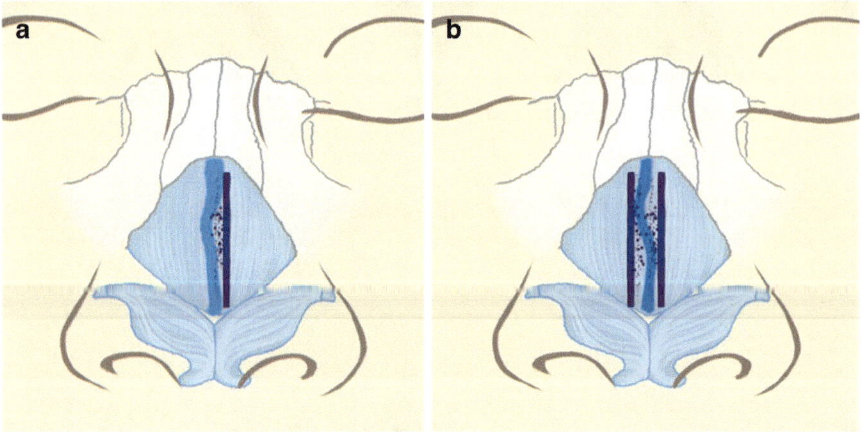

Fig. 6.12 (**a**) Unilateral (plus camouflaging graft) and (**b**) bilateral spreader graft schemes

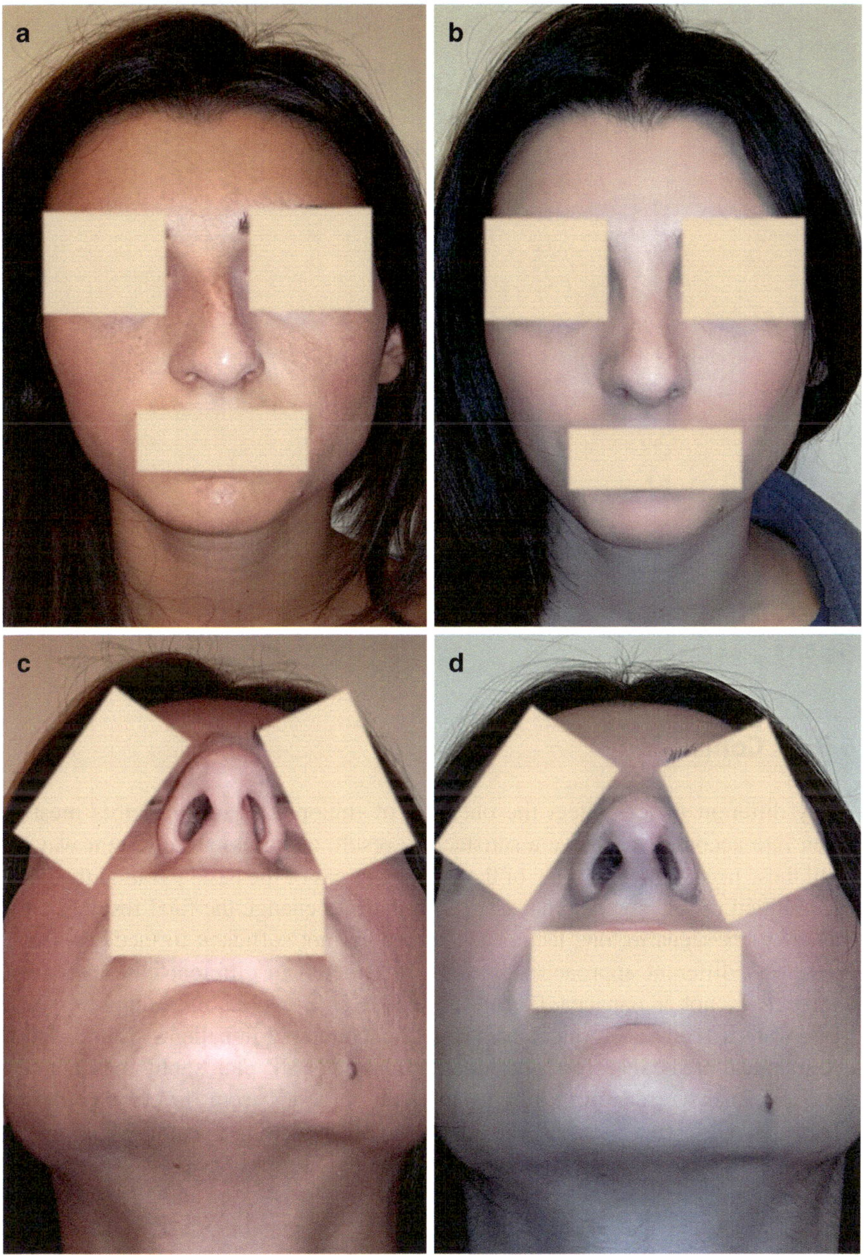

Fig. 6.13 Unilateral spreader graft (right side) for crooked nose correction. (**a**, **c**, **e**) Preoperative; (**b**, **d**, **f**) postoperative

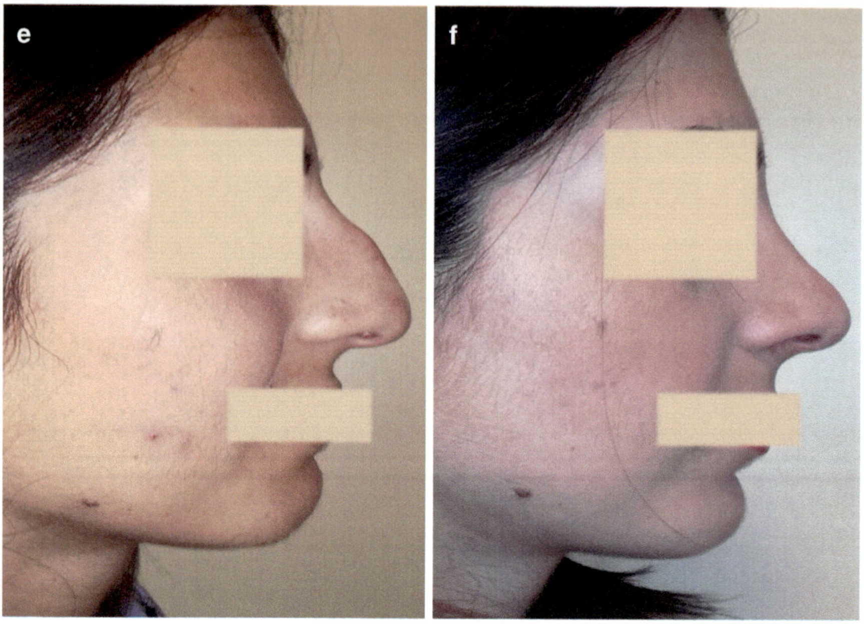

Fig. 6.13 (continued)

6.3 Conclusion

Many different factors affect the outcome of rhinoplasty: many factors must be taken into account to achieve a satisfactory result, and there are different ways to fulfil these needs. The interplay of the different areas of the nasal pyramid that must be modified during surgery may also contribute to change the final result. Due to this complex scenario, one technical approach is not sufficient to face every case [7–9], and different approaches must be considered in different cases. A single approach is not a panacea for all problems encountered in rhinoplasty [10]. Moreover, different anatomical cues can be encountered in patients from different geographical areas; therefore, the 'one-approach-fits-all' philosophy may not be a good choice when dealing with patients and surgeons from different countries. Therefore, a selective attention must be paid to the way of performing a rhinoplasty in different countries and a graduated and tailored approach seems to be the most successful policy [9, 11]. Each patient is individually assessed and allocated to the appropriate surgery based on the presenting anatomy, patient's desires and aesthetic goals that may change considerably from patient to patient, both from an anatomical and cultural point of view. Any effort must be done to reach pre-operatively defined goals shared with the patient, possibly in the simplest, most efficient way, while minimizing the extent of dissection and maintaining or fortifying structural support [10]. The closed rhinoplasty has proven to be a reliable tool to correct the vast majority of the defects encountered in patients from our area. It allows various techniques to be applied in the modification of the nasal dorsum and tip, in order to deal with the most common alterations present in these patients. A good deal of ability to plan and execute different surgical manoeuvers is felt advisable to obtain satisfactory results anyway [9, 12].

In conclusion, closed rhinoplasty reduces dissection to the strictly needed, unnecessary trauma is therefore avoided. A closed non-delivery approach with or without hemi transfixion incision is reserved for simpler cases [3, 13]. Greater exposure may be obtained when needed by extended closed tip delivery. Wide dissection may lead to increased scarring, if possible, it must be avoided since thick skin is frequent in our patients and it may lead to post-operative edema and scarring [12–15]. Finally, it seems worthy to manage conservatively the SMAS ligaments to reduce trauma to the tip region [16, 17].

References

1. Roe JO. The deformity termed "pug nose" and its correction by a simple operation. By John Orlando Roe, 1887. Arch Otolaryngol Head Neck Surg. 1989;115(2):156–7. https://doi.org/10.1001/ARCHOTOL.1989.01860260030010.
2. Palma P, Bignami M, Delù G, De Bernardi F, Castelnuovo P. Rhinoplasty for the Mediterranean nose. Facial Plast Surg. 2003;19(3):279–94. https://doi.org/10.1055/s-2003-43163.
3. Tebbetts JB. Open and closed rhinoplasty (minus the "versus"): analyzing processes. Aesthet Surg J. 2006;26(4):456–9. https://doi.org/10.1016/j.asj.2006.06.003.
4. Vartanian AJ. Basic closed rhinoplasty: background, history of the procedure, problem. 2020. https://emedicine.medscape.com/article/1291976-overview. Accessed 18 Feb 2021.
5. Voizard B, Theriault M, Lazizi S, Moubayed SP. North American survey and systematic review on caudal septoplasty. J Otolaryngol Head Neck Surg. 2020;49:38. https://doi.org/10.1186/s40463-020-00435-4.
6. Samaha M, Rassouli A. Spreader graft placement in endonasal rhinoplasty: technique and a review of 100 cases. Plast Surg (Oakv). 2015;23(4):252–4. https://doi.org/10.4172/plastic-surgery.1000944.
7. Dayan SH. Evolving techniques in rhinoplasty. Facial Plast Surg. 2007;23(1):62–9; discussion 70–79. https://doi.org/10.1055/s-2007-970166.
8. Adamson PA, Galli SKD. Rhinoplasty approaches: current state of the art. Arch Facial Plast Surg. 2005;7(1):32–7. https://doi.org/10.1001/archfaci.7.1.32.
9. Simons RL, Grunebaum LD. The endonasal approach to rhinoplasty. In: Stucker FJ, de Souza C, Kenyon GS, Lian TS, Draf W, Schick B, editors. Rhinology and facial plastic surgery. Springer; 2009. pp. 713–721. https://doi.org/10.1007/978-3-540-74380-4_68.
10. Röjdmark J, Mouchammed A. A modified closed-open approach as part of a graduated and integrative approach to rhinoplasty. Indian J Plast Surg. 2019;52(3):270–6. https://doi.org/10.1055/s-0039-3401472.
11. Cafferty A, Becker DG. Open and closed rhinoplasty. Clin Plast Surg. 2016;43(1):17–27. https://doi.org/10.1016/j.cps.2015.09.002.
12. Jordan JR. Dallas rhinoplasty: nasal surgery by the masters. By Jack P. Gunter, Rod J. Rohrich, William P. Adams, Quality Medical Publishing, Inc. St. Louis, 2002, 1200 pp, 2 volume set. Head Neck. 2003;25(6):511. https://doi.org/10.1002/hed.10248.
13. Sheen JH. Closed versus open rhinoplasty—and the debate goes on. Plast Reconstr Surg. 1997;99(3):859–62. https://doi.org/10.1097/00006534-199703000-00039.

14. Rohrich RJ, Janis JE, Kenkel JM. Male rhinoplasty. Plast Reconstr Surg. 2003;112(4):1071–85; quiz 1086. https://doi.org/10.1097/01.PRS.0000076201.75278.BB.
15. Guerrerosantos J. Open rhinoplasty without skin-columella incision. Plast Reconstr Surg. 1990;85(6):955–60. https://doi.org/10.1097/00006534-199006000-00022.
16. Cakir B, Oreroğlu AR, Doğan T, Akan M. A complete subperichondrial dissection technique for rhinoplasty with management of the nasal ligaments. Aesthet Surg J. 2012;32(5):564–74. https://doi.org/10.1177/1090820X12445471.
17. Giacomini PG, Boccieri A, Moretti A, Rosati V, Flora B, Di Girolamo S. Nasal tip rotation by exclusive superficial musculoaponeurotic system deep medial ligament management: an objective evaluation. Ann Plast Surg. 2020;85(1):12–7. https://doi.org/10.1097/SAP.0000000000002319.

Northern Mediterranean Nose Correction: Italian Experience—Open Approach

7

Armando Boccieri

7.1 Introduction

Several anthropometric studies have classified as typical Mediterranean facial features the darker shade of skin and eyes, black hair, not-too-wide forehead, strong lineaments and prominent nose [1]. In particular, the nose has a convex shape on the lateral view, while its upper third looks wider on the frontal view. It often shows tip ptosis and thick skin. In these patients such a prominent nose may catch the attention of the observer, offering a deformed look of the overall harmony of the face. In opposite cases, a saddle nose, often outcome of previous nasal surgery, might as well lead to a contrast between the nasal shape and the harmony of the rest of the face, with its other typically Mediterranean features. Therefore, rhinoplasty must always aim to re-establish the right proportions of the nose, in order to give back symmetry and beauty that belong to Mediterranean ethnicity.

When advising a patient, thus, it becomes of primary importance for the facial plastic surgeon to delineate a standard of beauty to refer to, in order to specifically assess every patient's nasal pyramid defect and to plan its correction. At this regard, it might be useful to observe famous portraits made by the artists of the past, or modern pictures of famed actors and other notorious people that are globally believed to be testimonials of Mediterranean beauty.

Such an aesthetic evaluation, for males, may take into consideration the statue of Augustus Caesar, which dates back to the first century BC, the face of Michelangelo's David, or the far more recent pictures of actors like Marcello Mastroianni and Antonio Banderas. All these examples share the same anatomical characteristics that express the Mediterranean beauty. They all show a nose with a straight profile, yet considerable dimensions that fits harmoniously amongst the other features of the face that are also strong and well defined. Another common element displayed in all

A. Boccieri (✉)
Italian Association of Facial Plastic Surgery (AICEFF), Rome, Italy

P. G. Giacomini (ed.), *Mediterranean Rhinoplasty*,
https://doi.org/10.1007/978-3-031-05551-5_7

the aforementioned examples is an open nasolabial angle, with a good tip rotation and tip projection.

Concerning feminine beauty standard, it can be detected in Nefertiti's face, Venus de Milo, Paolina Borghese's statue and in decidedly more recent pictures of actresses such as Sofia Loren or Penelope Cruz. Even in this case, the analysis of the celebrated faces reveals a rather long nose, with a straight profile, good tip projection and an open nasolabial angle. This last feature seems to be particularly frequent in most beautiful Mediterranean faces, probably because it enhances labial prominence and other facial landmarks which all-together increase the overall facial attractiveness.

Hence, it is of pivotal importance for facial plastic surgeons performing rhinoplasty on a Mediterranean patient to locate nasal pyramid defects that avert from the aforementioned facial beauty standard, in order to better correct them. One of the most common is tip ptosis and it is of great importance to evaluate also whether it is associated with a normal tip projection or to its under- or over-projection, since the technique needed to correct it would be different.

7.2 Rhinoplasty: Open Approach

The most common technique employed to correct Mediterranean nose defects is the open rhinoplasty, which exposes nasal pyramid and septum through a columellar "inverted V" incision. The current trend in modern open approach is prompted towards a conservative technique, aimed to the preservation and reinforcement of the nasal structures.

One of the most famous nasal surgeons worldwide, J. P. Gunter, defined his experience with the open rhinoplasty as follows: "*The more I work with the open approach the more I find there are things I can do through it that I cannot do through the endonasal approach (or can do a lot easier)*".

The open rhinoplasty can be considered not properly as a different surgical technique than the classical endonasal one, but as a different approach to nasal pyramid and septum. It doesn't have clear indications and each surgeon, knowing his/her own experience, should ask him or herself this question: "Am I able to guarantee the same result with the endonasal approach?" Being a less invasive technique, which allows the operator to feel the osteo-cartilaginous structures under his/her fingers and to imagine their anatomical correction, the endonasal approach has become one of the most challenging yet fascinating procedures in modern facial aesthetic surgery.

Nevertheless, during the last years the trend to better expose the anatomical structures has interested several surgical specialties, facial plastic one included, in order to guarantee, under a close visual control, a better result. The sequence exposure-correction-contention, which is borrowed from the maxillo-facial and orthopedic surgery, can be applied to the nasal pyramid open surgery with

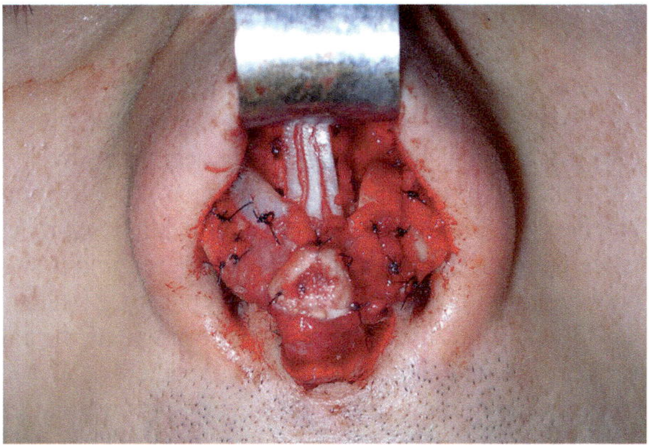

Fig. 7.1 Multiple grafts in open approach. Secondary rhinoplasty treated with spreader grafts, alar batten grafts, lateral crural grafts, tip onlay grafts sutured in inaccessible areas

interesting advantages. The possibility to expose the osteo-cartilaginous scaffold of the nose, without having to imagine it, is one of the principal benefits of the open approach, since it also eliminates the tension and distortions typical of the endonasal one. In fact, it allows a more precise diagnosis of the factors responsible for nasal deformity and, thus, their punctual correction under strict visual control, with the chance to use both hands and also the help of a second operator. At this regard, the second surgeon serving during the procedure has the chance to actively participate to the decisional process of the first operator, just like in every other open surgery. These advantages allow a simpler positioning and fixation of the grafts in places that are utterly inaccessible during a closed approach and this guarantees a more stable and long-lasting result (Fig. 7.1). Moreover, it is possible to remodel the cartilaginous nasal structure with sutures, with a direct visual feedback on the outcome, without tensions or distortions.

The goal of an "open structure rhinoplasty" is to remodel or rebuilt the nasal osteo-cartilaginous framework, in order to offer a valid support to the upper soft tissues. Little has changed in the old rhinoplasty techniques described by Joseph more than one century, in comparison with modern ones. What has evolved is the fact that nasal surgeons no longer proceed removing tissues, demolishing and interrupting anatomical structures; on the contrary, modern trends are to preserve these important structures, remodelling and rebuilding them, with respect of the existing osteo-cartilaginous scaffold. This applies perfectly to the Mediterranean nose, where rhinoplasty must give due consideration to the ethnic identity of the patient, aiming to preserve it. Excessive resections, in fact, have led in the past to a high rate of unsatisfying outcomes, not only because of the concave profile of the nasal dorsum but also due to the lack of harmony between the nose and the other facial landmarks, typical of Mediterranean ethnicity.

Open rhinoplasty can be therefore considered not just as an incisional approach but also and namely as a set of techniques aimed to increase surgical versatility, accuracy and predictability of the outcome.

7.3 Clinical Evaluation

When analysing of nasal parameters needed to plan surgery, it is convenient in clinical practice to use simple methods. Concerning tip rotation: It can be inferred calculating the nasolabial angle. Its ideal measure has been considered between 95°–105° in women and 90°–95° in men [2], but its range depends on the ethnicity and personal preference. Tip projection can be easily evaluated considering the distance between nasal tip and subnasal point, and it should be equal to the distance between the subnasal point and the upper lip [3]. Otherwise, it can be derived using the "3–4–5 rule", obtained drawing a triangle on the nasal profile [4]. The ideal ratio between the first cathetus, the second cathetus and the hypotenuse should be 3:4:5, indeed a major or a minor ratio involving the first cathetus leads respectively to overprojection or underprojection of the nasal tip.

Another important parameter to be acknowledged when approaching a Mediterranean nose is the position of the lateral crura of the lower lateral cartilages, which can be more vertical than horizontal [5]. A thorough clinical observation of the face in frontal view allows to assess the malposition of alar cartilages cephalically oriented leading to a deformity of the nasal tip known as "parenthesis deformity" [6, 7].

The evaluation of the frontonasal angle requires the localization, on the lateral view, of the deeper spot of this angle, called nasion: Its height is around 15 mm, when calculated from the inner canthus [8]. The assessment of this parameter is fundamental to define nasal dorsum: Dorsal hump can be disguised by a not too deep nasion, or it can be enhanced by a too deep one. This last possibility can also worsen tip overprojection.

Clinical evaluation can be completed with the assessment of two more parameters regarding nasal pyramid: Quality of the soft tissues covering it and the robustness of the osteo-cartilaginous structures underneath. Nasal pyramid palpation, in case of a Mediterranean nose, often highlights a considerable thickness of the skin, with a sebaceous aspect that gets more accentuated on the nasal tip. The osteo-cartilaginous framework is usually strong, yet it is important to identify patient with weak cartilages that might need the use of reinforcement grafts.

Only after the analysis of the results of this careful evaluation of the patient's face and of the defects identified on the nasal pyramid, the surgeon can choose the technique that better fits that patient's needs.

7.4 Most Frequent Surgical Techniques

The Mediterranean nose very often shows a too prominent nasal dorsum, with **osteo cartilaginous dorsal hump**. The correction of this defect, lowering the dorsal nasal line, must be carefully performed, with parsimony, in order to preserve ethnic identity of both male and female patients.

At this regard, a surgical rasp is the best tool to use to reduce the hump has it hardly allows too generous resections, even in more voluminous humps. Therefore, it is advisable to complete dorsum reduction with the rasp, after the use of common chisels. Sometimes the depth of the frontonasal angle also needs correction, especially when the nasion is not deep enough. This procedure as well must not be done too aggressively; median osteotomy isn't always required and when it actually is, it is advisable to perform it with a median-oblique direction, in order to preserve continuity and stability of the bony structure after the fracture. Given the frequent thickness of nasal bones, often it can be hard to close the open roof after lateral osteotomies. Therefore, when suspecting this possibility, it is advisable to remove two little triangular-shaped bony pieces between the bony nasal septum and the nasal bone, after the median osteotomies, in order to reapproach again the nasal bones after lateral osteotomies.

In most cases, one single lateral osteotomy per each side is enough, but when the width of the upper third of the nasal pyramid is larger, it may require two lateral osteotomies per each side. This kind of procedure, which is quite often employed in case of Mediterranean noses, offers the chance to tighten the nasal bone after the suture more than other techniques.

Once the resection of the dorsal hump has been carried out, it has proven useful to insert a graft of morselized septal cartilage to help camouflage remnant irregularities of the nasal bones after osteotomies, which otherwise would render the nasal dorsum some millimetres higher.

Though a too prominent nasal dorsum is a typical Mediterranean nose defect that needs correction, also a concave one very often needs to be surgically rectified in order to bring back the nasal profile into the correct beauty canons specific of this ethnicity. The clinical recognition of a **saddle nose deformity** can derive from old nasal traumas or, more frequently, it can be the result of previous nasal surgery. The best choice in these cases is the use of autologous grafts harvested from septal cartilage, auricular or costal one, tailored to fit the needs of the specific patient and sutured to the underlying structures (Fig. 7.2).

A too prominent nasal tip is also one of the most common nasal features in the Mediterranean area. During preoperative clinical evaluation, it is important to

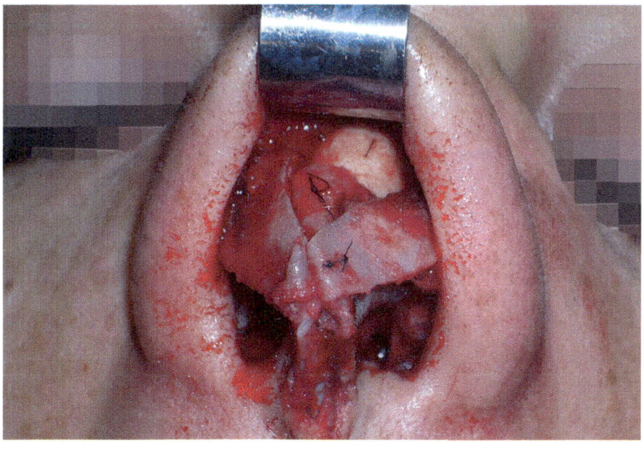

Fig. 7.2 Saddle nose deformity. Correction with conchal graft sutured on the nasal framework

estimate the degree of **tip rotation deficit** and also to assess if it comes with normal tip projection rather than with over or underprojection.

In case of mild tip rotation deficit, it can be sufficient to delicately trim the cephalic portion of the lateral crura of the lower lateral cartilages; the following cicatricial retraction of the remnant empty space will be enough, in time, to pull the tip slightly upwards. In case of more severe tip rotation deficit, the correction may require adding to the previous procedure a triangular resection of the caudal septum, with the apex pointing downwards, with preservation of the basal portion of the septum and its septo-columellar ligaments, which are responsible for tip support.

Another simple yet effective strategy is to put a plumping graft, made of diced or crushed cartilage harvested from the nasal septum, into a subcutaneous pocket crafted before the anterior nasal spina, in order to "plump" the nasolabial angle, hence giving the illusion of an increased tip rotation upward.

In case of tip ptosis, alone or associated with tip overprojection, it is advisable to use the lateral crural overlay technique [9]. The analysis of this defect in lateral view shows how it derives from an excessive length of the lateral crura of the lower lateral cartilages. In these cases, the lateral crural overlay technique associates the slight cephalic trimming of the lateral crura of the LLCs with the incision of the lateral crura in their posterior thirds, followed by the sliding of the anterior segment onto the posterior one, preserving the vestibular mucosa underneath (Fig. 7.3). Hence, the two segments are sutured with Nylon 5.0. This manoeuver creates an important tip rotation, reducing tip projection. On the other side, the lateral shift of the lateral crura of the LLC causes a widening of the domal region which almost always requires a double-dome unit technique in order to give the tip a better definition [10]. This technique is carried out with two horizontal mattress sutures combined with another transdomal suture that forces the two domes closer.

Another common problem most surgeons face in the Mediterranean area is the **nasal tip under-projection**. Usually, cartilaginous sutures or cartilaginous grafts are employed to correct this alteration. Lateral crural steal technique is frequently used as a starting procedure [11], and it can be followed by the use of combined

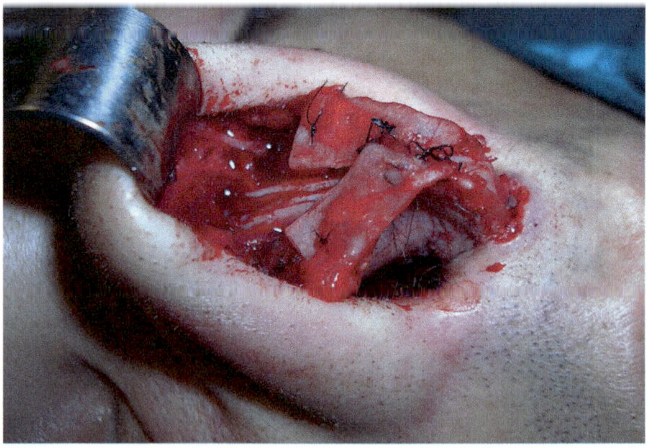

Fig. 7.3 Intraoperative view of the "lateral crural overlay technique"

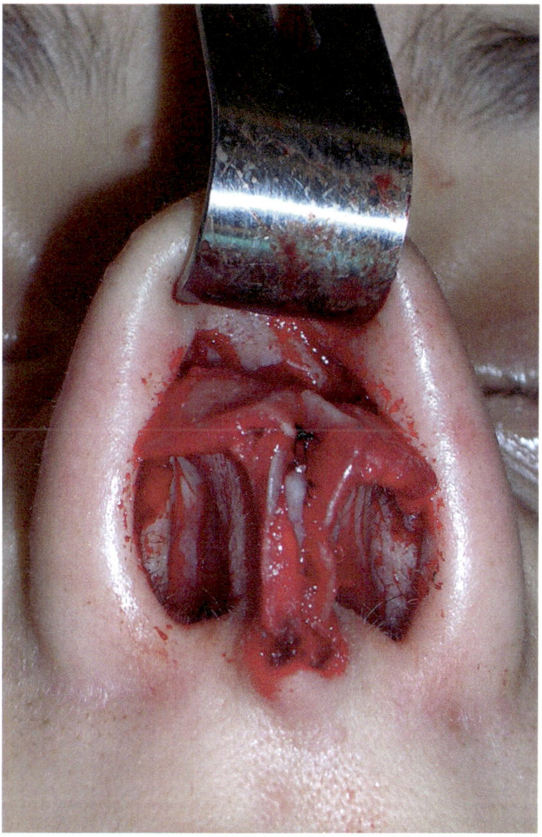

Fig. 7.4 Intraoperative view of the "lateral crural steal technique"

grafting if it is necessary. This steal is done in order to elongate the medial crura of the LLCs, shifting the domal region laterally (Fig. 7.4). The first step of this procedure is to detach the vestibular skin underneath the lateral crura in order to free them from any kind of traction when elevated with sutures and also to avoid the formation of adherences. The next step is to put two mattress stitches on the lateral crura, in order to create new domal regions, lateral to the previous ones and more projected. The last step is to put a final trans-domal suture to force the new domes closer. If the result isn't yet satisfying, a further augmentation of tip projection can be obtained using "*Peck onlay grafts*" positioned on the domal complex [12]. These grafts are made of whole or morselized septal cartilage; the previously trimmed cephalic portion of the lateral crura of the LLCs may also be used (Fig. 7.5).

Another very common cartilaginous graft used to preserve the newly obtained increased tip projection is the columellar strut [13]. It has a rectangular shape and it is harvested from the nasal septum, possibly from a robust and straight portion of it. It is sutured between the two medial crura of the LLCs and it is of paramount importance to give strength and support to the tip; it is also very effective to correct the asymmetry of the columella.

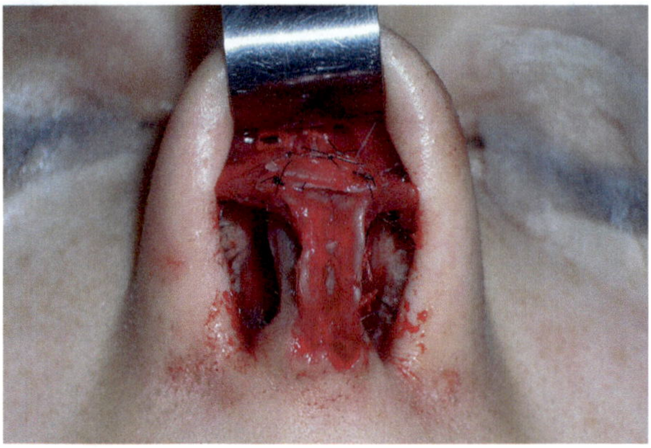

Fig. 7.5 Onlay Peck tip graft sutured onto the domes

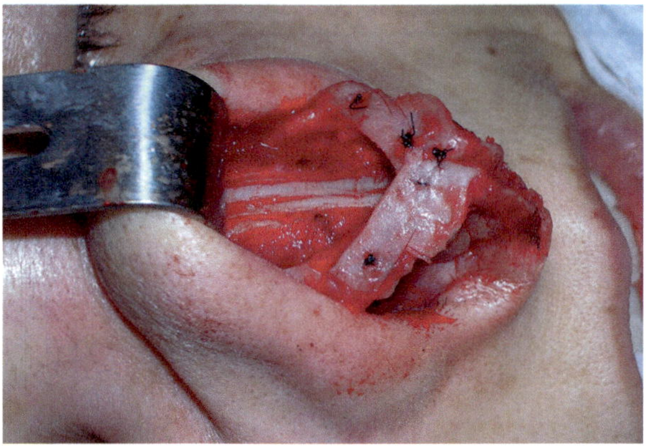

Fig. 7.6 Intraoperative view of the "stairstep lateral crural technique"

Tongue-in-groove technique can be used alternatively to the columellar strut. It substitutes the cartilaginous strut with the caudal portion of the basal septum, which is sutured between the medial crura of the LLCs [14]. The sutures in this technique may be positioned in a way that allows to increase tip projection and rotation, obtaining also a shortening of nasal length.

The analysis of nasal tip defects has led, during the last years, to the identification of a new parameter which holds important aesthetic and functional implications: The position of the lateral crura of the LLCs. The Mediterranean nose can often present a cephalic malposition of the lateral crura that causes a defect called "**parentheses deformity**" of the nasal tip [15]. This feature can be alone or associated with several degrees of tip projection and rotation alteration.

Alar malposition correction can be done with a variant of the lateral crural overlay technique, where the lateral crural incision is not performed vertically but with the aim to create a step. This variant, known as lateral crural stairstep technique [16], in fact, allows to move and fixate downwards the anterior segment of the lateral crura still keeping it anchored to the posterior segment (Fig. 7.6). The technique requires the complete detachment of the underlying skin from the crura, up to the

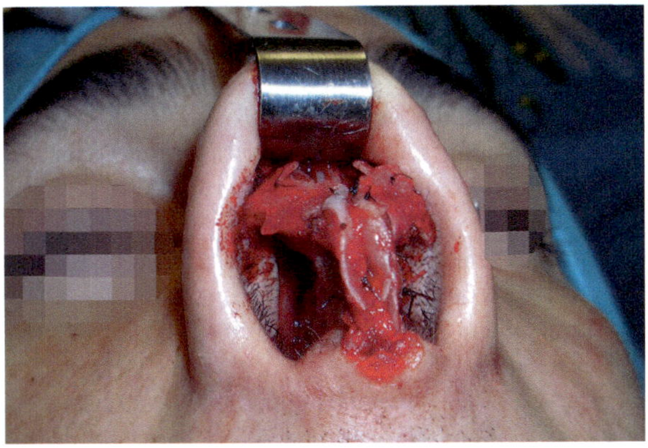

Fig. 7.7 Stairstep lateral crural technique combined with medial crural overlay technique

domal region, in order to free the anterior flap of the lateral crura. Hence, it is possible to reposition it, according to the needs of the specific case.

In case of parentheses deformity alone, the lateral crura are shifted downwards with the superior flap sliding onto the inferior one. In case of associated tip ptosis and over projection, the shifting downwards of the anterior lateral crural flap is associated with its sliding backward onto the posterior lateral crural flap, in order to reach the right degree of rotation and projection.

If the alar malposition is accompanied by a sever tip overprojection, a medial crural overlay can also be added to the previous procedure, sectioning and overlapping the two segments of the medial crura [17] (Fig. 7.7).

Another useful technique employed to correct lateral crura mispositioning, commonly used in case of Mediterranean nose correction, is the lateral crural strut graft [7]. This technique is carried out by an open approach and requires the removal of a cartilage strip from the cephalic portion of the lateral crura. Subsequently, the underlying vestibular mucosa is detached from the lateral crural cartilage and both lateral crura are completely mobilized by sectioning their ligamentous connections with the accessory cartilages. Two rectangular grafts are then harvested from the septal cartilage, hence remodelled and positioned on the inner face of the lateral crura and fixated with two or three Vycril 5.0 stitches. These struts are longer than the lateral crura, and they are lodged into a pocket before the pyriform aperture. This way the lateral crura of the LLCs are both shifted downwards. Lateral crural strut graft technique is therefore useful not only to correct alar malposition but also to flatten the lateral crura in order to reduce tip bulbosity.

As previously mentioned, a sebaceous thick skin is a typical feature of the Mediterranean nose. A **bulbous nasal tip with thick skin** is often associated with a week cartilaginous support. Thus, remodelling these cartilages must be a preservative procedure prompt to adding cartilaginous grafts rather than removing tissue. In these cases, surgical correction may employ shield grafts harvested from the nasal septum and sutured before the caudal margin of the medial crura of the LLCs with Nylon 6.0 [18]. When the bulbous thick skinned nasal tip is also underprojected, the superior margin of the shield graft must slightly surpass the domal regions; this way, the protruding pointy ends of the grafts, covered with thick skin, will give the tip better definition, improving its aspect even without reducing greatly its actual dimensions.

Thick skinned nasal tip can also require intervention on the lateral crura with double-dome unit technique or lateral crural steal suture technique, leaving the cartilaginous structures roughly sharp and overcorrected to increase final tip definition.

In some selected cases tip bulbosity can be reduced with a delicate tapering of the skin with prudent removal of subcutaneous fatty tissue. This particular procedure can lead to complications such as chronic edema, excessive scarring and cutaneous necrosis [19].

The use of subcutaneous injections of triamcinolone 3, 5 and 7 weeks after surgery is far more frequent and safer. These small injections must be done in the regions where a thinning of the skin is desired, especially on the supratip or nasal tip.

7.5 Discussion

Surgical correction of Mediterranean nose defects needs to give due consideration to the beauty canons typical of the cultural and artistic tradition of this specific ethnic group. The surgeon that decides to perform a rhinoplasty on a patient belonging to this ethnicity must correct major defects in order to reach a more harmonic aspect of the nose among the rest of facial landmarks, without altering the ethnic identity of the patient. Nasal defects in this geographic area are, in fact, mostly recurring and they derive mostly from the exasperation of some of the typical features of the Mediterranean nose. Generally, surgeons in this area have to deal with long noses with large prominent dorsum; tip ptosis with over or underprojection and thick skin. Four types of conformation of the Italian-Mediterranean nasal pyramid have been described, which group together some of the alterations described: the drooping nose, the strong prominent nose, the heavy nose and the northern nose [20]. A cephalic malposition of the lateral crura of the LLCs is quite common in this region, with poor definition of the nasal tip [15].

The open rhinoplasty, with its new concept of preservation and reinforcement of pre-existing structures, well fits the needs of these patients. Nowadays the tendency to the excessive demolition of nasal tissues has changed into the trend towards reconstruction and remodelling of the osteo-cartilaginous structures. Moreover, the modern increased use of grafts and particular suture techniques allows correction of several kinds of nasal defects, even more severe ones; therefore, surgeons need, today more than ever, to acknowledge the ethnic peculiarities of each patient, together with a higher visual control on the surgical field that only the open approach can guarantee.

Mediterranean nose correction mostly involves dorsal hump resection with the aim to straighten the nasal profile without exaggerating, especially in male patients. A concave nasal profile, in fact, wouldn't melt in very well with the rest of the typically strong and well-defined lineaments of the Mediterranean face. Concerning female patients, on the other hand, a very mild concavity of the nasal dorsum would improve the over-all harmony of the face, giving it a more feminine aspect, even if the rest of facial features preserve stronger lineaments. It must be told, anyway, that modern requests tend more and more towards a straighter nasal profile, even in women, rather than a concave one, like it was in the past decades.

The presence of noses with overprojection of the tip associated with marked ptosis is very frequent in the Mediterranean ethnic group but it is not as frequent to find situations of overprojection associated with normo or overrotation as happens for other ethnic groups such as the Nordic ones.

Concerning tip ptosis, correction depends on its severity and therefor requires different kind of techniques, from the easier ones to more challenging ones, like the lateral crural overlay, which is capable of achieving a high degree of tip rotation. A plumping graft can often be needed, since this simple cartilaginous graft added before the anterior nasal spine opens the nasolabial angle, creating the optic illusion of increased tip-rotation. The final effect is that of a rejuvenated and more good-looking face. It isn't surprising, in fact, that a wider nasolabial angle can be seen in the faces of the most attractive Mediterranean celebrities of both current and past times.

The lateral crural stairstep technique can be considered as a recent variant of the lateral crural overlay, meant to correct lateral crura malposition. This particular recently described tip deformity is quite common in Mediterranean patients and must be therefore thoroughly assessed. It can be recognized on the frontal view because the caudal margin of the lateral crura of the LLCs is oriented cephalically, causing the so-called "parenthesis deformity". The stairstep-like incision followed by the detachment of the vestibular mucosa from the anterior segment of the lateral crural cartilage allows to slide it caudally in order to correct the malposition without the use of cartilaginous grafts.

Another valid alternative might be the lateral crural strut graft technique, which uses a cartilaginous rectangular graft fixed underneath the lateral crura, in order to shift its insertion downwards.

Mediterranean nose tip projection must be modified carefully, always keeping in mind the height of the nasal dorsum and its relationship with the supratip area.

While a thin, well-rotated nasal tip with a little depression at the supratip break point is common in the Anglo-Saxon ethnicity, together with sweeter face lineaments, the same characteristics do not fit well with the stronger features of a typical Mediterranean face.

Therefore, during surgical planning, the surgeon must give the right importance to his/her aesthetic view of the harmony of the face in its ethnic context, in order to modify nasal shape accordingly, rather than simply analysing facial features objectively, calculating parameters like tip projection and rotation and nasal angles.

Figures 7.8 and 7.9 illustrates two cases of Mediterranean nose correction using some of the aforementioned open techniques.

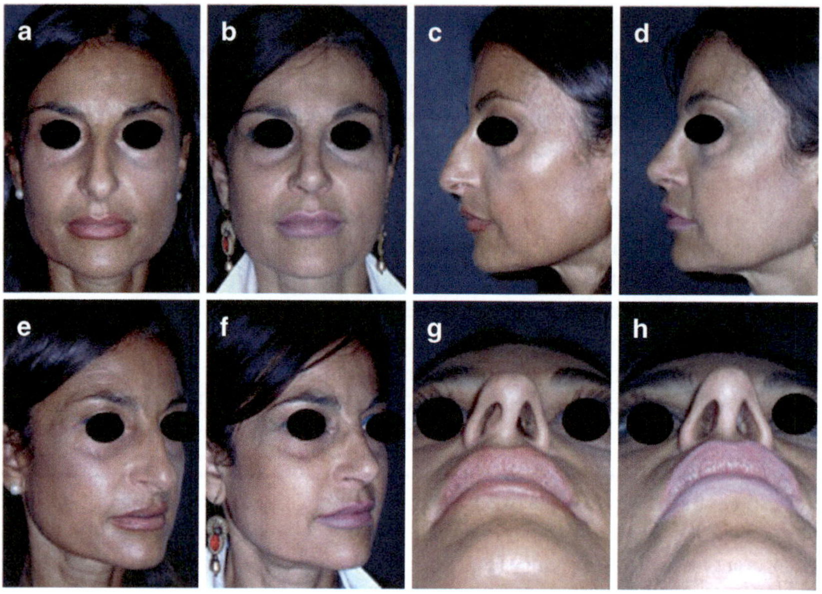

Fig. 7.8 Case 1: Patient with osseocartilaginous dorsal hump, tip ptosis with over-projection and acute nasolabial angle. (**a**, **c**, **e**, **g**) Preoperative views. (**b**, **d**, **f**, **h**) Postoperative views following hump removal, lateral crural overlay technique, double dome sutures and columellar strut

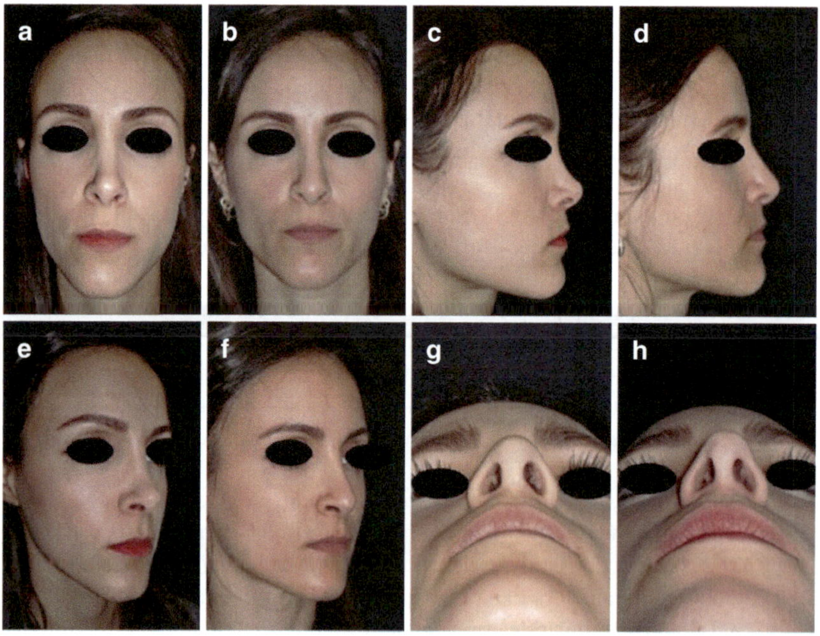

Fig. 7.9 Case 2: Patient with saddle deformity, bulbous tip with over-projection. (**a**, **c**, **e**, **g**) Preoperative views. (**b**, **d**, **f**, **h**) Postoperative views following conchal dorsal graft, columellar strut, dome division and suture of the domal arch, placement of shield graft

7.6 Conclusions

Mediterranean nose correction must acknowledge the typical ethnic characteristics of this population and rhinoplasty must aim to modify nasal parameters in order to increase the overall harmony of the face. From this modern point of view, the tendency towards preservation of the ethnic identity of the patient overcomes the research of an abstract ideal of beauty based only on the mere analysis of numerical values.

Following this philosophy, it is advisable to straighten the nasal dorsum, both in male and female patients, seeking for a widening of the nasolabial angle. Regarding the nasal tip, its ptosis is quite frequent in Mediterranean noses; therefore, surgeons have to choose the best technique to increase tip rotation, from the simpler to the more complex ones, which require section and overlapping of the segments of the lateral crura. A useful algorithm would suggest starting with a simple trimming of the cephalic portion of the lateral crura, followed by the removal of a thin strip of the caudal septum, the use of plumping grafts and eventually the lateral crural overlay technique in the most severe cases. Depending on the degree of underprojection, also to obtain an increase in tip projection it is preferable to start with cartilage suturing techniques and then move on to the use of various types of grafts. Alar malposition is another typical Mediterranean feature which can be dealt with using techniques aimed to mobilizing and repositioning the lateral crura of the LLCs like lateral crural stairstep technique or lateral crural strut graft one.

The hardest phase of Mediterranean rhinoplasty is to harmonize the tip projection with the nasal dorsum. This goal can only be obtained keeping clear in mind the ethnic elements that characterize the face and using surgical technique able to spare tissues rather than demolishing them, in order to guarantee better and longer-lasting results.

References

1. Howells WW. Carleton Stevens Coon 1904–1981. A biographical memoir.
2. Gunter JP. Facial analysis for the rhinoplasty patient. 12th Annu Dallas Rhinoplasty Symp. 1995.
3. Simons RL. Adjunctive measures in rhinoplasty. Otolaryngol Clin North Am. 1975;8(3):717–42. https://doi.org/10.1016/S0030-6665(20)32750-X.
4. Crumley RL, Lanser M. Quantitative analysis of nasal tip projection. Laryngoscope. 1988;98(2):202–8. https://doi.org/10.1288/00005537-198802000-00017.
5. Friedman O, Akcam T, Cook T. Reconstructive rhinoplasty: the 3-dimensional nasal tip. Arch Facial Plast Surg. 2006;8(3):195–201. https://doi.org/10.1001/archfaci.8.3.195.
6. Gunter JP, Friedman RM. Lateral crural strut graft: technique and clinical applications in rhinoplasty. Plast Reconstr Surg. 1997;99(4):943–52.
7. Toriumi DM. New concepts in nasal tip contouring. Arch Facial Plast Surg. 2006;8(3):156–85. https://doi.org/10.1001/archfaci.8.3.156.
8. Goldman IB. Principles in rhinoplasty. Minn Med. 1967;50(6):833–6.
9. Kridel RW, Konior RJ. Controlled nasal tip rotation via the lateral crural overlay technique. Arch Otolaryngol Head Neck Surg. 1991;117(4):411–5. https://doi.org/10.1001/archotol.1991.01870160065011.

10. McCollough EG, English JL. A new twist in nasal tip surgery. An alternative to the Goldman tip for the wide or bulbous lobule. Arch Otolaryngol. 1985;111(8):524–9. https://doi.org/10.1001/archotol.1985.00800100072010.
11. Konior RJ, Kridel R. Controlled nasal tip positioning via the open rhinoplasty approach. Facial Plast Surg Clin North Am. 1993;1:53–62.
12. Peck GC. The onlay graft for nasal tip projection. Plast Reconstr Surg. 1983;71(1):27–39. https://doi.org/10.1097/00006534-198301000-00007.
13. Fomon S, Goldman IB, Neivert H, Schattner A. Management of deformities of the lower cartilaginous vault. AMA Arch Otolaryngol. 1951;54(5):467–72. https://doi.org/10.1001/archotol.1951.03750110003001.
14. Kridel RW, Scott BA, Foda HM. The tongue-in-groove technique in septorhinoplasty. A 10-year experience. Arch Facial Plast Surg. 1999;1(4):246–56; discussion 257–258. https://doi.org/10.1001/archfaci.1.4.246.
15. Boccieri A. The surgical approach to the Mediterranean nose. Facial Plast Surg. 2010;26(2):119–30. https://doi.org/10.1055/s-0030-1253498.
16. Boccieri A, Raimondi G. The lateral crural stairstep technique: a modification of the kridel lateral crural overlay technique. Arch Facial Plast Surg. 2008;10(1):56–64. https://doi.org/10.1001/archfacial.2007.7.
17. Soliemanzadeh P, Kridel RWH. Nasal tip overprojection: algorithm of surgical deprojection techniques and introduction of medial crural overlay. Arch Facial Plast Surg. 2005;7(6):374–80. https://doi.org/10.1001/archfaci.7.6.374.
18. Sheen JH. Achieving more nasal tip projection by the use of a small autogenous vomer or septal cartilage graft. A preliminary report. Plast Reconstr Surg. 1975;56(1):35–40. https://doi.org/10.1097/00006534-197507000-00007.
19. Cobo R. Mestizo rhinoplasty. Facial Plast Surg. 2003;19(3):257–68. https://doi.org/10.1055/s-2003-43161.
20. Palma P, Bignami M, Delù G, De Bernardi F, Castelnuovo P. Rhinoplasty for the Mediterranean nose. Facial Plast Surg. 2003;19(3):279–94. https://doi.org/10.1055/s-2003-43163.

Northern Mediterranean Nose Correction: Italian Experience: Preservation Approach

8

Valerio Finocchi and Valentino Vellone

8.1 Introduction

The history of the Mediterranean area sees the migration of many people from various parts of the world with the consequent development of what we now call the Caucasians. According to our experience, the vast anatomical variability of this ethnic group is such that it does not allow the surgeon to apply one and only one philosophy in the aesthetic/functional approach to the nose.

It is essential that the rhino-surgeon has numerous techniques in his arsenal, in order to apply the one that is most suitable for the clinical case.

The surgeon must therefore be able to mold and "sacrifice" himself rather than "forcing" the patient to undergo the same surgical approach.

The philosophy and surgical techniques of Preservation Rhinoplasty (PR) has had a profound impact on rhinoplasty surgery and continues to evolve [1].

In our clinical experience, the Preservation approach, contrary to what one might think, turns out to be very heterogeneous and varied, allowing the treatment of different types of nose and at the same time guaranteeing natural results with rapid postoperative recovery. In recent years, thanks to the experience gained, several

V. Finocchi (✉)
MySelf Clinic, Rome, Italy
e-mail: info@valeriofinocchi.com

V. Vellone
Maxillofacial Surgery Unit, Santa Maria Hospital, Terni, Italy

P. G. Giacomini (ed.), *Mediterranean Rhinoplasty*,
https://doi.org/10.1007/978-3-031-05551-5_8

authors have been able to evaluate when this technique was successful, when to associate it with a structural technique, or when, on the contrary, it is better to avoid it.

The preoperative analysis and planning of the technical project is essential for the result. The number of publications relating to Preservation Rhinoplasty has grown exponentially, so much that it has been defined by Rollin K. Daniel as a "revolution" in this field [1].

This philosophy has three cardinal principles: the soft tissues, the dorsal, and the alar cartilages preservation.

From our point of view, there is another fundamental structure that must not be put aside, the nasal septum. In 1905, Killian [2] had attributed it a key role in supporting the nasal pyramid.

Jankowsky [3, 4] also revealed that the triangular cartilages and the septum represent a single unit from an embryological point of view.

According to this point of view, the dorsal deformity would derive mainly from a disorder caused by the centrifugal growth of the quadrangular cartilage [5] that comes into conflict posteriorly with the perpendicular lamina of the ethmoid bone and with the vomer and anteriorly with the maxilla.

For the nasal tip, the primary causes of deformity are multifactorial, and, as already seen in cleft lip [6], may depend on bony defects such as maxillary displacement, alveolar gap, a depressed piriform margin, as well as aberrant muscular attachment of the orbicularis oris and other muscles of the nasal complex or by a push of the quadrangular cartilage.

Therefore, to correct a nasal deformity it is mandatory to understand the causes and processes that led that structure to acquire a given shape with the aim of choosing a technique able to reverse the evolutionary process. The result is a philosophy which, depending on the case, can be purely preservative or balancing preservation (manipulation, remodeling, etc.) with resection/restructuring/structuring. In conclusion, authors aim to correct the deformities presented trying, as much as possible, to preserve the normo-conformed structures by repositioning them in their right position and changing their angles (e.g., dorsal ROM of the Key Stone Area or Resting Angle for the lateral crus) and resecting/altering/reconstructing those that cannot be modulated/remodeled (e.g., deformity of the triangular or septum).

The ultimate goal is to create a correct structure where every component is placed in the right anatomical position, occupying the right place without leaving dead spaces.

Preservation of the ligaments reduces the postoperative fibrosis, which is often responsible for the modification of a well-constructed framework [7].

In the Mediterranean population, anatomical variability is really important not only as osteo-cartilaginous structures but also as soft tissues (e.g., thin skin and thick subcutis).

The aim of this chapter is to focus on the dorsal-septal unit and to describe the extreme anatomical variability showing the key points that need to be analyzed when choosing the best technique (Fig. 8.1).

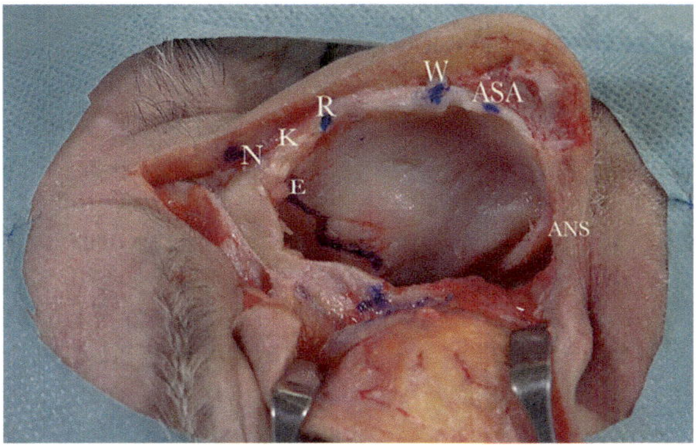

Fig. 8.1 N, Nasion; K, Kyphion; R, Rhinion; ANS, Anterior Nasal Spine; ASA, Anterior Septal Angle, W-point, upper lateral cartilages septal junction (approximately 10 mm cephalic to the ASA)

8.2 Relevant Surgical Anatomy

The shape and size of the nasal dorsum remain the primary reason why Caucasian patients seek aesthetic nasal surgery.

The studies by Lazovich et al. [8] have allowed to understand the key stone area and the intrinsic curvatures of the bony cap in the sagittal plane.

In our opinion, although this represents a great step forward in the understanding of the dorsum joint and in the development of more or less conservative techniques (Saban [9], SPQR [10], Ishida [11], Spare Roof [12]), more studies are still needed taking into account the deformity not from a two-dimensional point of view but from a three-dimensional point of view. This is mandatory because the surgical techniques must consider all projections as patients will judge the nose from every angle.

An in-depth evaluation of three relevant anatomical areas—the keystone area, the subdorsal septum, and the nasal walls—allows one to understand dorsal hump configuration and to select appropriate surgical techniques.

8.2.1 The Key Stone Area

Palhazi et al. [13] introduced the concept of the cartilaginous vault being composed of a dorsal keystone area (DKA), which consists of the T-shaped dorsal septum, and a lateral keystone area (LKA), which reflects the cephalic portions of the upper lateral cartilages. The anatomy of the osseocartilaginous junction and in particular its area of overlap (8–9 mm on average) [13] at the keystone area (KA) is a direct reflection of its embryological development. As shown histologically [14], there is a juxtaposed layer of periosteum and perichondrium wherever there is osseous-cartilaginous overlap. Another important feature of the keystone is the pyriform aperture ligament which consists of perichondrial/periosteal fibers joining the ULC and nasal bone [15–18]. This ligament can be as thick as 1 mm and attaches directly to the bone at its distal edge, confirming its anchoring role. On the dorsal keystone area, the ligament is very thick (more than 1 mm) and is made of multiple layers of fibrous periosteum and perichondrium going in different directions [15]. As emphasized by Saban [19], the keystone area is not a rigid fixed structure, but rather a flexible chondro-osseous joint, thus allowing changes of the dorsal shape. Histological studies of the keystone area (KA) indicate that the periosteum on the deep surface of the bony cap, fuses with the perichondrium on the superficial surface of the cartilaginous vault. The result is a flexible dorsum which allows the convexity of the dorsum to be modified by reducing the underlying cartilaginous septal support. Thus, the vault can be changed from convex to concave without losing its continuity.

8.2.2 The Subdorsal Septum

The subdorsal segment of the cartilaginous septum is a critical area, both in a longitudinal and vertical direction. Longitudinally, the sub-dorsal junction of the cartilaginous and bony septum is highly variable, often extending quite cephalically towards the radix. According to East et al. [14] and confirmed by Ferreira [20], the mean distance from Transverse Radix Osteotomy Plane (TROP) to the junction between the perpendicular plate of the ethmoid (PPE) and quadrangular cartilage (E-point) is −7.25 mm (range: −19.2 to 5.22 mm). A negative value denotes that the subdorsal septal junction between quadrangular cartilage and PPE (E point) is located posterior to the TROP, meaning that cartilaginous septum underlies the keystone area in the majority of cases. Thus, the direct septal support of nasal humps is usually cartilaginous rather than bony. With experience, release of the subdorsal cartilaginous septum from the junction point (E) to the rhinion pivot point (R) can be achieved with careful dissection.

8.2.3 Lateral Bony Nasal Walls

The lateral bony walls are formed by the nasal bone and the ascending process of the maxillary bones, which represent the lateral dorsal pillars. In cross section, the maxillary ascending branch is thicker compared to nasal bones. In contrast to hump modification which is directly influenced by resection of the subdorsal septum, reduction of dorsal height is achieved by osteotomies at the base of the lateral wall, thus allowing preservation of the dorsum. The head of the inferior turbinates is often in close contact with the caudal portion of the lateral walls in the area of Webster's triangle.

8.3 Hump Analysis/Classification

To date, there have been relatively few articles detailing analysis and classification of both the dorsal hump and the dorsal profile. Subsequent to Topinard's five basic profiles, there were attempts made to measure profile angles and components of the nose. At the present time, two articles are of particular relevance. Recently, Saban [21] presented the concept of a combined reduction—hump reduction and dorsal height reduction—which is a particularly valuable concept for dorsum preservation (DP) procedures.

In the traditional Joseph resection rhinoplasty, both goals were achieved in one major reduction. If one is not directly resecting the hump, then the dorsal hump must be eliminated by reducing its direct support (septal strip excision) and allowing flexion at the chondro-osseous joint. These DP methods work well on cartilaginous structures, but not on intrinsic bony vault contour deformities, especially in the bony cap. Dorsal height reduction is then achieved with either a cartilage vault or bony vault impaction maneuver. Thus, the surgeon needs to analyze the shape and composition of the nasal hump as well as to select an operative technique for the desired aesthetic profile changing. The second critical paper is by Lazovic et al. [8], who classified the dorsal profile into V-shaped and S-shaped based on profile analysis of bony hump anatomy (Fig. 8.2).

The V-shaped dorsum has a flat bony cap starting at the level of the Nasion (N) and finishing at the level of the Rhinion (R). The nasion is defined as the deepest point in the radix area of the bony vault on profile view. The Rhinion is defined as the most caudal point of the paired nasal bones and marks the midline junction of the bony and cartilaginous vaults. The S-shaped dorsum has a curved bony cap. The line starts at the level of the Nasion, passes to a distinct point called Kyphion (K, the most prominent point of the nasal bones) before continuing to the Rhinion. The intersection of the two lines N-K and K-R creates the Kyphion angle (KA). Studies

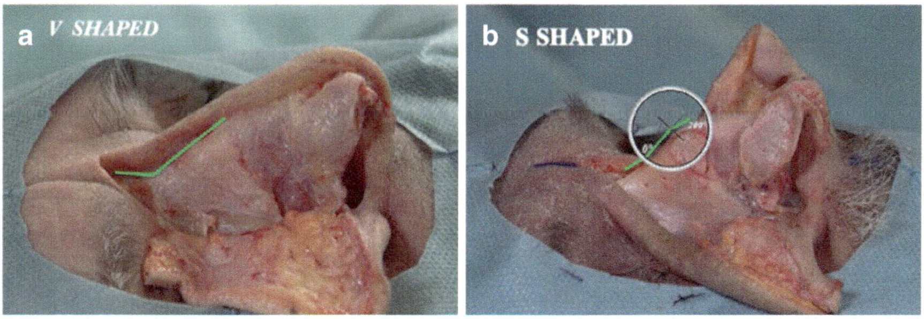

Fig. 8.2 Cadaver dissections. (**a**) A V-Shaped bony dorsum with a straight line from nasion (N) to Rhinion (R) with absence of the Kyphion point and thus no Kyphion angle. (**b**) S-Shaped bony dorsum with a distinct Kyphion point (K) and therefore a Kyphion angle (KA)

by Lazovic [8] and Palhazi [13] were done on cadavers, and the application of their findings to patients seeking rhinoplasty can be challenging. With the increasing use of preoperative cone beam CT scans (CBCT), it has become clear that the soft tissue envelope (STE) can modify clinical presentation of the bony vault anatomy. For this reason, one can often have a hidden S-shaped dorsum in which the bony vault has an intrinsic Kyphion angle, but a V-shaped clinical dorsal profile (Fig. 8.3).

The diagnosis can be made on palpation as a distinct Kyphion point (K) and can be felt cephalic to the Rhinion junction (R) within the bony cap. Although not essential, the diagnosis can be confirmed with a CBCT.

Moreover, it is our opinion that the anatomy of the cartilaginous vault has to be taken into account in the final operative decision because even if dorsal aesthetic lines are considered ideal, the ULCs length and R-ASA segment profile line must be considered in order to choose the right technique. Ultimately, the surgeon must analyze dorsal composition to determine the optimal operative plan.

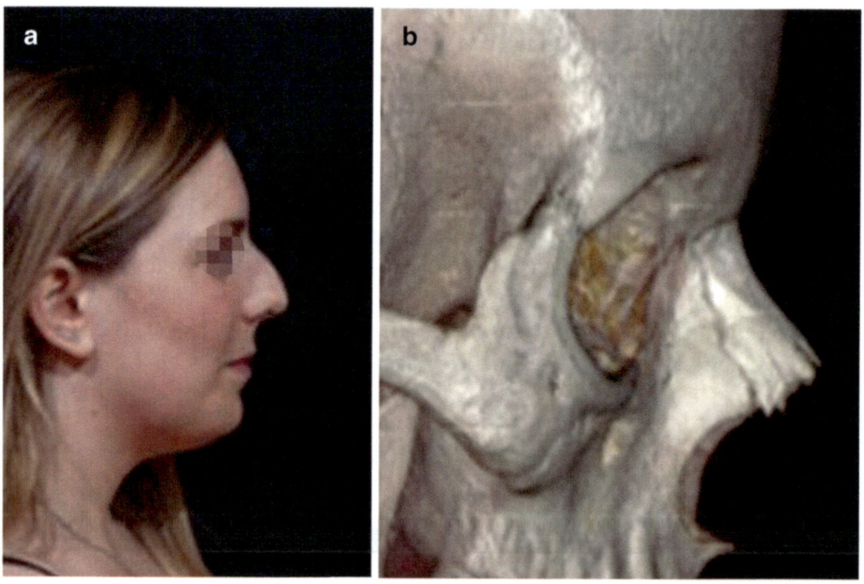

Fig. 8.3 Range of dorsal deformities. (**a**, **b**) 26-year-old female patient with a V-shape dorsum. The Bony vault is flat therefore no need for bony vault shaping. (**c**, **d**) 28-year-old female patient with an S-shape dorsum. The palpable bony cap curvature indicates the need for bony cap reshaping. (**e**, **f**) 28-year-old female patient with hidden S-shape dorsum. Clinically seams a V-shape but it isn't. Palpation diagnosis is confirmed by CT scan. This case requires bony vault reshaping

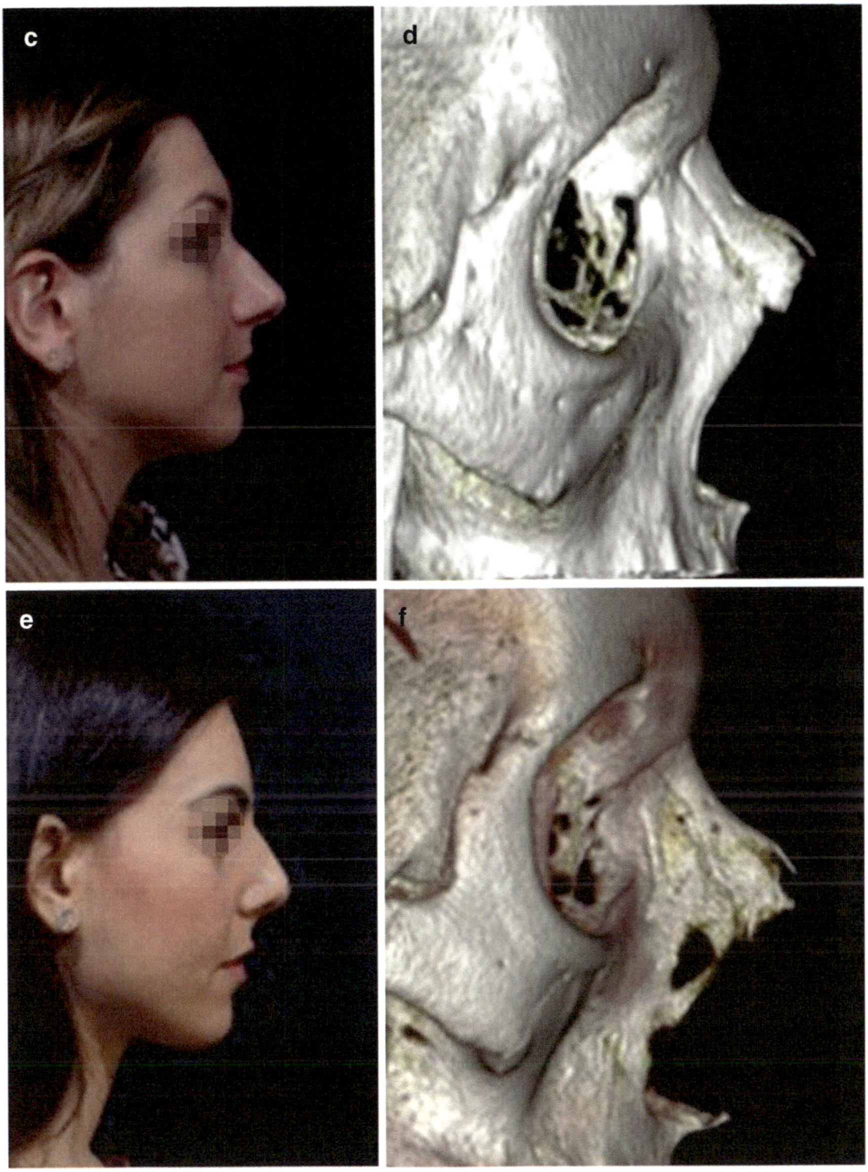

Fig. 8.3 (continued)

8.3.1 Nasal Dorsum Variability and Surgical Approach

Usually, dorsum deformities can be divided into two large groups: V- and S-shaped, but this classification does not take into account the three-dimensionality of the dorsum (e.g., narrow or wide, bony cap curved from side to side but flat profile) nor the cartilaginous dorsum that can also present numerous variables (Fig. 8.4).

According to Fig. 8.4, a thorough anatomical analysis can be done:

(a) Straight dorsum with good relationships between bone and cartilage and normal Key Stone area. It is possible to reduce dorsal height by impacting the nasal pyramid on its foundations, preserving all anatomical structures.

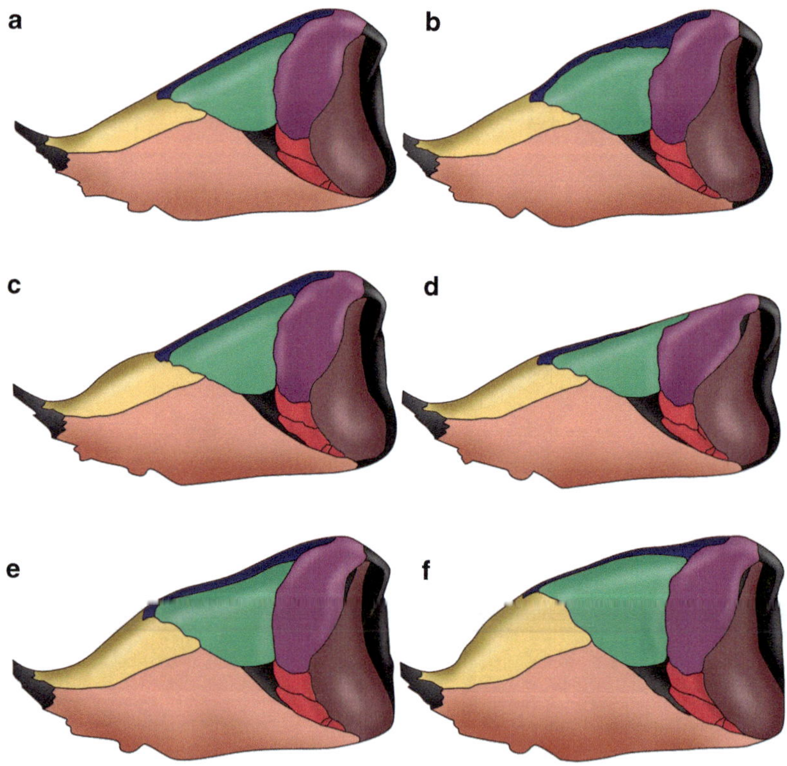

Fig. 8.4 Extreme profile anatomical variability where DALs are assumed to be fine: Pink nasal bones; green ULCs; brown maxillary bone; purple LLCs. (**a**) Straight dorsum with good relationships between bone and cartilage and normal Key Stone area. (**b**) Flat bony cap (V-shaped) with abnormal relationship with the cartilaginous vault (**c**) Curved nasal bone (S-shaped) with the presence of a Kyphion at the level of the most prominent part of the bony cap. (**d**) Both bony and cartilaginous vault are well shaped, but they are not well articulated and form an angle. (**e**) Malformed keystone area, the bony vault is well shaped but over-projected and the ULCs are therefore altered. (**f**) The whole osseocartilaginous vault is malformed and therefore preservation is not indicated

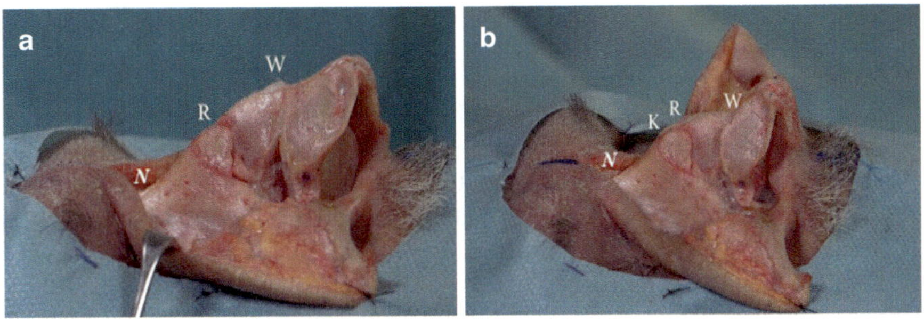

Fig. 8.5 The V-shaped dorsum (**a**) has a flat bony cap starting at the level of the Nasion (N) and finishing at the level of the Rhinion (R). The nasion is defined as the deepest point in the radix area of the bony vault on profile view. The Rhinion is defined as the most caudal point of the paired nasal bones and marks the midline junction of the bony and cartilaginous vaults. The S-shaped dorsum (**b**) has a curved bony cap. The line starts at the level of the Nasion, passes to a distinct point called Kyphion (K, the most prominent point of the nasal bones) before continuing to the Rhinion. The S-shaped dorsum has a distinct angulation from Nasion to Kyphion and then a plateau from Kyphion to Rhinion. The bones have a sharp takeoff of the hump from the Nasion (N) resulting in a high Kyphion (K) point and a second locus of angulation

(b) Flat bony cap (V-shaped) with abnormal relationship with the cartilaginous vault, where the nasal profile is convex from the Rhinion to the anterior septal angle, and the ULCs and the anterior septum are malformed. Bony vault can be preserved while cartilaginous vault must be remodeled (Fig. 8.5a).
(c) Curved nasal bone (S-shaped) with the presence of a Kyphion at the level of the most prominent part of the bony cap. Bony vault must be remodeled while the Cartilginous vault is well shaped and can be preserved (Fig. 8.5b).
(d) Both bony and cartilaginous vault are well shaped, but they are not well articulated and form an angle. It is possible to preserve both vaults, but it is important to work on their foundation to flat the angle.
(e) Malformed keystone area, the bony vault is well shaped but over-projected and the ULCs are therefore altered. Preservation is not indicated.
(f) The whole osseocartilaginous vault is malformed and therefore preservation is not indicated.

8.4 Preoperative Analysis

The surgeon must do a thorough preoperative analysis of the patient's nose, in order to personalize the operative planning.

1. **Inspection.** Are the aesthetic dorsal lines good looking? Is it possible to keep this dorsum intact or partially intact? Is it a V-shaped or an S-shaped dorsum?
2. **Rhinoscopy.** A detailed internal exam is mandatory, and the following questions must be answered. Is the septum in the midline? In the case of septal deviation, is it a low septal deviation, high septal deviation, or a mixed deformity? The position of the deviation can also be assessed following Cottle principles,

considering the septal areas involved (Area 1,2,3,4,5a,5b), premaxillary spurs, and posterior bony septal deviation.

3. **Palpation.** It is important to touch the keystone area and feel the osseocartilaginous components. The evaluation of the degree of flexibility of the KA joint is important when planning to eliminate the dorsal hump. In addition, palpation can provide a relative indication of the location of the PPE-QC junction (E POINT) – hard resistance indicates that the junction is at the same location while a soft response indicates that the junction is located cephalic to the KA. Every keystone area is different due to its bony component and connective tissue adherence. For example, in case of major bony component with S-shaped dorsum, it will be necessary to reshape the bony dorsum, and the Ishida or Ferreira techniques may be more suitable. It is also important to palpate the bony cap to appreciate its three-dimensional shape.
4. **Cone Beam CT Scans.** CBCT is an X-ray computed tomography where the X-rays are divergent thus forming a cone. Total radiation doses from 3D dental CBCT exams are 96% lower than conventional CT exams and are comparable to the radiation of a chest X-ray. During the exam, the CBCT scanner rotates around the patient's head providing nearly 600 distinct images.

   CBCT has been described as the gold standard imaging for the maxillofacial area. It provides valuable insight into the anatomy of the septum and the relationship between the nose, skull base, and maxilla. The areas evaluated include the following: nasal bone length, bony cap shape, anterior nasal spine position, and QC-PPE (E POINT) relationship with the keystone area. In the asymmetric nose, these findings are very important for planning septoplasty and asymmetric osteotomies\ostectomies (Fig. 8.6).

   Digital image files of each patient are exported in Digital Imaging and Communication in Medicine (DICOM) format. Scanning software collects the data and reconstructs it, producing what is termed a *digital volume* composed of three-dimensional voxels of anatomical data.

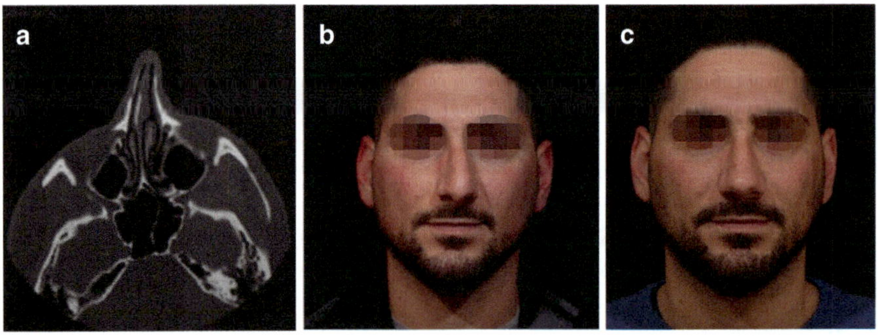

Fig. 8.6 (**a**) Preoperative CT scan shows a high septal deviation at the level of the PPE. (**b**) preoperative presentation. (**c**) As seen at 6 months postoperative, a swinging door septoplasty allows direct access to treat the PPE deviation which facilitates alignment of the pyramid onto the midline. With an L strut procedure, the PPE deviation would have been more difficult to treat and perhaps limit centralization of the pyramid

The great innovation is the distribution of open-source software that can read and manipulate DICOM files.

Each surgeon can thus independently visualize and reconstruct in three dimensions the area to be investigated.

Moreover, thanks to the presets already present, it is possible to emphasize the bone rather than the cartilage in the 3d reconstruction.

Authors use HOROS software (FOSS, Horosproject.org, NIMBLE Co LLC, Annapolis, MD) or OsiriX Lite software for MacOS.

Horos is a free and open-source code software (FOSS) program that is distributed free of charge under the LGPL license at Horosproject.org and sponsored by Nimble Co LLC d/b/a Purview in Annapolis, MD USA.

HOROS PROJECT has the same virtual environment of OsiriX Lite software (open-source PixMeo Sarl).

5. **Photographic Analysis**. Preoperative photographs are important not only for medical-legal matters, but also during surgery to visualize anatomical details that can be hidden by edema. Computer morphing is done to determine the amount of dorsal reduction and to simulate the range of motion that the KA joint must have to change the nasal profile from convex to straight to concave. Moreover, it is important to discover those cases of hidden S-shaped dorsum, which present clinically as a V-shaped one, but show the presence of a Kyphion during the anthropometric studies on the CT scan.

8.5 Decision-Making Algorithm

After analyzing the dorsum, authors start a mental process to choose the right technique for each case (Fig. 8.7). The first important crossroad feature is the DALs in the frontal view.

Classically, the nose is shown in frontal view with two divergent concave lines that extend from the supraorbital rim through the radix area and then continue as paired lines to the nasal tip. However, these traditional dorsal aesthetic lines are slightly different when viewed through the nasal polygon aesthetic unit concept.

As seen in Fig. 8.8, the dorsal aesthetic lines should have a fusiform pattern starting at the brows with the nasal radix area being narrow, the keystone area wider, and the supratip region narrow again before ultimately diverging at the tip. This fusiform pattern is important to create a natural-looking aesthetic dorsum. The dorsal aesthetic lines are formed when the skin softens the lines that join [22] the glabellar, the dorsal bone, the dorsal cartilage, and the lateral edges of the dome polygons.

If the DALs are not ideal or the dorsum is very wide, the dorsal preservation approach should be avoided, and a structured approach would be more suitable.

What guides us in choosing the correct technique is the combination of the dorsal characteristics, the septal anatomy, and finally the nasal bony lateral walls.

The analysis should be done on the single Dorso-Septal unit rather than on each structure alone, yet we will present them separately for a better comprehension.

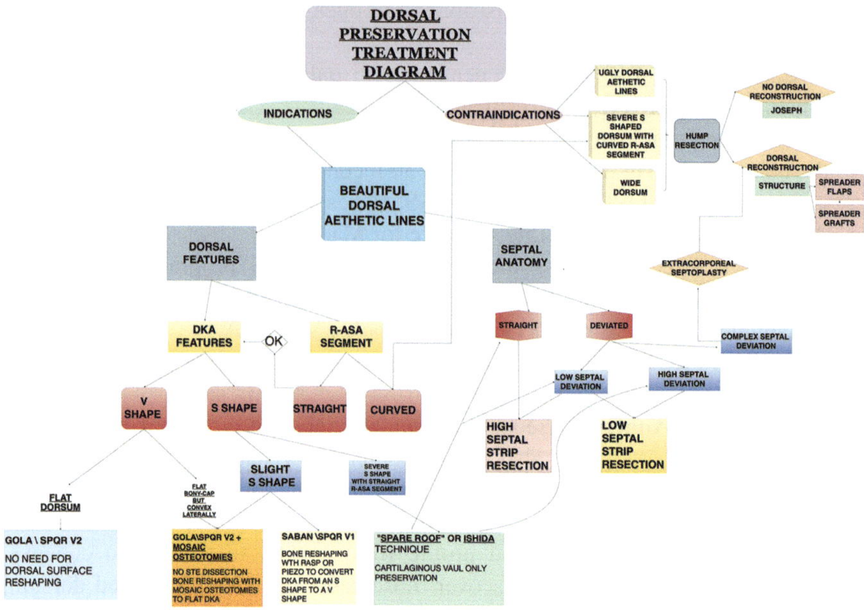

Fig. 8.7 Dorsal preservation treatment diagram

Dorsal profile analysis: Composition and position of all the important key points (NASION, KYPHION if present, RHINION, W-POINT, ANTERIOR SEPTAL ANGLE), 3-D bony cap shape and R-ASA segment anatomy.

Septal anatomy: Straight, low or high septal deviation. The septum is the most important pillar of the nasal pyramid and therefore septal correction is paramount for the final aesthetic-functional result. The septoplasty thus influences the surgeon on which dorsal preservation technique should be employed.

In case of high septal deviations, the swinging door septoplasty is more suitable, and this technique can be associated with Ishida and SPQR techniques.

In case of straight and low septal deviations an L strut septoplasty is more appropriate, and this technique can be associated with Saban and Ferreira's techniques.

Bony lateral walls: In case of crooked noses, the pyriform aperture is asymmetric, and therefore the distance between the Webster triangle and the Rhinion is asymmetric. These cases require asymmetric treatment of the bony pyramid ("PISA TOWER CONCEPT"; Fig. 8.9).

The possible anatomical variables are unlimited; therefore, it is difficult if not impossible, to draw a perfect guideline.

Authors describe the most used techniques in their practice.

- Saban's technique (5% in our clinical practice):
  - Indications: straight septum or low septal deviations with perpendicular plate of the ethmoid on the midline (Fig. 8.10), V-shaped dorsum with good aesthetic dorsal lines (type A, B, slight C, and D seen in Fig. 8.4, with straight or with low septum deviation).

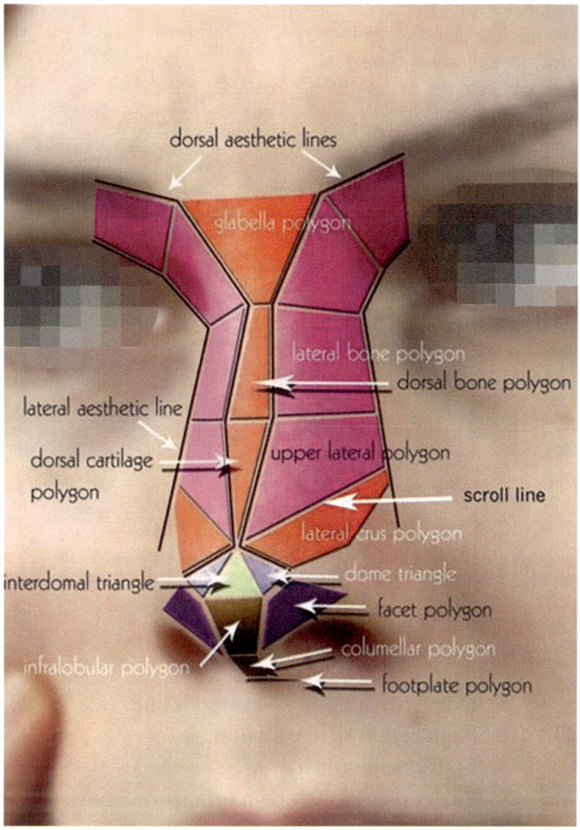

Fig. 8.8 Nasal surface aesthetics can be analyzed in terms of these geometric shapes: glabella polygon, dorsal bone polygon, dorsal cartilage triangle, lateral bone polygons, upper lateral polygons, dome triangles, lateral crus polygons, interdomal triangle, facet polygons, infralobular polygon, columellar polygon, and footplate polygons. (From Çakır et al. (Rhinoplasty: surface aesthetics and surgical techniques. Aesthetic Surg J. 2013;33(3):363–375.) Reprinted with permission from Sage Publications)

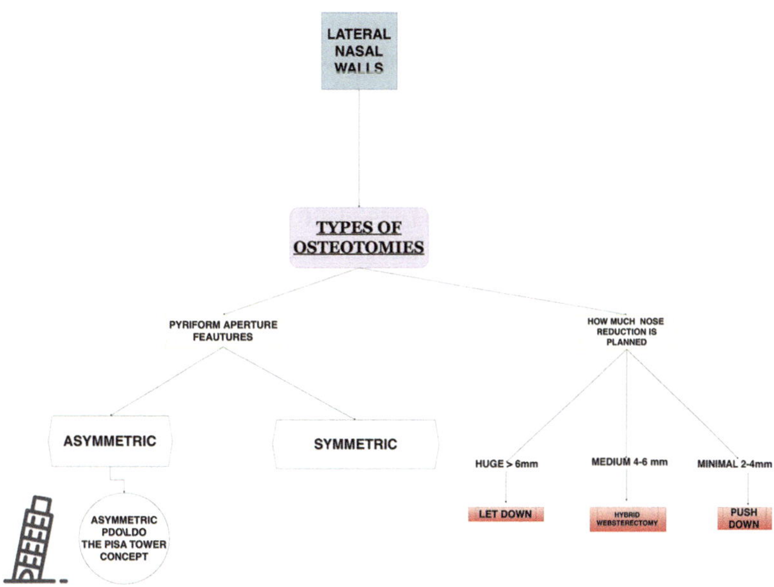

Fig. 8.9 "Pisa tower concept"

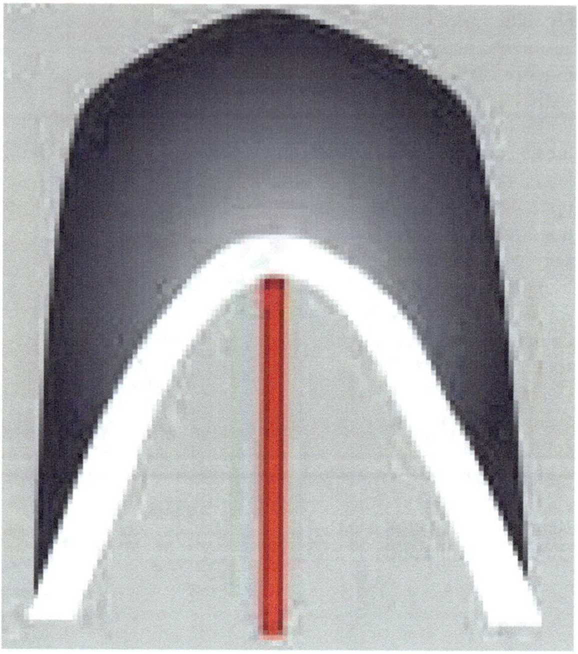

Fig. 8.10 The PPE is on the midline therefore an L strut septoplasty is enough to correct the septal deviation

1. Dorsal dissection and remodeling
2. High septal strip excision
3. L-strut septoplasty
4. Push down or let down impaction consists in dorsal impaction performing a high septal strip excision associated with a total nasal pyramid mobilization with a push down or let down maneuver.

The cartilaginous strip excision consists of an incisional curved subdorsal cut first and then a straight excisional cut through the septum to remove the so-formed cartilaginous strip. It is important that the cartilaginous cut doesn't start at the ASA point, but rather at the W-point. The W-point represents the point of separation of the ULCs from the septum. From the surgeon's viewpoint, looking from caudal to cephalic, it resembles the letter W. Anatomically, the W-point will be 4.4 mm (range: 1–8 mm) (Palhazi et al. 2015) from the ASA. However, we recommend clinically to place the incision at the actual W-point, which should be at least 6–8 mm cephalic to the ASA. The incisional cut then continues subdorsally, keeping intimate contact between the scissor tips and the undersurface of the dorsum. The incision proceeds cephalically until bone is encountered at the junction of cartilaginous septum and the perpendicular plate of ethmoid (PPE).

The excisional cut is performed using straight scissors, and it begins 2–4 mm below the W-point. It then continues until the bony septum is encountered. It is good practice to preform it carefully, removing little strips at a time, with the possibility of adding incremental excisions until the desired outcome is reached.

- Golà's technique [23]: (2% in our clinical practice).

- Indications: straight septum or low septal deviations, straight dorsum with good aesthetic dorsal lines without any need of dorsum remodeling (type A and D seen in Fig. 8.4, with straight or low septum deviation).
  1. No dorsal soft tissue envelope (STE) dissection
  2. High septal strip
  3. L strut septoplasty
  4. Push down or let down impaction

  Basically, this technique is similar to the Saban approach but without dorsal STE dissection; and therefore, it ensures faster recovery from surgery.

- The Spare Roof—Ferreira's technique [24]
  - Indications: straight septum or low septal deviations, S-shaped dorsum with good aesthetic dorsal lines. (type C seen in Fig. 8.4. Slight to severe S-Shaped dorsum with straight septum or with low septum deviation)

    It is another method of dorsal modification and consists of the following:
    1. A longitudinal septal strip excision for dorsal reduction,
    2. Resection or contouring of the bony cap to set the ideal profile line
    3. Suturing the cartilage vault down to the underlying septum
    4. Routine lateral low to low and medial osteotomies as indicated
- SPQR (Simplified Preservation Quick Rhinoplasty)
  - Indications: high or complex septal deviations, V or slight S-shaped dorsum with good aesthetic dorsal lines (type A, B, slight C, and D, seen in Fig. 8.4, with PPE deviation—Fig. 8.11)

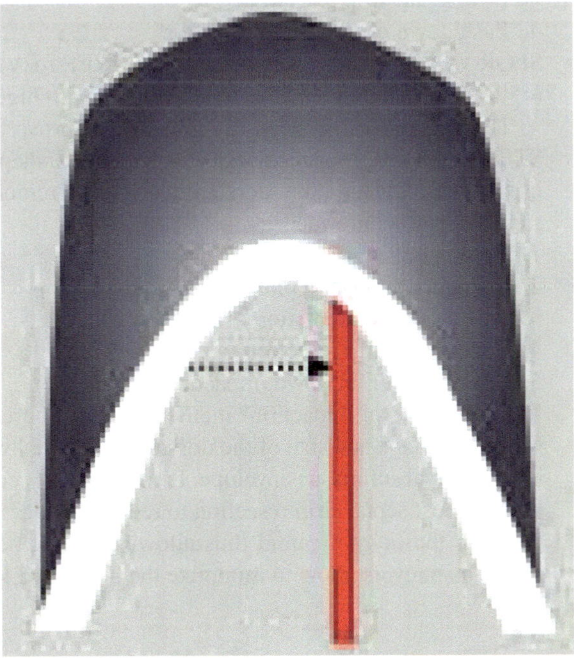

Fig. 8.11 In the high septal deviation the PPE is not on the midline therefore an L strut septoplasty is not enough to correct the septal deviation and a swinging door septoplasty is more indicated

Finocchi's SPQR operation has updated the Cottle procedure with its inferior strip excision. Multiple surgeons have validated the role of the modified Cottle operation for severely deviated noses with complex septal deformities. "Swinging door" septoplasty, as described by Wright [25], consists in the detachment of the cartilaginous septum from its base, going from posterior to anterior at the chondro-osseous junction, and the vomer bone, from the base until the dorsal nasal region, using the sharp end of the elevator. The septal flap (quadrangular cartilage—QC flap) is hence mobilized and can be displaced to approach to the posterior septum. QC flap is connected to the dorsum from the Rhinion to the Anterior septal angle and can be rotated forward to change the profile dorsal line. After new position is set, a 5/0 polydioxanone suture (PDS) is used to fix the quadrangular cartilage flap to the anterior nasal spine.

SPQR V1: (30%) is indicated when dorsum needs to be remodeled and consists of:

1. Dorsal STE dissection and remodeling
2. Low septal strip resection
3. Swinging door septoplasty
4. Push down or let down impaction

SPQR V2: (5%) (type A, and D seen on Fig. 8.4 with high septal/PPE deviation) is indicated when dorsum does not need to be remodeled (basically corresponds to Golà approach [23] but the septoplasty changes according to the septal deviation and so does the septal strip resection).

1. No dorsal STE dissection
2. Swinging door septoplasty
3. Low septal strip resection
4. Push down or let down impaction

- SPQR V2 and mosaic osteotomies or "THREE LEVEL IMPACTIONS" [26, 27] (45%) (Type slight C or D seen in Fig. 8.4, with high septal/PPE deviation)

This technique has been developed to improve the indication for no dorsal STE dissection approach in case of V or slight S-shaped bony dorsum. Therefore, it is indicated when bony dorsum needs to be remodeled but cartilaginous dorsum is normo-conformed.

1. No dorsal STE dissection
2. Swinging door septoplasty
3. Inside-out fragmentation of the bony cap
4. Low septal strip resection
5. Push down or let down impaction

The "Three Level Impaction" method is a dorsal preservation (DP) technique in which the shape and size of the dorsum is changed without the need for dissecting the dorsal soft tissue envelope. In most DP procedures, impaction is achieved in two steps: septal strip resection to reduce the dorsal hump and osteotomies to mobilize the bony pyramid thus allowing dorsal height reduction. These integrated maneuvers allow to minimize the hump and lower the nasal profile while preserving the anatomical integrity of the dorsum. The three-level impaction technique incorporates a series of multiple micro-osteotomies of the bony cap, resulting in a mosaic fragmented configuration which flattens the intrinsic curve of the bony cap. Leaving intact the periosteum connection avoids fragments collapse. Since the micro-osteotomies are done from an endonasal approach, there is no need for dorsal skin dissection. The operative sequence is as follows:

- Step #1 Septoplasty and septal strip removal

  A swinging door septoplasty is performed via bilateral mucoperichondral flap exposure followed by release of the quadrangular cartilage (QC) from the anterior nasal spine, premaxilla, vomer, and perpendicular plate of the ethmoid (PPE) [10].

  Next, the subdorsal segment of the cartilaginous septum is released and the dorsal pivot point is located; it usually corresponds to the Rhinion (Fig. 8.12a). Any posterior septoplasty is completed as indicated at this time. In order to create space for future impaction, two septal strips are removed—(1) a subdorsal strip cephalic to the pivot point, and (2) a triangular septal strip at the base of the QC (Fig. 8.12b). The shape of the subdorsal strip resection can be either triangular or rectangular and is done with a rongeur instrument. A triangular strip resection allows a hinge movement on dorsal impaction which avoids radix descent. In contrast, a rectangular strip resection is chosen for patients with high nasal radix, where a radix drop is desired.

  Next, a limited low septal strip resection is performed to allow mobilization. An additional definitive resection of the inferior septum is done after the circumferential osteotomies. The quadrangular cartilage remains attached to the cartilaginous vault, but it is freed from the influence of the bony septum and can be moved in three dimensions.

- Step #2 Mosaic micro osteotomies of the bony cap

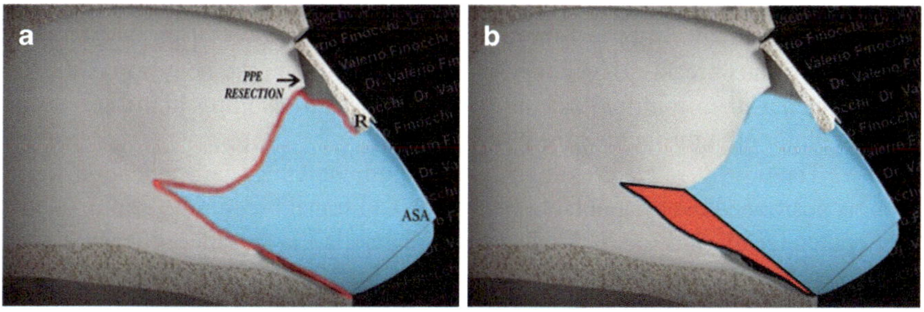

Fig. 8.12 Swinging Door Septoplasty with Bipartite Septal Resection. (**a**) A "swinging door" septoplasty is achieved by total mobilization of the quadrangular cartilage from its bony attachments. The subdorsal dissection releases the QC-PPE junction and then turns caudally towards the Rhinion. (**b**) The excisional cuts to remove the inferior strip should be done in a triangular fashion, less anteriorly and more posteriorly

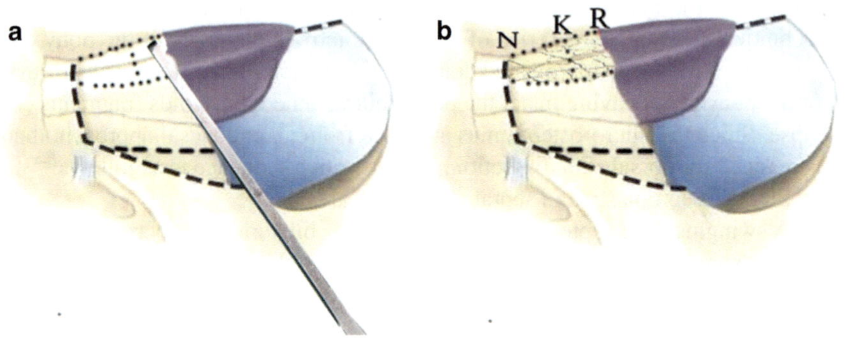

Fig. 8.13 (**a**, **b**) Mosaic Micro Osteotomies of the Bony Cap. (**a**) Markings for bony cap osteotomies indicated by small dots. It is shaped as the letter H with the bilateral longitudinal bony cap osteotomies passing along the to DKA from the Rhinion up towards the Nasion. Transverse osteotomies interrupt the Kyphion in order to break its angle. Circumferential osteotomies for complete mobilization are indicated by heavy dash lines. In such case, transverse, radix and LDO osteotomies. (**b**) final effect of micro mosaic osteotomies with complete bony cap flattening

- Micro osteotomies of the bony cap in a mosaic configuration allow flattening of a curved bony cap without the need for dorsal skin dissection (Fig. 8.13a).

  The osteotomies are performed endonasally with a 2 mm osteotome inserted between the muco-perichondral flaps in an oblique direction. Multiple fractures are created in the bony cap, and at the level of the Kyphion angle to break the intrinsic curvature of the bony cap (Fig. 8.5b). This portion of the bony vault is usually very thin and easy to break with the resulting fragments creating a mosaic. The fragments are not displaced as the periosteum keeps them in position. It should be noted that a range of bony cap deformities are encountered in three dimensions: vertical bone thickness, transverse width, and longitudinal angulation. Therefore, the micro-osteotomies most frequently have a longitudinal H-shape with the parallel lines along the desired dorsal aesthetic lines and the transverse bar at the level of the Kyphion (K point), thus breaking the bony Kyphion angle. When the bony cap is thicker or wider, then multiple osteotomies are required resulting in a true mosaic configuration throughout the bony cap.

  The postoperative dressing is very important. After tape application, a pad is positioned over the dorsum to provide additional pressure to minimize any potential displacement. A thermoplastic cast is then applied to ensure even more stability for the mosaic micro-osteotomies.
- Step #3 Push down operation or let down operation

  The choice between a Push Down Operation (PDO) and a Let Down Operation (LDO) depends on the size of the desired dorsal reduction. A PDO is performed if the reduction is less than 5 mm while a LDO is preferred for reductions greater than 5 mm. In both procedures, percutaneous transverse and radix osteotomies are performed first using a 2 mm osteotome. The radix osteotomy direction can change according to the case—oblique for a hinge motion or vertical for radix reduction. In the PDO procedure, the lateral low to low osteotomy is done with a 3 mm guarded osteotome. It is placed endonasally and continues from the piriform aperture up to the level of the transverse osteotomy. Special attention must be paid to the blocking points that can prevent impaction. The blocking points are often created by the internal periosteum and the medial canthal tendon, both of which should be released to prevent a "spring effect" after impaction [11].

If a major reduction (>5 mm) is required, then a LDO procedure is performed. Following the transverse and radix osteotomies, an inferior wedge of bone is resected from the piriform aperture up to the transverse osteotomy (Fig. 8.14a). The resection can be done employing a guarded osteotome or a small Rongeur. When osteotomes are used, the superior osteotomy is done first to ensure stability and resistance. The LDO procedure is the most common procedure performed and has (in the authors' opinion) multiple advantages including the following: (1) minimizes narrowing at the level of internal nasal valve area, (2) precludes narrowing at the level of the piriform aperture, and (3) facilitates release of the piriform ligament with improved osseocartilaginous joint flexion. The resection can be done employing a guarded osteotome or a small Rongeur (Fig. 8.14b, c).

When osteotomes are used, the superior osteotomy is done first to ensure stability and resistance. The LDO procedure is the most common procedure performed and has (in the authors' opinion) multiple advantages including the following: (1) minimizes narrowing at the level of internal nasal valve area, (2) precludes narrowing at the level of the piriform aperture, and (3) facilitates release of the piriform ligament with improved osseocartilaginous joint flexion.

- Final fixation

  After the three impaction maneuvers are performed, the septoplasty is completed by advancing and rotating the quadrangular cartilage (QC) flap in order to obtain final flattening of the dorsal profile. The QC flap should reach the anterior nasal spine (ANS) without tension. Special attention should be given to the final trimming of the QC base in order to ensure solid contact of the septum along the premaxilla and the ANS. If pushing downward on the dorsum results in a curve in the QC flap, then the QC size is excessive and additional 1 mm inferior strips are resected until the cartilage becomes straight. Once all these key points are addressed, the QC Flap is fixed to the ANS periosteum with a 4/0 PDS figure of eight suture.

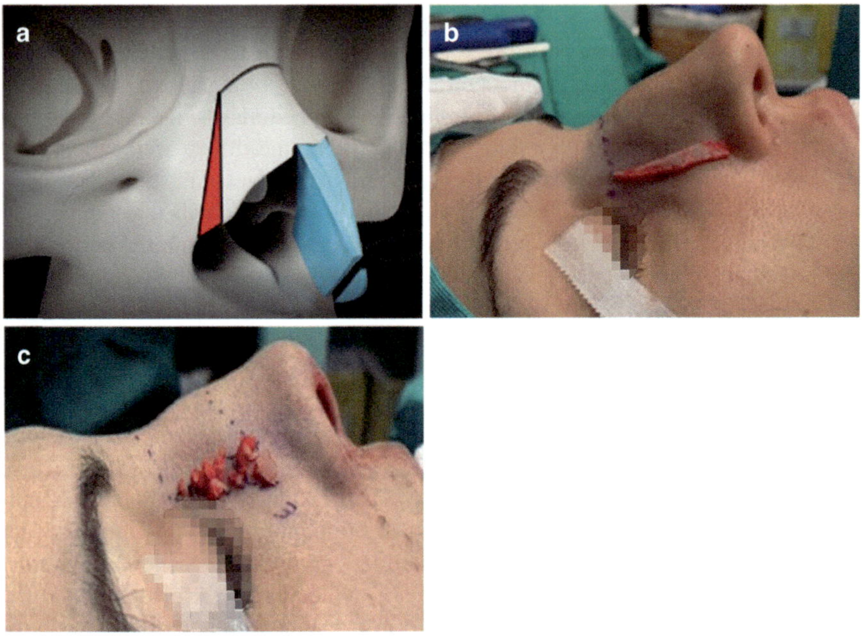

Fig. 8.14 (**a**) 3-D model showing the shape and position of the bony wedge to resect in let down technique. (**b**) LDO: Bony wedge resection performed with a 4 mm osteotome. The inferior osteotomy is always performed after the superior one. (**c**) Bony wedge resection can be done with the help of a Rongeur instrument taking care to avoid any twisting motion during small bony fragments resection. This allows to avoid any unwanted fracture lines

- Ishida cartilaginous vault preservation [28] (25%)
  - Indications: high or complex septal deviations, S-shaped dorsum with good aesthetic dorsal lines. Luiz Carlos Ishida has modified his father's concept of removing the bony hump following lowering of the cartilaginous hump subsequent to excision of an intermediate septal strip [29].
  - Type 1:
    1. Dorsal STE dissection
    2. Dorsal bone removal and preservation of the cartilaginous vault
    3. Swinging door septoplasty
    4. Low septal strip resection

    Type 2: This modified technique retains a triangular portion of the dorsal bony cap, thus maintaining the integrity and smoothness of the keystone area.
    1. Dorsal STE dissection
    2. Dorsal bone and dorsal cartilaginous vault preservation
    3. Removal osseous LKA
    4. Low septal strip resection
    5. Swinging door septoplasty

- Pisa Tower Concept
  - Indications: severe asymmetric dorsal deformities.
    1. "Swinging door" septoplasty, as described by Wright [25].

       The cartilaginous septum is dissected from its base and from the vomer bone, from posterior to anterior at the chondro-osseous junction and from the base until the dorsal nasal region, using the sharp end of the elevator. The septal flap is mobilized and can be displaced to approach to the posterior septum. A 5/0 polydioxanone suture (PDS) is then used to fix the quadrangular cartilage flap to the anterior nasal spine. After the septoplasty, the quadrangular cartilage is left attached to the cartilaginous vault and is free from perpendicular plate influence.
    2. Performe the transverse and radix osteotomies, with a Tastan-Cakir convex saws or with a 2-mm osteotome percutaneously. For the bony vault, authors usually apply the Pisa Tower concept [30], consisting of an asymmetric let down/push down operation, in order to obtain dorsal preservation. A bony wedge was excised from the ascending maxillary process to obtain greater impaction on the longer side compared to the shorter, based on preoperative measurements. The amount of bone to be resected laterally is valuated and planned preoperatively taking into account the amount of hump to be reduced and the level of the deviation to be corrected. The final goal is to obtain two lateral bony walls of equal length. The average bone resected is 9 mm, range: 3–14 mm. Rongeur is the ideal instrument to perform a bony wedge resection after a wide internal periosteal dissection. The authors, removing the bony wedge, avoid internal nasal valve narrowing during the nasal impaction because the nasal wall will not slide in towards the inferior turbinate head. The treatment on the shorter side depends on the amount of nose reduction expected: if minimal, then a Push down operation (PDO) is necessary because this side acts as a pivot point; in case of major nose reduction a minimal LDO may be necessary because a simple PDO would not be enough to allow a correct impaction. In combination with swinging door septoplasty, it is possible to correct very severe crooked noses without the need for an extracorporeal septoplasty. The association with the swinging door septoplasty allows to free the quadrangular cartilage (QC) flap from the perpendicular plate of the ethmoid (PPE) and this allows the repositioning of a total bony cartilaginous vault.

Each case must be evaluated externally and internally to choose the right technique. In Table 8.1 is possible to analyze nine different cases (all with good dorsal aesthetic lines in frontal view) all treated with nine different techniques. The table shows how to choose the technique after analyzing the anatomical deformity.

Table 8.1 Analysis of 9 cases of nasal dorsum deformities with normal dorsal aesthetic lines (DALs), with the proposed surgical technique for each case

Dorsal features	Septal features	Lateral view	3D imaging	Clinical case	CT coronal view	Surgical technique	Dorsal STE dissection	Molding	Preservation	Indication	Septal technique	%
S-shaped dorsum with straight R-ASA	Straight septum or with low deviation	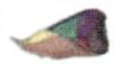	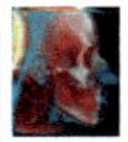	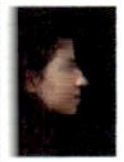	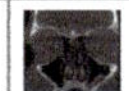	Ferreira's technique	Yes	Dorsum (bone)	Cartilaginous dorsum	S shaped dorsum with straight septum or low septal deviation Rhinion to anterior septal angle should be straight	L-strut	5
S-shaped with straight R-ASA	High septal deviation	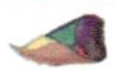	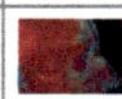	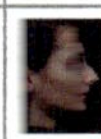	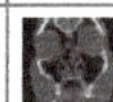	Ishida's technique	Yes	Dorsum (bone)	Cartilaginous dorsum	Severe S shaped dorsum with high or complex septal deviation	Swinging door	27

Hidden S- shape	High septal deviation		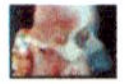	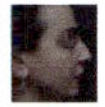	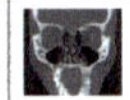	SPQR V2 with mosaic osteotomies	No	Dorsum (bone)	Cartilaginous dorsum	Slight S shape bony dorsum with high septal deviation	Swinging door	14
V-shaped dorsum with straight R-ASA	High septal deviation	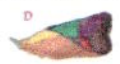	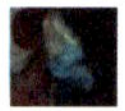	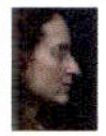	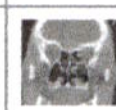	Low strip SPQR V2	Just tip and septum	In most of cases is not necessary to model any component of the dorsum if the bony dorsum is well formed	Dorsum-septal unit	V shape dorsum with high septal deviation	Swinging door	20
V shaped dorsum with straight R-ASA	Low septal deviation	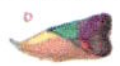	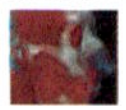	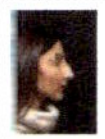	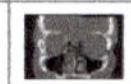	High strip (Saban)	Yes	Dorsal modifications if possible if necessary	Cartilaginous dorsum	V shape or shlight S shape dorsum with straight or low deviated septum	L strut	10

(continued)

Table 8.1 (continued)

Dorsal features	Septal features	Lateral view	3D imaging	Clinical case	CT coronal view	Surgical technique	Dorsal STE dissection	Molding	Preservation	Indication	Septal technique	%
Straight dorsum	Straight septum	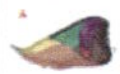	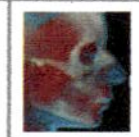	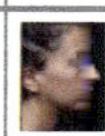	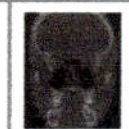	GOLA'	No	X	Whole dorsum and STE connection	Straight profile cases with straight or low deviated septum	L strut	4
Straight dorsum	High septal deviation	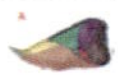	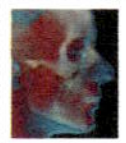	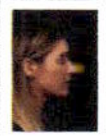	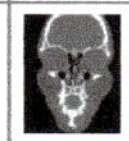	SPQR V2	No	X	Whole dorsum and STE connection	Straight profile cases with high or complex septal deviation	Swinging door	6
S shaped dorsum with curved RASA segment and long nasal bones	Low septal deviation	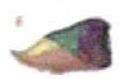	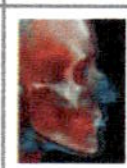	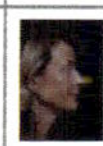	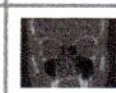	Spreader grafts	All	Total dorsal re-configuration	X	All the dorsum is curved on the profile. Therefore is better to reconstruct alle the vault instead of preserving	L strut or extracorporeal septoplasty	5

S shaped dorsum with curved RASA segment and short nasal bones	Low septal deviation	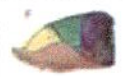	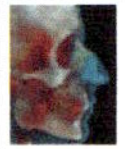	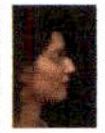	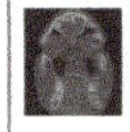	Spreader flaps	All	Total dorsal re-configuration	X	All the dorsum is curved on the profile. Therefore is better to reconstruct alle the vault instead of preserving	L strut or extracorporeal septoplasty	8

Note to add: All the types of noses described in the table have good dorsal aesthetic lines in frontal view. The scheme below analyzes this population only

8.6 Clinical Cases

Some clinical cases are shown, describing the decision-making algorithm.

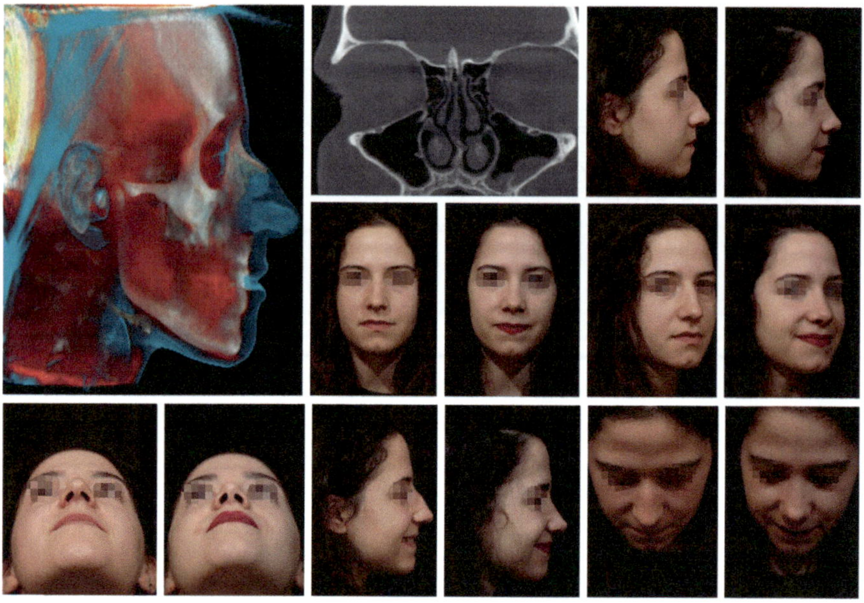

Clinical Case 8.1 S-shaped dorsum with straight R-ASA (Ferreira)—straight septum

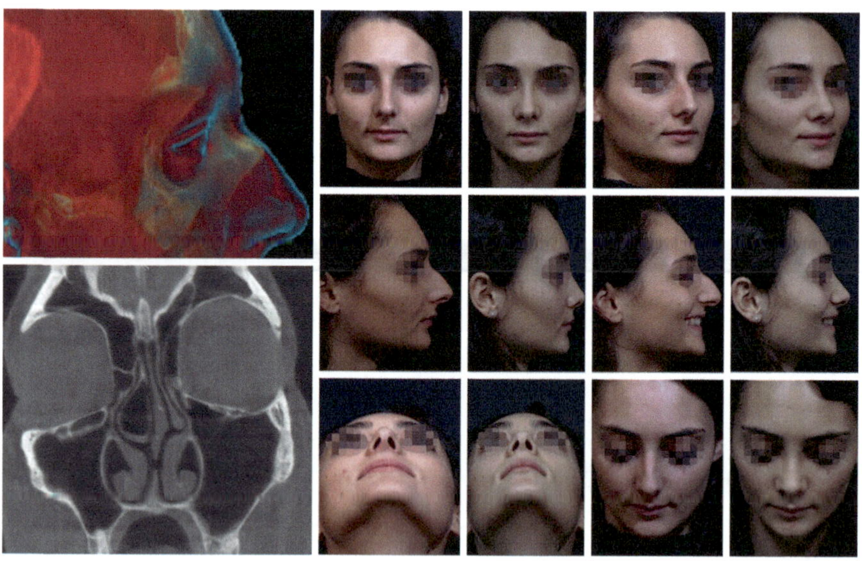

Clinical Case 8.2 S-shaped with straight R-ASA (Ishida)—high septal deviation

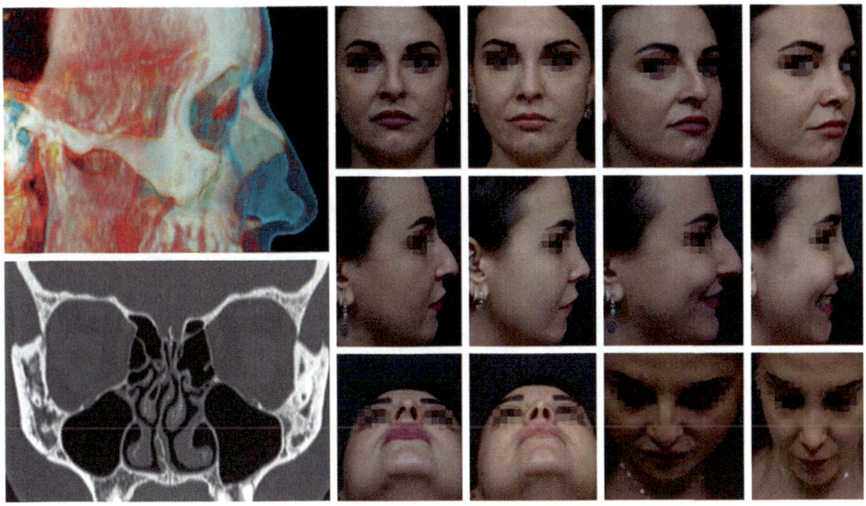

Clinical Case 8.3 Hidden S-shape (SPQR V2 with mosaic osteotomies)—high septal deviation

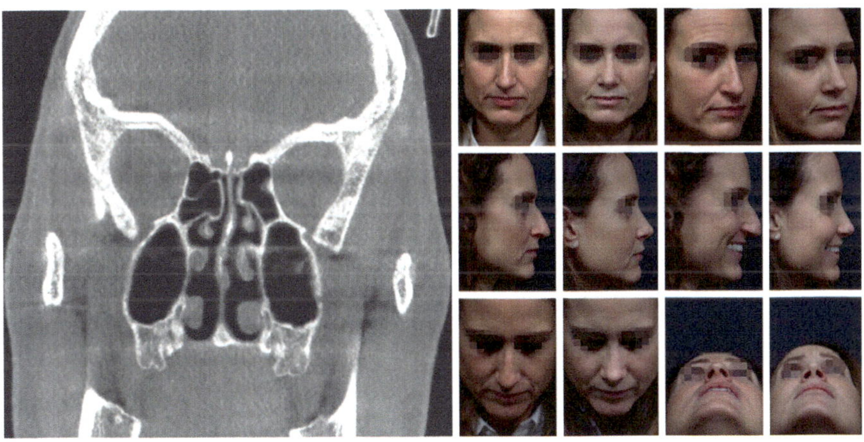

Clinical Case 8.4 V-shaped dorsum with straight R-ASA (low strip SPQR V2 ± mosaic)—high septal deviation

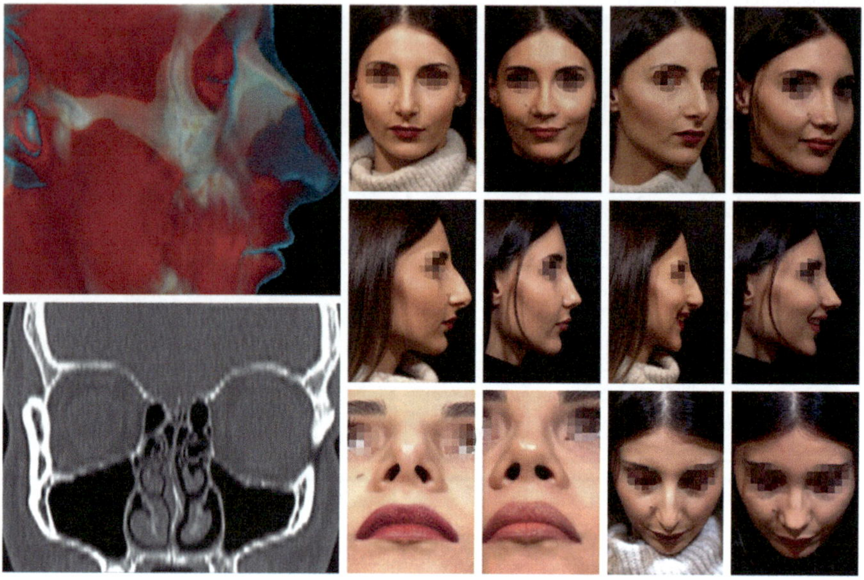

Clinical Case 8.5 V-shaped dorsum with straight R-ASA (Saban)—low septal deviation

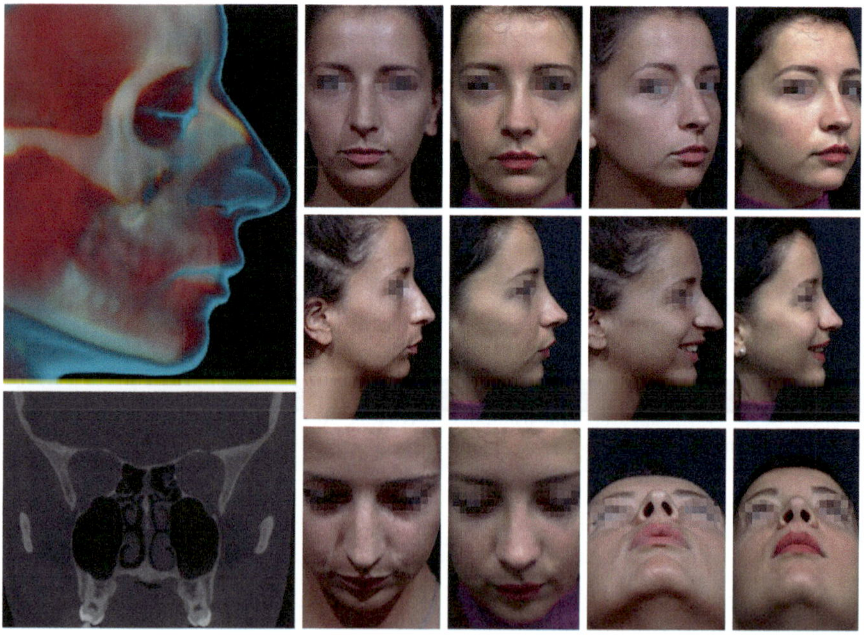

Clinical Case 8.6 Straight dorsum (Golà)

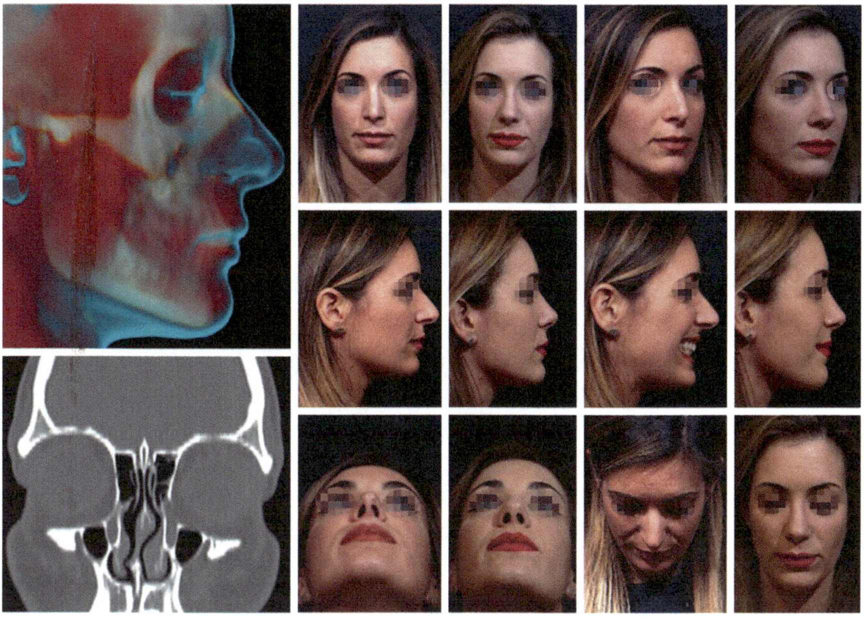

Clinical Case 8.7 Straight dorsum (SPQR V2)—high septal deviation

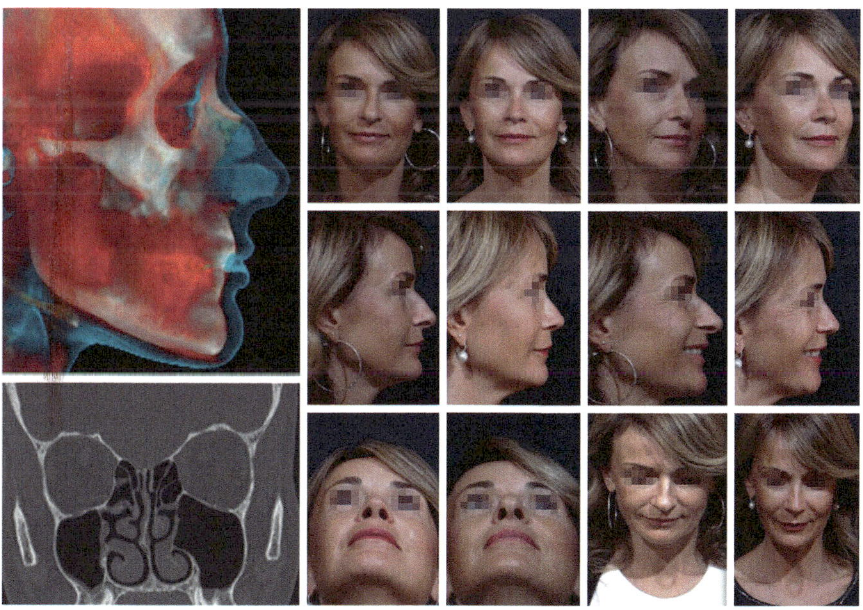

Clinical Case 8.8 S-shaped dorsum with curved R-ASA segment and long nasal bones (spreader graft)—low septal deviation

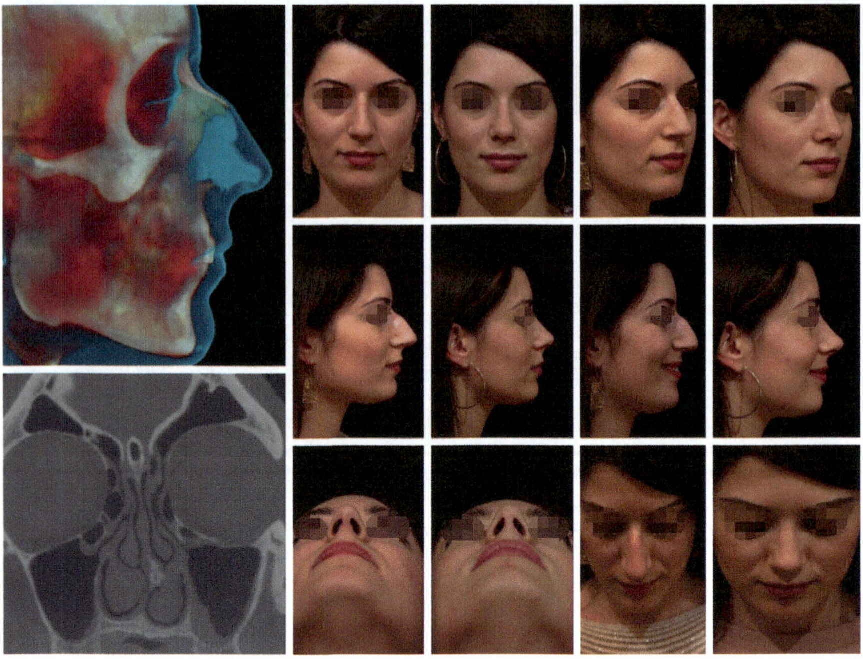

Clinical Case 8.9 S-shaped dorsum with curved R-ASA segment and short nasal bones (spreader flaps)—low septal deviation

8.7 Conclusions

The necessary and essential requirements for a correct rhinoplasty are the understanding of embryology, the analysis of the anatomical deformity, and the creation of a preoperative project based on the evaluation of the present deformity. The difficulty lies in being "multi-tasking"; our "brain computer" must be able to enter data, process them, and then combine all the concepts together to perform a technique that takes into account all the pieces of the puzzle and how each of these also affects the others (for example the septum has an influence on the tip support but also on the dorsal and tip asymmetries in frontal view).

References

1. Daniel RK. The preservation rhinoplasty: a new rhinoplasty revolution. Aesthet Surg J. 2018;38(2):228–9. https://doi.org/10.1093/asj/sjx258.
2. Killlan G, Foster EE. XXIII. The submucous window resection of the nasal septum. Ann Otol Rhinol Laryngol. 1905;14(2):363–93. https://doi.org/10.1177/000348940501400210.
3. Jankowski R, Márquez S. Embryology of the nose: the evo-devo concept. World J Otorhinolaryngol. 2016;6(2):33. https://doi.org/10.5319/wjo.v6.i2.33.

4. Varoquier M, Rumeau C, Vuissoz PA, Perez M, Hossu G, Jankowski R. Do the upper lateral nasal cartilages exist? The concept of septolateral cartilages. Eur Ann Otorhinolaryngol Head Neck Dis. 2021;138:77–81. https://doi.org/10.1016/j.anorl.2020.06.017.
5. Jankowski R. Septoplastie et Rhinoplastie Par Désarticulation. In: Elsevier Masson, editor. Elsevier Masson SAS; 2016.
6. Nicksic PJ, Pfaff MJ, Ayeroff JR, Lee JC. Management of the cleft nasal tip: an overview of classic techniques and strategies. Ann Plast Surg. 2018;80(5):581–6. https://doi.org/10.1097/SAP.0000000000001334.
7. Çakir B, Öreroğlu AR, Doğan T, Akan M. A complete subperichondrial dissection technique for rhinoplasty with management of the nasal ligaments. Aesthet Surg J. 2012;32(5):564–74. https://doi.org/10.1177/1090820X12445471.
8. Lazovic GD, Daniel RK, Janosevic LB, Kosanovic RM, Colic MM, Kosins AM. Rhinoplasty: the nasal bones—anatomy and analysis. Aesthet Surg J. 2015;35(3):255–63. https://doi.org/10.1093/asj/sju050.
9. Saban Y, Daniel RK, Polselli R, Trapasso M, Palhazi P. Dorsal preservation: the push down technique reassessed. Aesthet Surg J. 2018;38(2):117–31. https://doi.org/10.1093/asj/sjx180.
10. Finocchi V, Daniel RK, Palhazi P. Modified SPQR cottle rhinoplasty. In: Preservation rhinoplasty. 3rd ed. Istanbul: Septum; 2020. p. 256–81.
11. Ishida LC. Cartilage vault push down with optional bony cap preservation. In: Preservation rhinoplasty. Istanbul: Septum; 2020. p. 354–63.
12. Santos M, Rego ÂR, Coutinho M, e Sousa CA, Ferreira MG. Spare roof technique in reduction rhinoplasty: prospective study of the first one hundred patients. Laryngoscope. 2019;129(12):2702–6. https://doi.org/10.1002/lary.27804.
13. Palhazi P, Daniel RK, Kosins AM. The osseocartilaginous vault of the nose: anatomy and surgical observations. Aesthet Surg J. 2015;35(3):242–51. https://doi.org/10.1093/asj/sju079.
14. East C, Badia L, Saban Y. Cone beam CT analysis for dorsal preservation surgery. In: Preservation rhinoplasty. Istanbul: Septum; 2020. p. 44–55.
15. Daniel RK, Palhazi P. The nasal ligaments and tip support in rhinoplasty: an anatomical study. Aesthet Surg J. 2018;38(4):357–68. https://doi.org/10.1093/asj/sjx192.
16. Popko M, Verlinde-Schellekens SAMW, Huizing EH, Bleys RLAW. Functional anatomy of the nasal bones and adjacent structures. Consequences for nasal surgery. Rhinol J. 2018;56(1):89–95. https://doi.org/10.4193/Rhin17.189.
17. Natvig P, Sether LA, Gingrass RP, Gardner WD. Anatomical details of the osseous-cartilaginous framework of the nose. Plast Reconstr Surg. 1971;48(6):528–32. https://doi.org/10.1097/00006534-197112000-00002.
18. Craig JR, Bied A, Landas S, Suryadevara A. Anatomy of the upper lateral cartilage along the lateral pyriform aperture. Plast Reconstr Surg. 2015;135(2):406–11. https://doi.org/10.1097/PRS.0000000000000918.
19. Saban Y, Braccini F, Polselli R, Micheli-Pellegrini V. Rhinoplasty and narrow pyriform aperture. In: Rhinoplasties; the monographs of Cca group N°32. Paris: C.V. Mosby; 2002. p. 251–5.
20. Ferreira MG, Dias DR, Cardoso L, et al. Dorsal hump reduction based on the new ethmoidal point classification: a clinical and radiological study of the keystone area in 138 patients. Aesthet Surg J. 2020;40(9):950–9. https://doi.org/10.1093/asj/sjaa030.
21. Saban Y, De Salvador S, Polselli R. Revision following dorsal preservation rhinoplasties. In: Preservation rhinoplasty. 3rd ed. Istanbul: Septum; 2020. p. 404–29.
22. Çakir B, Öreroğlu AR, Daniel RK. Surface aesthetics and analysis. Clin Plast Surg. 2016;43(1):1–15. https://doi.org/10.1016/j.cps.2015.09.004.
23. Gola R, Nerini A, Laurent-Fyon C, Waller PY. [Conservative rhinoplasty of the nasal canopy]. Ann Chir Plast Esthet. 1989;34(6):465–475. http://www.ncbi.nlm.nih.gov/pubmed/2482688.
24. Ferreira MG, Monteiro D, Reis C, Sousa CAE. Spare roof technique: a middle third new technique. Facial Plast Surg. 2016;32(1):111–6. https://doi.org/10.1055/s-0035-1570503.
25. Wright WK. Principles of nasal septum reconstruction. Trans Am Acad Ophthalmol Otolaryngol. 1969;73(2):252–5. http://www.ncbi.nlm.nih.gov/pubmed/4890426.

26. Mattioli R. Surgery of the nasal tip: a personal approach. Facial Plast Surg. 1996;12(04):357–66. https://doi.org/10.1055/s-2008-1064506.
27. Finocchi V, Vellone V, Mattioli RG, Daniel RK. A 3-level impaction technique for dorsal reshaping and reduction without dorsal soft tissue envelope dissection. Aesthet Surg J. 2022;12;42(2):151–65. https://doi.org/10.1093/asj/sjab261. PMID: 34175938.
28. Ishida LC, Ishida J, Ishida LH, Tartare A, Fernandes RK, Gemperli R. Nasal hump treatment with cartilaginous push-down and preservation of the bony cap. Aesthet Surg J. 2020;40(11):1168–78. https://doi.org/10.1093/asj/sjaa061.
29. Ishida J, Ishida LHC, Ishida LHC, Vieira JC, Ferreira MC. Treatment of the nasal hump with preservation of the cartilaginous framework. Plast Reconstr Surg. 1999;103(6):1729–33; discussion 1734–5. http://www.ncbi.nlm.nih.gov/pubmed/10323714.
30. Finocchi V, Vellone V, Ramieri V, De Angelis F, Marianetti T. Pisa tower concept: a new paradigm in crooked nose treatment. Plast Reconstr Surg. 2021;148(1):66–70. (Epub Ahead of Print).

Northern Mediterranean Nose Correction: The Italian Experience: Tip Surgery

9

Marianetti Tito Matteo

9.1 Introduction

The North Mediterranean includes populations with extremely varied phenotypes. Its coasts include Spain, France, Italy, Slovenia, Croatia, Bosnia, Albania, Greece, and Turkey. Looking for a clear morphological correlation between the inhabitants of these nations is difficult. Even the comparison between the "Italian nose" and the "French nose," does not hold, although the two nations share a border and are lapped by the same sea. The term "Mediterranean race" was coined by William Z. Ripley [1] in "The Races of Europe," describing their main physical characteristics as having dark eyes and hair, an elongated face, narrow nose and dolichocephalic skull, slender build, and olive skin. Today it is more correct to speak of the Mediterranean civilization, in order to emphasize the cultural and historical unity of different peoples who have looked out over the Mediterranean Sea over the centuries and who formed the cradle of humanity. In regard to the Italian population, despite the fact that the Greek-Roman origin of Italian culture has certainly influenced aesthetic canons over the centuries, it is currently difficult to identify an aesthetic ideal of reference and a classic Italian nose. Even the stereotype of the face of southern Italy with features that are more markedly "Mediterranean" and those of northern Italy that are more "northern European" are gradually giving way to a mixture of somatic traits due to the continuous movement of people from North to South and vice versa throughout the peninsula since the last post-war period until today. The classic Italian patient who goes to a surgeon requesting a rhinoplasty procedure may now be blond, blue-eyed with a fair complexion and thin skin, or a brunette with dark eyes, olive complexion, and thick skin. The criterion of personalizing the surgical treatment and attempting to create the most suitable nose for the patient's face—by

M. T. Matteo (✉)
Assunzione di Maria Santissima Clinic, Rome, Italy

MarianettiMed Clinic, Avezzano, Italy

P. G. Giacomini (ed.), *Mediterranean Rhinoplasty*,
https://doi.org/10.1007/978-3-031-05551-5_9

taking their individual, somatic, and family characteristics into account—is the most important parameter when analyzing a face and planning surgery. "To change, without distorting," to obtain a natural result as if the patient had been born with that nose, to operate on the nose in such a way that no one can tell it has been "redone," and to avoid creating noses that are all the same: these should be our guidelines in planning and carrying out rhinoplasty surgery.

Our idea of beauty has always been influenced by art. It is therefore worth making a brief digression into the history of art to look at the evolution of the canons of beauty of the nose in Italy and the North Mediterranean. The common nose throughout the Mediterranean basin in the history of art has always featured a high dorsum and a normal/hypo-rotated tip. Fayum portraits, highly realistic funeral portraits from the Roman era of a mixed Greek/Egyptian population, feature typically Mediterranean aesthetic traits (Fig. 9.1). These paintings dating back to the first century A.D, together with the frescoes of Herculaneum and Pompeii, those of the "Tomb of the Diver" in Paestum and certain tomb representations in Verghina in Central Macedonia, are among the best preserved examples of painting of antiquity. The beauty ideal for men and women's faces and noses is provided by the synthesis of a series of picturesque and sculptural images that would be produced over the centuries. A male example of ideal beauty of the body and face that we find in the Mediterranean, which was actually recovered from the very same sea, is embodied by the "Bronzi di Riace," the Riace bronze statues, in particular Bronze "B," the younger one, whose nose is particularly realistic with a

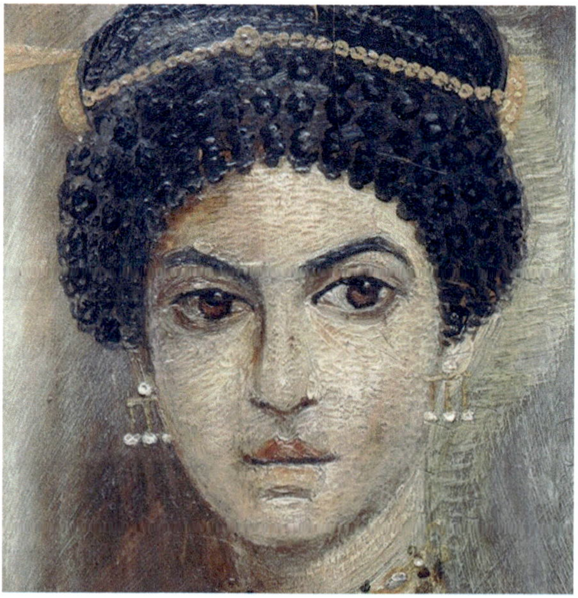

Fig. 9.1 Portrait of a woman (Mummy-portrait or Fayum portrait), detail, circa 110–130 AD, Edinburgh, National Museum of Scotland

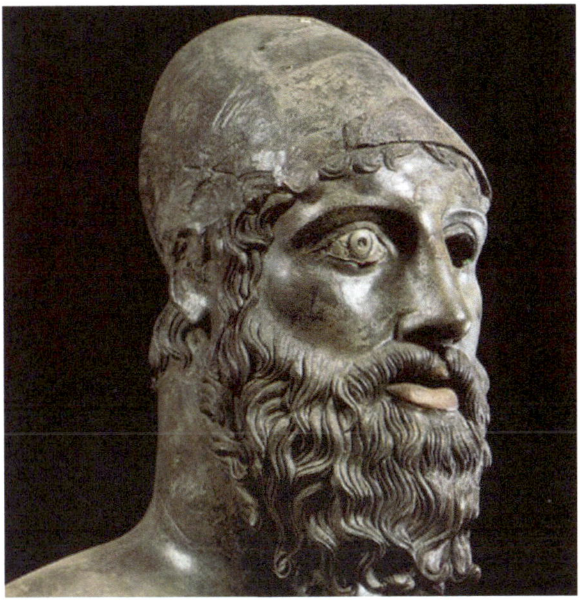

Fig. 9.2 Bronze of Riace Statue B: note the elegance and the strong, masculine profile of the typically Mediterranean nose. (National Archaeological Museum of Reggio Calabria)

high dorsum and a strong, chiseled profile (Fig. 9.2). The "Doryphoros" of Polykleitos (second century B.C) is an example of refinement and balance, which actually uses the head as the measure and "canon" for the entire body (Fig. 9.3). In the faces of "Apollo and Daphne" (1600) by Gian Lorenzo Bernini, we find an ideal of beauty for the nose that is more akin to our modern day aesthetic ideal. Apollo's nose is largely straight in profile with a thin and balanced tip; Daphne has a slightly more pronounced nose, yet also has a small, balanced tip (Fig. 9.4). The thin and elegant nose of "Paolina Borghese" (1804) by Canova is the protagonist of the sculpture that favors and focuses on the profile of the woman (Fig. 9.5). Canova is perhaps the artist who represented an ideal of the nose that is closest to our current ideal of beauty in his sculptures.

What has revolutionized the culture of contemporary beauty is the spread of images on modern media and on television, and the internet in particular. Today, we are continuously and literally bombarded on TV, social media, and in advertising of any form with images of models, singers, and influencers, who have disrupted the classic aesthetic canons at a speed hardly imaginable in the pre-internet era, thereby dictating the law. Thus, the Renaissance profile with its receding chin and delicate nose has gradually given way to maxillo-mandibular biprotrusion and straight noses, even in women, with stronger and more marked profiles. Thus, the classic "Mediterranean nose," i.e., an ethnic nose with a non-sagging dorsum, a defined, yet strong profile, an open, yet not obtuse nasolabial angle, and a nose-frontal region that is not overly deep, is back not only as suitable for an "ethnicity," but as a predominant modern-day aesthetic ideal.

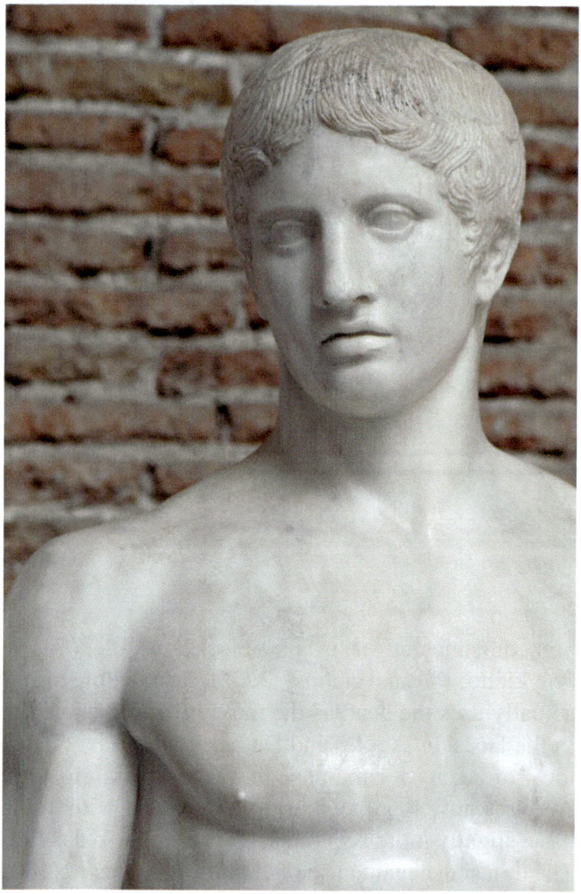

Fig. 9.3 Detail of the face of the statue "The Doryphoros" by Polykleitos, from the second century B.C, kept at the National Archaeological Museum of Naples

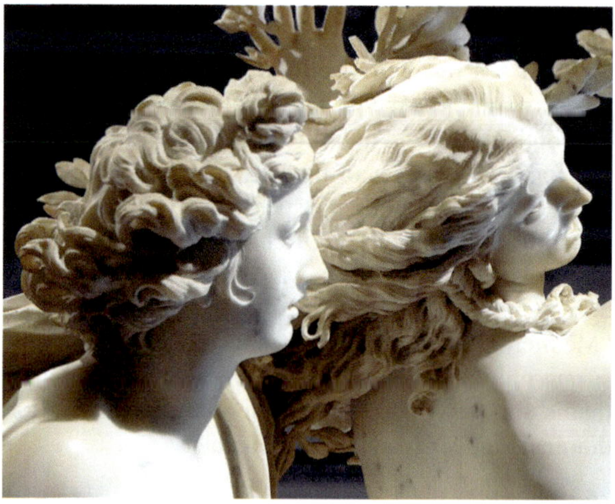

Fig. 9.4 Detail of the nose of Apollo and Daphne in "Apollo and Daphne," a sculpture created by the famous artist Gian Lorenzo Bernini between 1622 and 1625 and exhibited in the Galleria Borghese in Rome

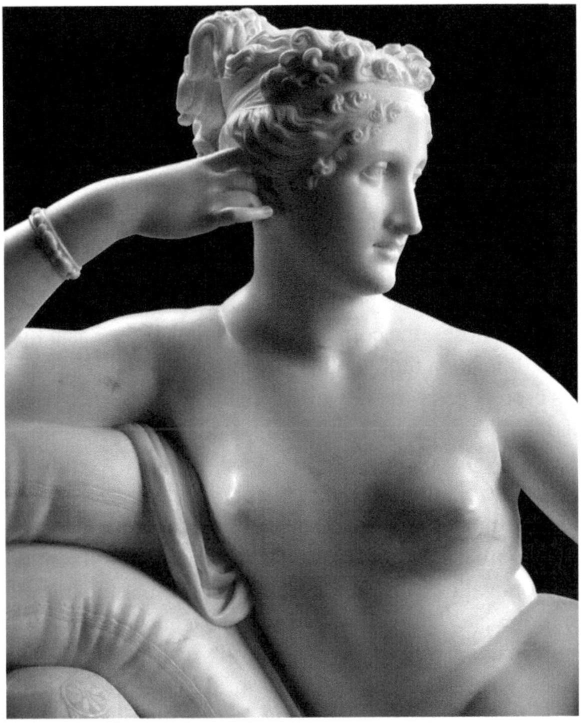

Fig. 9.5 Detail of the bust of "Paolina Borghese," a neoclassical sculpture from 1804 to 1808, made by Antonio Canova and preserved in the Galleria Borgese in Rome

9.2 Nasal Tip Assessment and Classification

Before proceeding with any surgical procedure, and especially in the case of rhinoplasty, a preoperative assessment is essential. The nasal tip can present various dysmorphisms in the case of a nose that has never been operated on, and an extremely wide range of deformities in the case of a revision rhinoplasty. Defects of the nasal tip can be grouped into several macro-areas:

1. Deviation from the midline
2. Projection alterations (overprojected or underprojected tip)
3. Rotational alterations (overrotated or underrotated tip)
4. Volume alterations (globular or excessively narrow tip)
5. Malposition or malformation of the lateral crura.

Although all combinations of the above malformations may be present in the North Mediterranean nose, the most frequent are underprojection combined with under-rotation of the tip, globularity, and cephalic malposition of the lateral crura [2, 3].

9.3 Deviation of the Nasal Tip: How to Correct It

Most of the studies in the literature focus on the correction of the deviation of the middle third and upper third of the nose [4–6]. Several osteotomy techniques have been proposed for treating the upper third of the nose and many surgical techniques, now in daily use, have been described for the treatment of middle third deviations. These include spreader grafts [7], spreader flaps [8], crossbar grafts [9], and extracorporeal septoplasty [10]. However, there are not many scientific papers in the national and international literature that focus on deviations of the lower third of the nose, except for those describing caudal septum correction [11, 12]. Yet, in the treatment of crooked noses, the correct repositioning of the nasal tip plays an extremely important role. It is often thought that if you correct the nasal septum, the tip will also return to its correct position; however, common experience demonstrates that correcting considerable asymmetries of the tip is not so simple. Sometimes as surgeons, we attempt to justify ourselves when faced with residual asymmetries of the tip and excuse ourselves by blaming cartilage memory and the sub-optimal management of the postoperative practices the patient was prescribed, such as massages or pressure to be applied to the nose; however, sometimes the problem is caused by a failure to correct anatomical defects. We must not forget that the nasal tip is made up of the medial, middle, and lateral crura of the alar cartilages, ligaments, SMAS, and skin. If the nose has developed asymmetrically, we must consider that the alar cartilages, the SMAS, the skin, and the width of the nostrils will also be asymmetrical, greater in length, width or thickness on one side, and lesser on the other. In this case, repositioning alone is not enough, but rather the conformation of these structures must be modified to achieve proper symmetrization of the nasal tip. The structural component most often altered in cases of nasal tip deviation is the lateral crus, which is generally more developed longitudinally on the side opposite the deviation. After repositioning the nasal septum on the nasal axis, it then becomes essential to shorten the longer crus with unilateral interruptive techniques. The dome truncation or lateral crural overlay techniques can be used, as described respectively in 1990 and 1991 by the same author, RW Kridel [13, 14], and then subsequently by many other authors [15–20]. They are usually performed bilaterally in order to define the projection and rotation of the nasal tip and are particularly useful when you want to reduce nasal tip projection. Their unilateral application, on the other hand, is crucial for correcting nasal tip deviation, thereby allowing the length of the hyperplasic alar cartilage to be reduced. If the intention is to shorten the alar cartilage anteriorly, monolateral dome truncation should be performed; while if the intention is to shorten the alar cartilage posteriorly, the monolateral crural overlay technique can be performed with the same rationale. Depending on the surgeon's preference, the nasal tip can be supported by a SEG (septal extension graft), by a columellar strut graft or even by the medial crura alone in the rare cases in which they are strong enough to support themselves without the help of a graft. Once the nasolabial angle has been re-established and the medial crura have been placed in the correct position, having sutured them to the septal extension graft or to the columellar strut graft, we then define the shape of the domes and the lateral crura. The goal is to shorten the longer cartilage. If we opt to use the monolateral crural overlay technique, the surgical procedure is as follows: at the border between the middle and posterior thirds of the lateral crus, the vestibular mucosa is disconnected without injury for an extension equal to the length of the segments to be overlapped. The cartilage is then interrupted at full thickness and the two segments are overlapped. The extent of the overlap is clinically assessed in the operating room, but is usually equal to the difference in length of the shorter contralateral lateral crus. The overlapping segments are sutured with a two-point polydioxanone (PDS) 5.0 in the cephalic and caudal portions of the overlapping cartilage. When suturing, we can also change the orientation of the lateral crus, which is often different to the contralateral, making it symmetrical with the other. Another method to shorten the long lateral crus is to use monolateral dome truncation. First, the dome prominence of the long lateral crus is accentuated using a lateral crural steal technique. In this intraoperative phase, a symmetrical tip can be appreciated in the posterior portion of the alae, yet is absolutely asymmetrical anteriorly, with the dome of the long side much higher than the contralateral one. We then proceed with the section of the dome of the hyperplasic side, after also having freed the vestibular mucosa underlying the domal cartilage. The amount to be resected is clinically evaluated, and it is recommended that you proceed in small steps, gradually removing the cartilage to avoid removing too much. When the right excision has been achieved, the medial and lateral crus, previously separated by the dome truncation, are sutured with two "figure-of-8" PDS 6.0 sutures, paying attention to reconstruct a shape that is as similar and symmetrical as possible to the contralateral dome.

Once a correct and satisfactory nasal osseocartilaginous scaffold has been obtained, the soft tissues must be considered, which should also not be underestimated if proper symmetrization is to be achieved. In this regard, the three areas to focus on predominately are the site of previous caudal deviation of the septum, the vestibular lining mucosa of the longer side, and the width of the nostrils. Proceeding in order, when the caudal septum is extremely deviated on one side, it will have expanded the skin over the deviation period (in most cases for many years) and there will certainly be more subcutaneous and cutaneous tissue on that side than on the contralateral side, where the eversion determined by the septum is not present. It is therefore important to remove the excess skin and subcutis in this region with a simple lozenge-shaped excision to avoid subsequent residual swelling of the region that could require a small revision and reduce patient satisfaction. The second area where the mucosa may be overextended following median repositioning of the nasal tip is the vestibular region below the longer alar cartilage. Again, excision of an appropriate amount of mucosa is necessary to avoid subsequent thickening in the region of the marginal incision on that side, which could also result in obstruction issues and breathing difficulties. It is essential not to exaggerate with excision because you risk retracting the nasal alae. Finally, particular attention must be paid to dealing with the shape of the nostrils. As the tip moves toward the midline, the shape of the nostril changes. The change is not always the same and cannot always be controlled in the same way; however, what happens most frequently is a lateral widening of the nostril on the long side (contralateral to the deviation); before the deviation was corrected, the nostril appeared elongated in the direction of the deviation and, after correction, it becomes wide and round. In this case, the nostril must be reshaped with a unilateral Weir resection, making the shape as symmetrical with the contralateral nostril as possible. It is advisable to proceed in small steps when excising the skin and subcutaneous wedge at the base of the wider nostril because it is easy to remove too much. Even small excisions in this area produce significant changes in the nostril contour. Figures 9.6, 9.7, 9.8, and 9.9 show two clinical cases

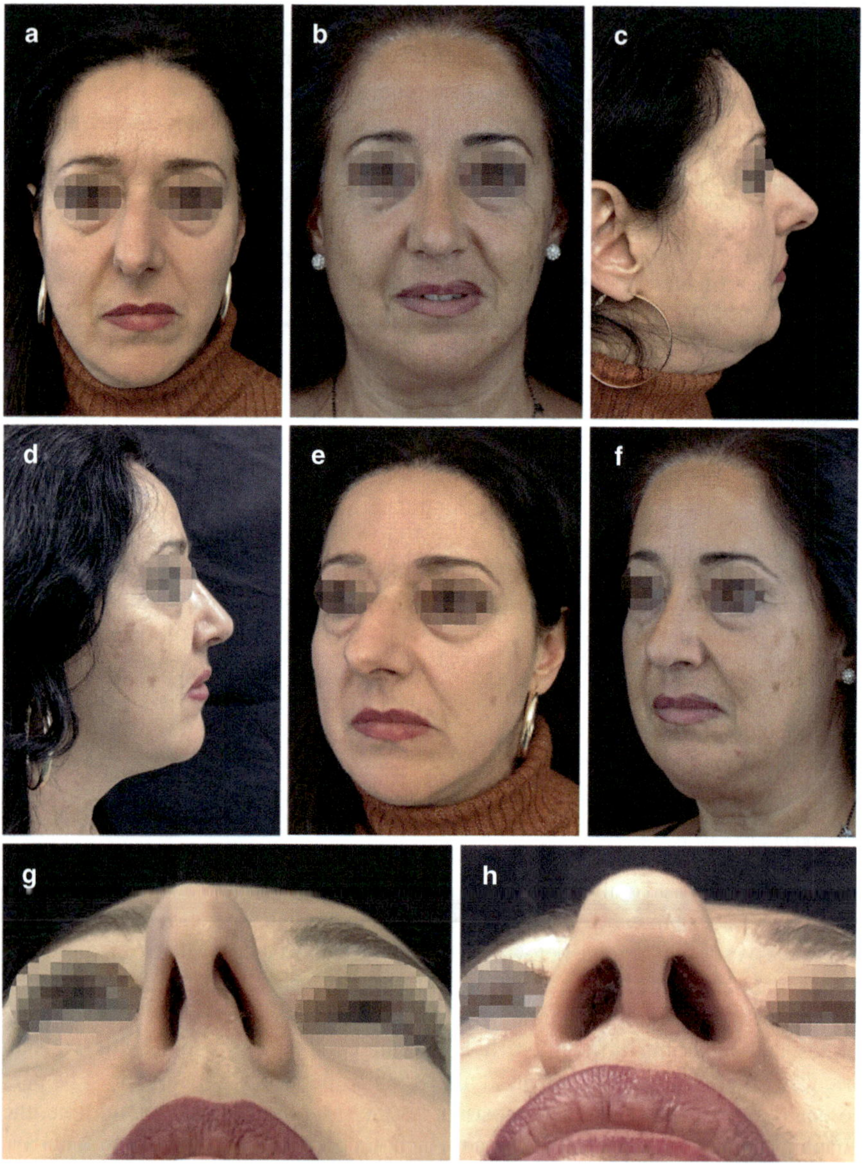

Fig. 9.6 Woman with severe nasal tip deviation. (**a**, **c**, **e**, **g**, **i**, **k**) Preoperative images. (**b**, **d**, **f**, **h**, **j**, **l**) corresponding post-op images. In this clinical case, the nasal pyramid was repositioned in axis using the Tower Pisa technique, septoplasty, removal of the anterior nasal spine, reconstruction of the caudal septum by septal extension graft, and asymmetrical shortening of the lateral crura to obtain deprojection associated with median tip repositioning

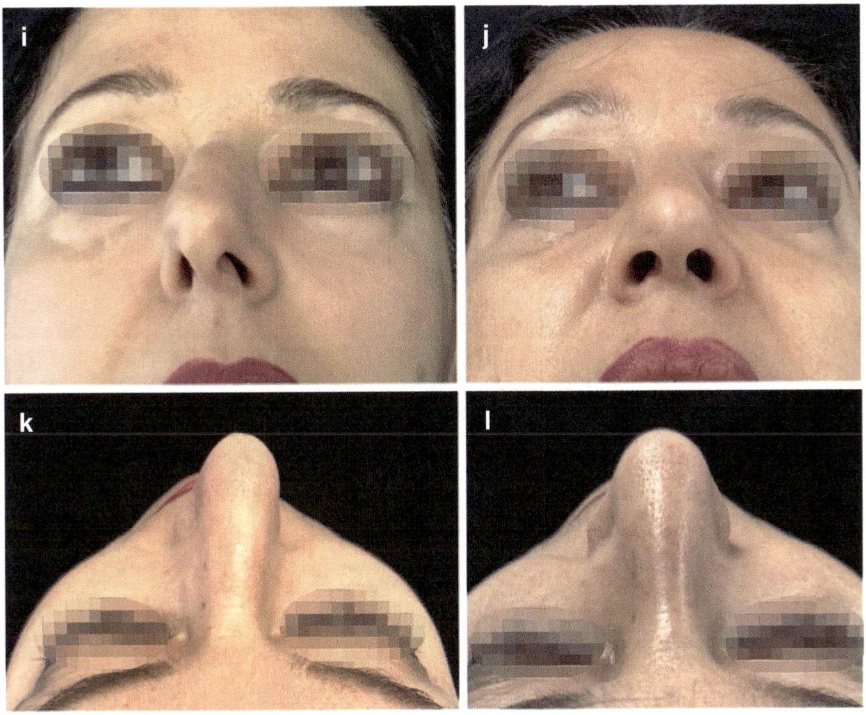

Fig. 9.6 (continued)

with their relative intraoperative photos illustrating the techniques described in this section.

9.4 Tip Rotation and Support

In the Mediterranean nose, a lack of nasal tip support is often present, resulting in the aquiline appearance of the tip, as well as a respiratory deficit at times. Although the not overly rotated tip and the acute nasolabial angle are ethnic characteristics of the Mediterranean nose, most patients who come to surgeons for corrective rhinoplasty request precisely the resolution of the ptosis of the tip. During the appointment, it is crucial to carry out a lateral previsualization to understand the real needs and expectations of the patient, as well as emphasize your vision and philosophy during this communication phase. The rotation of the nasal tip is what can most enhance the result in profile, but what can also make it appear most unnatural. The rotation of the nasal tip is well determined by the nasolabial angle that in the "Mediterranean nose" can range between 95 and 105° in women and between 90 and 95 in men. Extreme caution must be exercised in finding the right nasolabial angle, avoiding excesses, but ensuring the problem is resolved for the patient.

In addition, the support that must be guaranteed to the nasal tip must be stable over time to avoid ptosis of the tip forming and patient dissatisfaction a few months

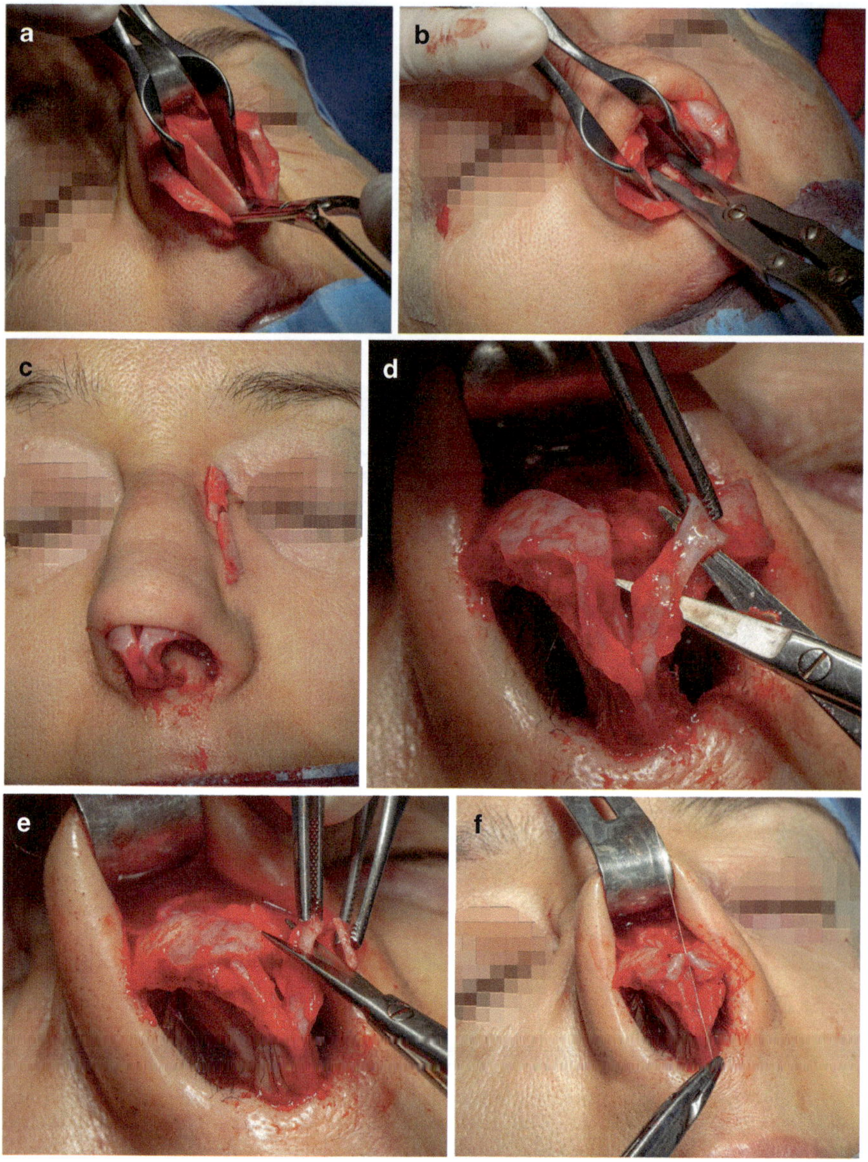

Fig. 9.7 Intraoperative images of the patient shown in Fig. 9.6. (**a**) Removal of the caudal portion of the deviated nasal septum; (**b**) Removal of the deviated anterior nasal spine; (**c**) Removal of a bone wedge at the level of the upright branch of the left maxilla to obtain a straightening of the bone pyramid using the Tower Pisa technique; (**d**) Detachment of the left intermediate and lateral crus; (**e**) Section of a portion of the left intermediate and lateral crus in order to shorten the longer lateral crus. The same section was performed, but to a lesser extent on the right also to deproject the tip. (**f**) Interdomal suture and final appearance of the tip

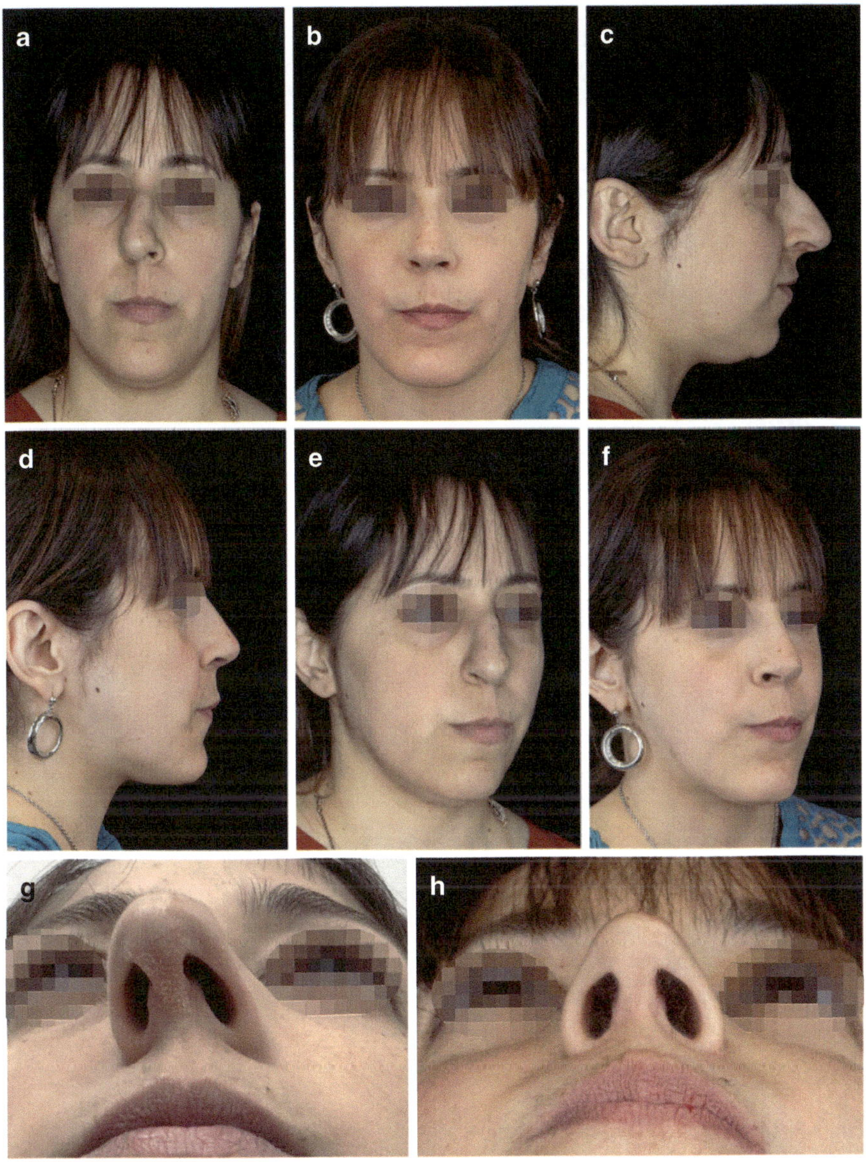

Fig. 9.8 Patient with severe nasal tip and nasal pyramid deviation. (**a**, **c**, **e**, **g**) Preoperative images. (**b**, **d**, **f**, **h**) corresponding post-op images. In this clinical case, the nasal pyramid was repositioned on axis using the Tower Pisa technique. The tip and middle third were straightened using a modified extracorporeal septoplasty, left spreader graft, asymmetric lateral crural steal, and left lateral crus section to achieve median tip repositioning

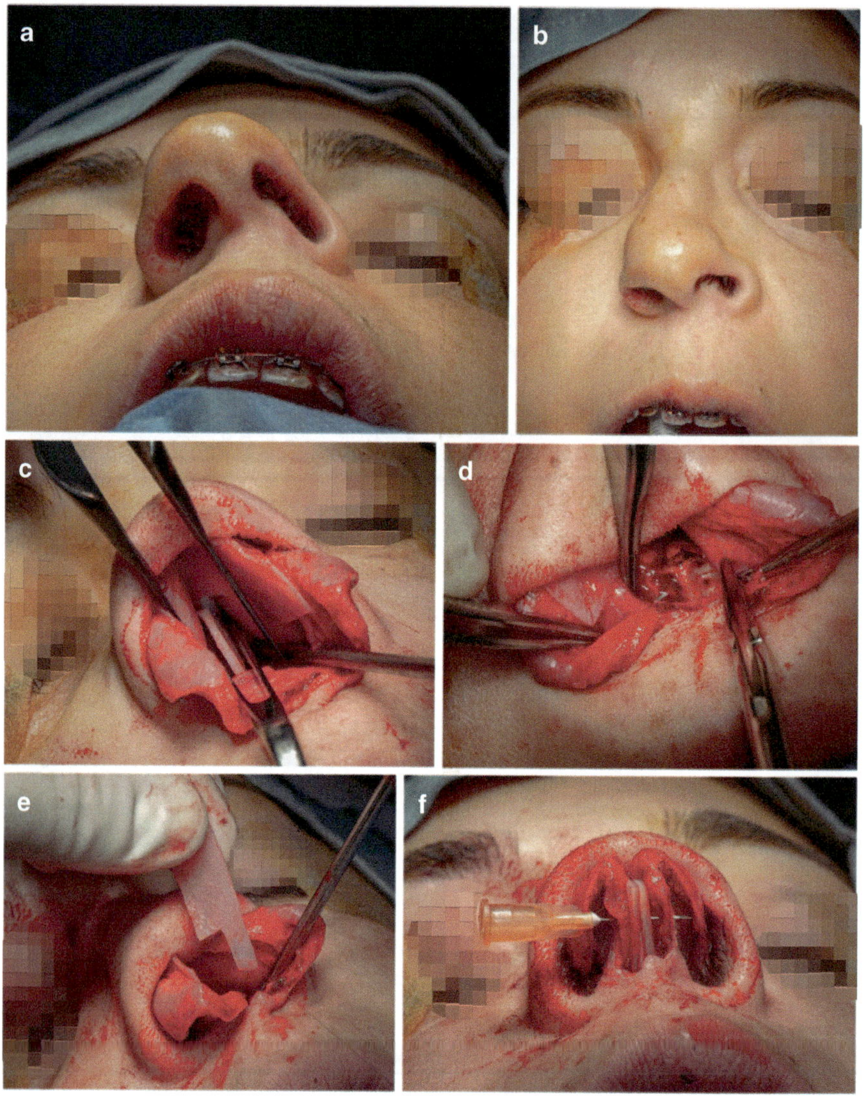

Fig. 9.9 Intraoperative images of the patient shown in Fig. 9.8. (**a**, **b**) Basal and mid-basal view of the severe deviation of the nasal tip; (**c**) Excision of the severe deviation of the nasal septum; (**d**) Fixation of the caudal pillar of the septum to the anterior nasal spine through a hole drilled on the spine; (**e**) Reconstruction of the caudal pillar of the septum; (**f**) Anchorage of the medial crura on the neoseptum; (**g**) Resection of the excess cephalic portion of the left lateral crus; (**h**) Resection of the excess cephalic portion of the left lateral crus; (**i**) Very lateralized left lateral crural steal in order to obtain traction on the tip toward the left; (**j**) Right lateral crural steal; (**k**) Desired asymmetry in the lateral crural steal between the two sides; (**l**) Detachment and section of the excess left medial/lateral crus. Subsequent suturing of the interrupted segments and interdomal suture results in tip symmetrization

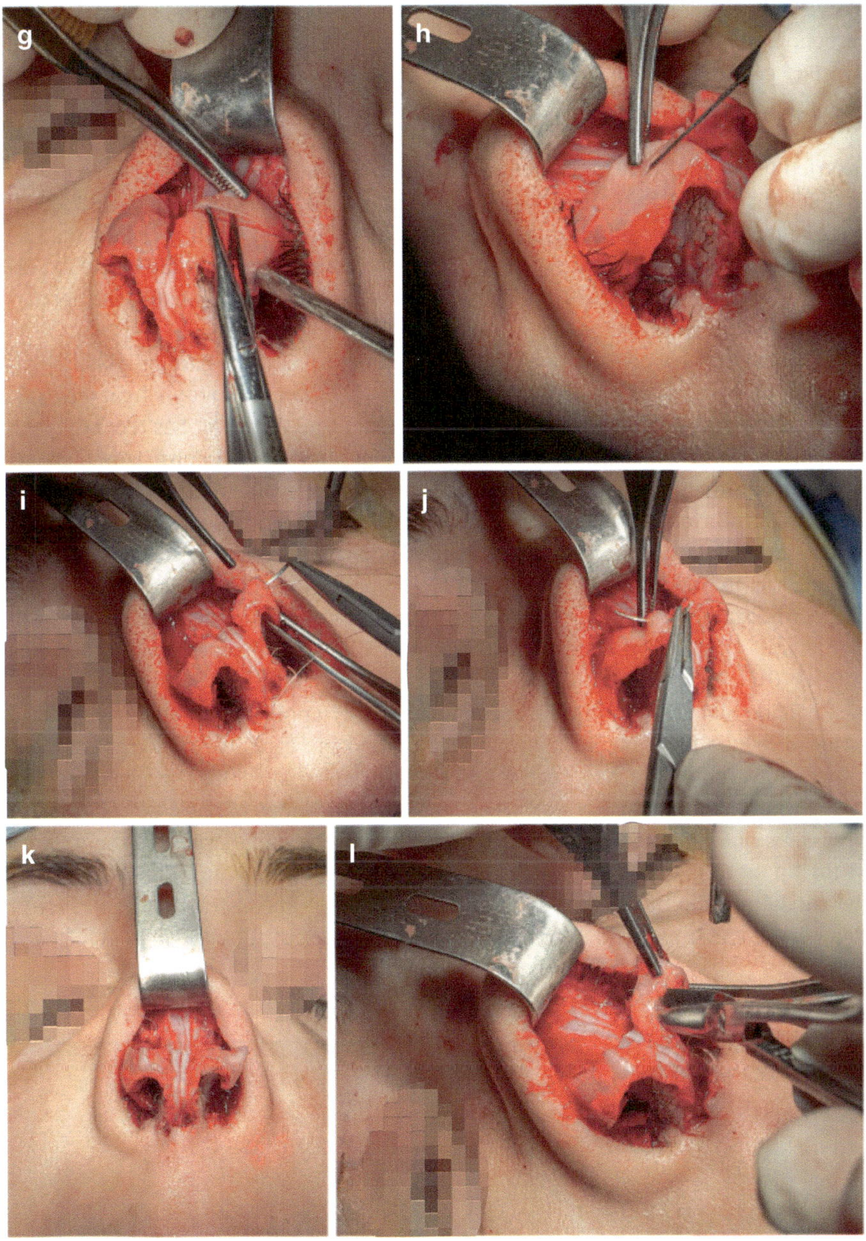

Fig. 9.9 (continued)

after surgery. Surgical techniques for rotating the nasal tip include caudal septal resection, Pitanguy's ligament shortening, cephalic alar resection, lateral crural overlay, columellar strut graft, the tongue-in-groove technique, and septal extension graft.

Caudal septal resection is a surgical technique that consists in removing an inverted triangle of the caudal and anterior portions of the septum, taking care not to touch the basal portion, which plays a structural role. This technique is effective, but requires proper healing for the stabilization of the nasal tip. It is crucial that we avoid removing too much of the caudal septum because the tip could rotate excessively or lose support and, after a few months, become ptotic and cause the appearance of a cartilaginous supratip.

Tip elevation by reworking Pitanguy's ligament has been particularly emphasized by proponents of preservation rhinoplasty [21, 22]. Pitanguy's ligament, initially described by Pitanguy [21] and considered a true ligament, has recently been reevaluated and considered an extension of the nasal SMAS. It consists of a superficial portion that passes superiorly to the interdomal ligament and a deep portion that passes inferiorly to it and continues with the nasal septal depressor muscle. Its preservation or sectioning and repositioning or disconnection is considered by some surgeons as an important mechanism for nasal tip support. Although, surgeons using it describe stable long-term results with this method, for surgeons accustomed to "structural" thinking, it becomes difficult to apply these ligament-based concepts (Fig. 9.10).

Cephalic alar resection is a procedure frequently applied in rhinoplasty, both in order to reduce the globular nature of the tip and increase its rotation. This technique is favored by the scar contraction resulting from the empty space created by the excision. It can be performed when small modifications of nasal tip rotation are necessary, but it is a technique aimed at modifying the globularity and the volume of the tip more than its rotation. If carried out along with a controlled resection of the caudal portion of the triangular cartilages and the reconstruction of the scroll ligament, it can offer valid, stable results over time (Fig. 9.11).

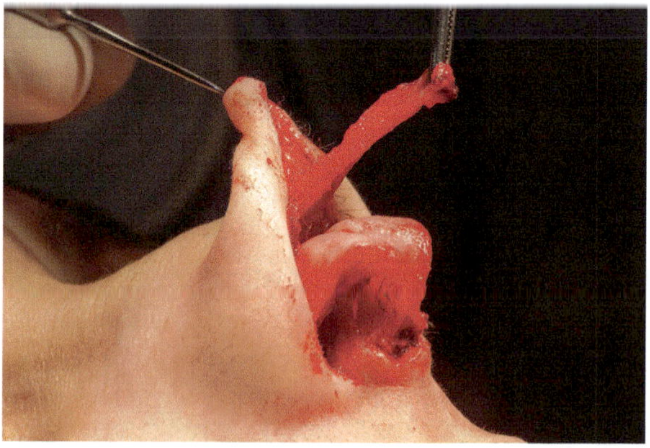

Fig. 9.10 Intraoperative image showing Pitanguy's ligament

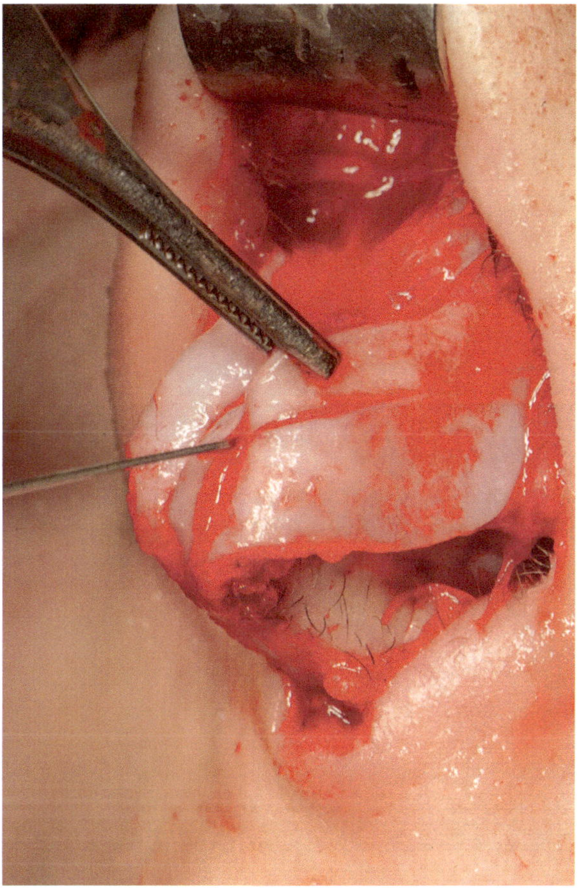

Fig. 9.11 Intraoperative view of cephalic resection of lateral crura

The lateral crura overlay is an extremely effective technique for nasal tip rotation, best indicated when there is also a hyperprojection of the tip [14]. This technique is performed by detaching the vestibular skin inferior to the lateral crura and cutting the latter at the border between the middle and posterior thirds. The two segments are then sutured with PDS 5.0. By restoring proper lateral crus length, this maneuver simultaneously causes significant tip rotation with reduced projection. As a side effect, there may be associated reduced definition of the domes region and widening of the alar base, which will need to be corrected accordingly (Fig. 9.12a–d).

The columellar strut is one of the most widely used grafts in both closed and open rhinoplasty [23, 24]. It provides support to the tip in proportion to the length, thickness, and consistency of the strut. It is inserted between the medial crura and anchored to them with transfixed or direct stitches. It can be attached to the anterior nasal spine, but is usually placed in a pocket between the base of the medial crura and the prespinal region. The problem that the columellar strut can sometimes present is a displacement of it in the caudal region, caused by the weight of thick skin or the excessive tension exerted on it, and this can sometimes result in the torsion of

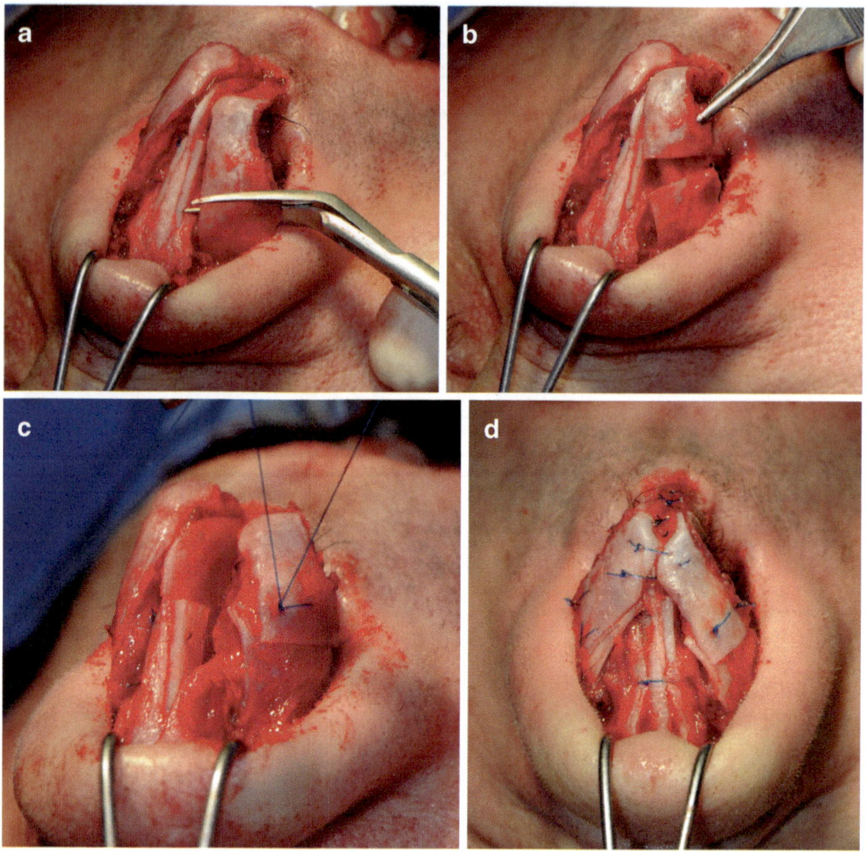

Fig. 9.12 Lateral crural overlay. (**a**) Lateral crus section bordering middle third and posterior third; (**b**) Lateral crus sectioned; (**c**) Lateral crus overlay and suture; (**d**) Lateral crural overlay performed bilaterally

the entire tip creating a deviated tip (Fig. 9.13). In the case of severe ptosis of the nasal tip, the most effective techniques to solve the problem are the tongue-in-groove technique and the septal extension graft [18, 25]. The tongue-in-groove technique consists in advancing the medial crura to the desired position on the caudal septum (Fig. 9.14). It is performed by detaching the caudal septum and separating the intercrural tissue until the medial crura are completely free. After regularizing the shape of the caudal septum to obtain a correct nasolabial angle, we proceed to stabilize the medial crura on the caudal septum using PDS 5.0 sutures. This technique allows to precisely adjust the projection and rotation of the tip with extremely high stability over time. It can be used to both project and deproject the tip, and to both increase and decrease rotation. However, it can only be done if the caudal septum is well represented and is on the midline. In the case of caudal septum deviation, the latter must be corrected first, otherwise the whole tip would follow the deviation of the septum. The downside of this technique is the tip stiffness it causes.

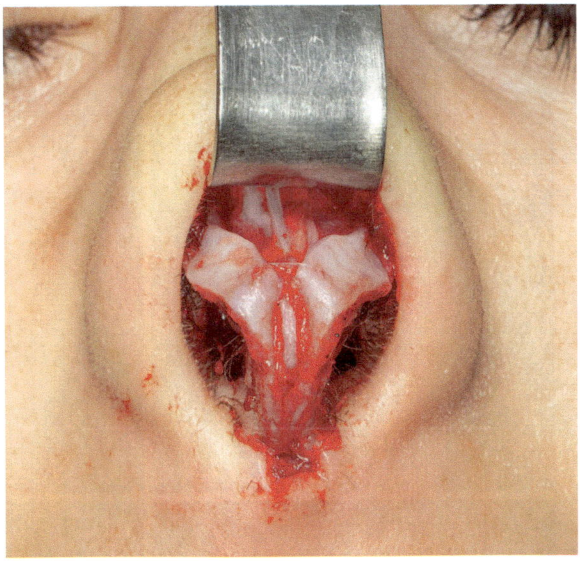

Fig. 9.13 Columellar strut inserted to support medial crura

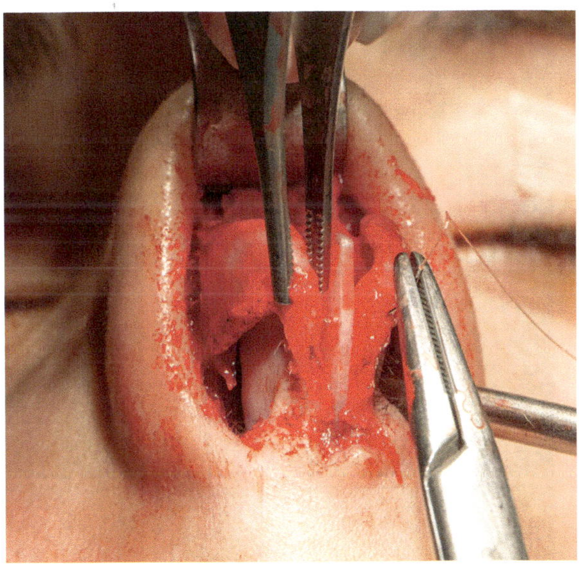

Fig. 9.14 Example intraoperative image of tongue-in-groove technique

However, this aspect is not considered a big problem by patients, who often willingly tolerate a certain stiffness of the nasal tip in exchange for a stable and defined result over time. Figures 9.15 and 9.16 show a clinical case in which support and rotation of the tip is provided by the tongue-in-groove technique.

The same concepts of the tongue-in-groove technique can be applied to the septal extension graft. In fact, the caudal septum does not always have the right length to be exploited with the tongue-in-groove technique. It is then possible to "extend"

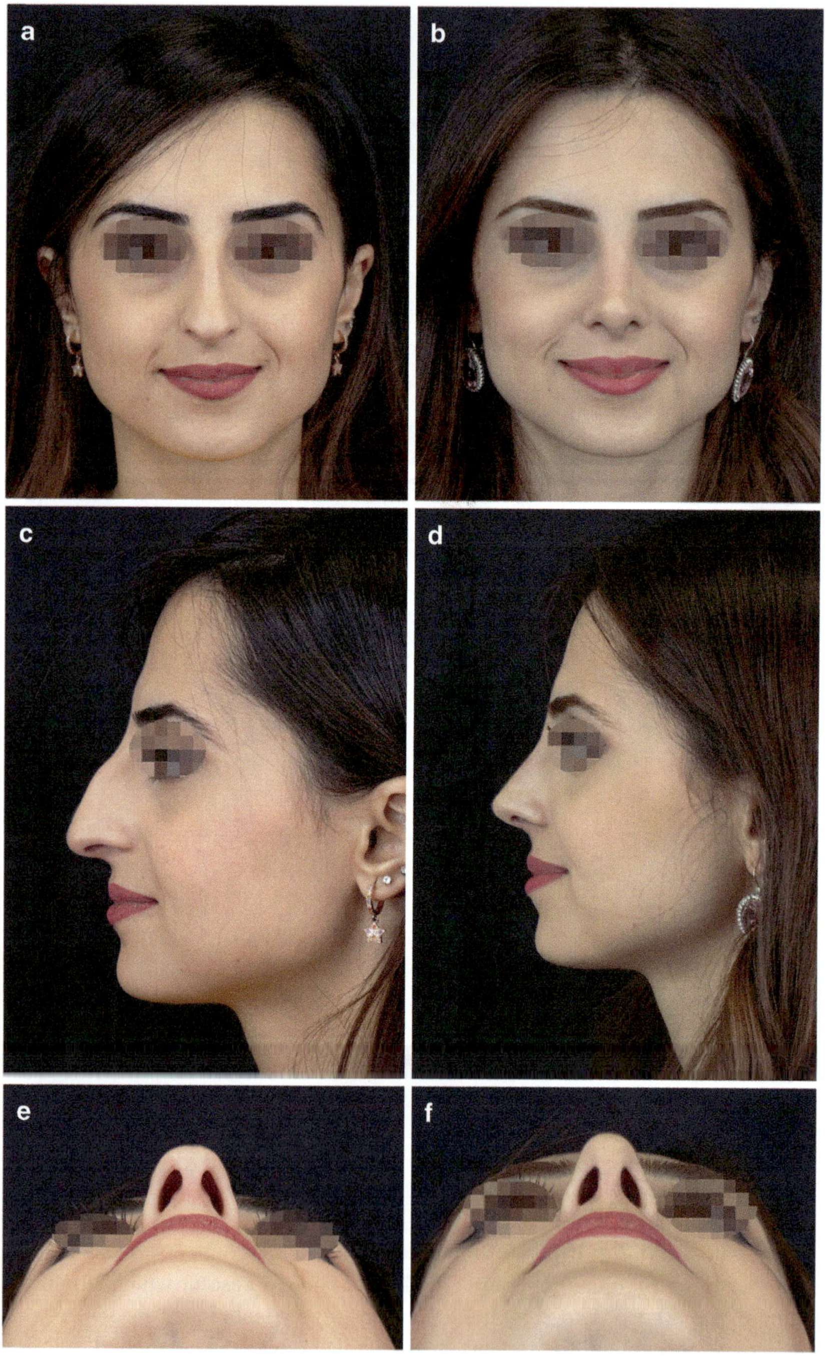

Fig. 9.15 Patient with a Mediterranean nose suffering from ptosis of the nasal tip combined with slight globularity. (**a**, **c**, **e**) Preoperative images; (**b**, **d**, **f**) corresponding post-op images

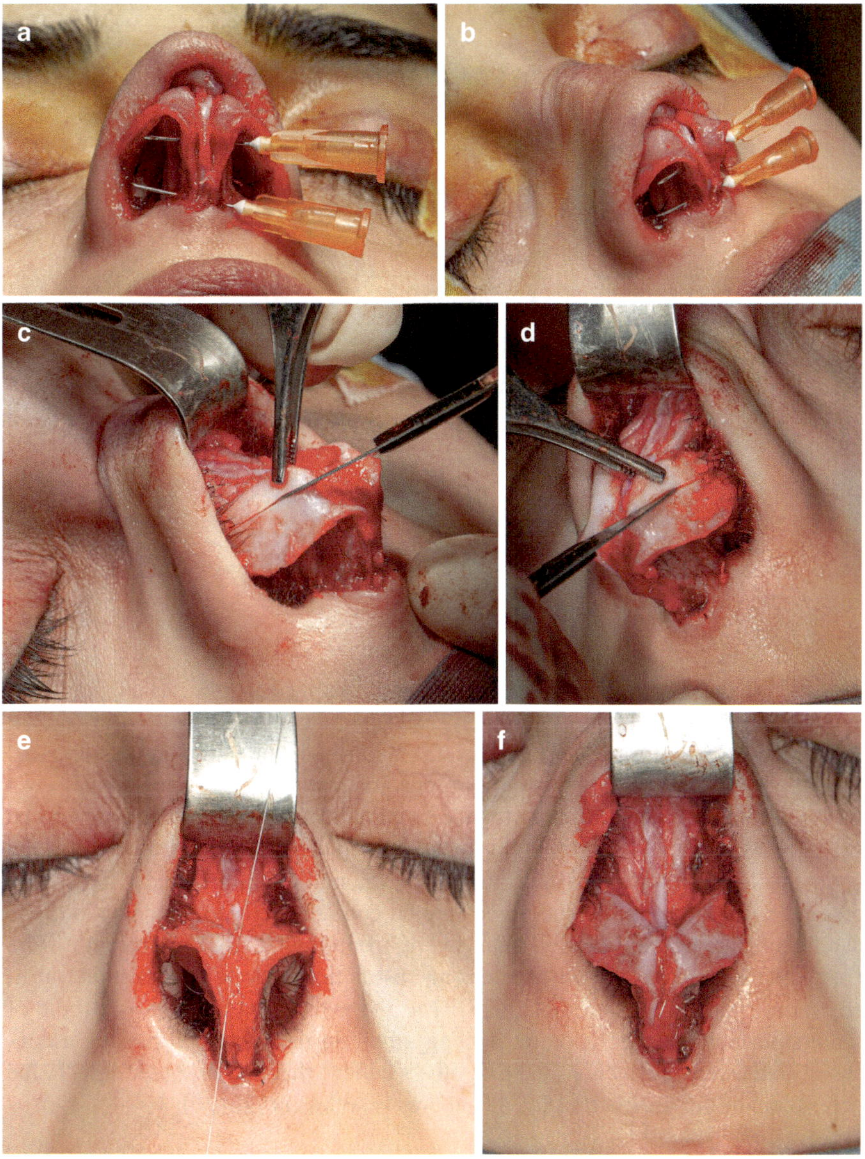

Fig. 9.16 Intraoperative images of the clinical case shown in Fig. 9.15. (**a**) Tongue-in-groove technique shown in axial view; (**b**) Tongue-in-groove technique shown in lateral view; (**c**) Right lateral crus cephalic resection; (**d**) Left lateral crus cephalic resection; (**e**) Interdomal suture; (**f**) Final intraoperative appearance of nasal tip

the septum with a graft taken from the intermediate portion of the septum itself (Fig. 9.17). This graft was first described by Byrd et al. in 1997 [25] and its ability to obtain precise control of rotation, projection, and definition of the nasal tip was emphasized even in the original publication. The two problems related to the use of

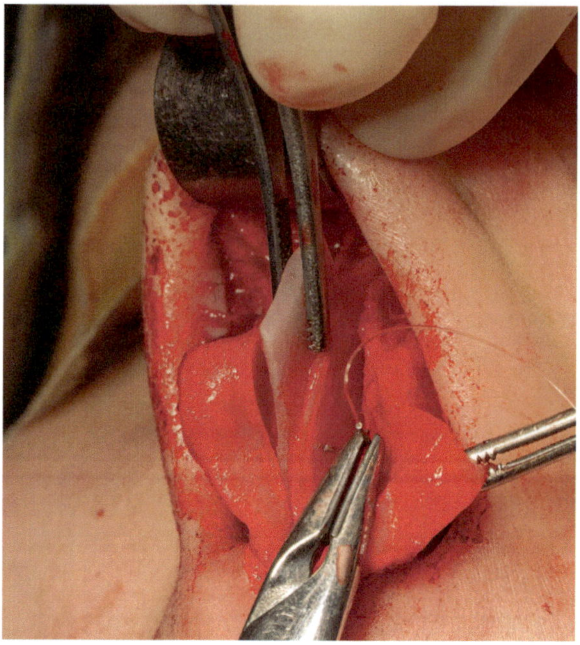

Fig. 9.17 Intraoperative image showing septal extension graft placement

the SEG are the need for a significant amount of cartilage and the nasal tip stiffness it causes. Fixation of the graft to the original septum can be either "end-to-end" or "side-to-side." The former requires several "figure-of-8" fixation sutures to avoid overlap. This fixation method saves cartilage and prevents excessive thickness, yet is more difficult to perform. Side-to-side fixation is easier to perform, but must be managed well to avoid abnormal thickness or caudal deviations occurring. It is the optimal solution when small deflections from the midline of the caudal septum are present; and in this case, it should be sutured contralaterally to the deviation. The overlapping area should be well managed by trimming the graft to prevent it from protruding into the nasal fossa and causing obstruction. Side-to-side fixation is usually more rigid. The fixation of the SEG to the anterior nasal spine is a topic of discussion. Some surgeons prefer drilling a hole in the spine and passing a non-absorbable sutures to anchor the SEG; others believe that anchoring the SEG to the periosteum of the spine with PDS 4.0 sutures is sufficient [26–30].

9.5 Modification of Nasal Tip Projection

The projection of the nasal tip can be determined using several methods. One of the simplest and most effective is that proposed by Simons RL [31], according to which the distance between the nasal tip and the subnasal point should be equal to the distance between the latter and the upper lip. Another method is proposed by Crumley and Lanser [32], according to whom, the ideal ratio between the first cathetus, the second cathetus, and the hypotenuse should be 3:4:5 when drawing a right triangle on the profile of the nose. A value greater to or less than 3 of the first cathetus determines the hyperprojection or hypoprojection of the nasal tip. Hypoprojection of the nasal tip combined with hyporotation is a frequent feature of the Mediterranean nose, but it is not uncommon to encounter patients presenting with a hypoprojected or hyper-rotated nose. Numerous surgical techniques have been described for modifying the projection of the nasal tip. The most commonly used surgical techniques for achieving tip deprojection make use of the Anderson tripod concept [33]. Sectioning and overlaying the medial crura (medial crural overlay) also causes a reduction in rotation, in addition to deprojection. Lateral crural overlay, on the other hand, results in increased tip rotation associated with reduced tip projection. As mentioned in the previous paragraph, tip projection can also be reduced by suturing the medial crura further back from the caudal septum in a tongue-in-groove deprojection technique or by anchoring the medial crura more caudally than originally positioned when using a septal extension graft. This deprojection technique with a suture on the caudal septum makes the tip quite rigid, but "locks" it permanently in that state of deprojection that is decided at the time of suturing. When this deprojection is performed, it classically happens that the most caudal portion of the medial crura widens and can occupy the nasal opening, together with the mucosal excess resulting from the deprojection. In order to resolve this problem, there are two possibilities: in the first hypothesis, a portion of excess mucosa is removed together with the excess medial crura component; in the second hypothesis, the septum is disconnected from both sides, medially and posteriorly, and the mucosa is distributed posteriorly, suturing it with vicryl rapide 4.0 transfixed mattress stitches, bringing the lateralized foot of the medial crura closer to the midline. This deprojection technique was performed in the clinical case shown in the Figs. 9.18 and 9.19.

Another extremely good technique when dealing with over-projected noses is dome truncation or dome division. This technique, as described by Kridel in 1990 [13], is still extremely current and consists in the section of the domes, after having freed the vestibular mucosa underlying the domal cartilage. The amount to be resected is clinically evaluated, and it is recommended that you proceed in small steps, gradually removing the cartilage to avoid removing too much. When the right excision has been achieved, the medial and lateral crus, previously separated by dome truncation, are sutured with two "figure-of-8" PDS 6.0 sutures.

If you want to increase the projection of the tip, you can use many surgical techniques. Some of them rely on the use of sutures, while others make use of grafts. The lateral crural steal is a common suturing technique, which involves "stealing" the lateral crus by creating a neo-dome in a more lateral position. The two neo-domes are then sutured together, anteriorizing the lateral crus and allowing for increased projection [17].

Anterior suturing techniques of the medial crura on the caudal septum (tongue-in-groove technique or septal extension graft) are by far the most stable and effective techniques when we want to effectively and significantly increase the projection of the nasal tip.

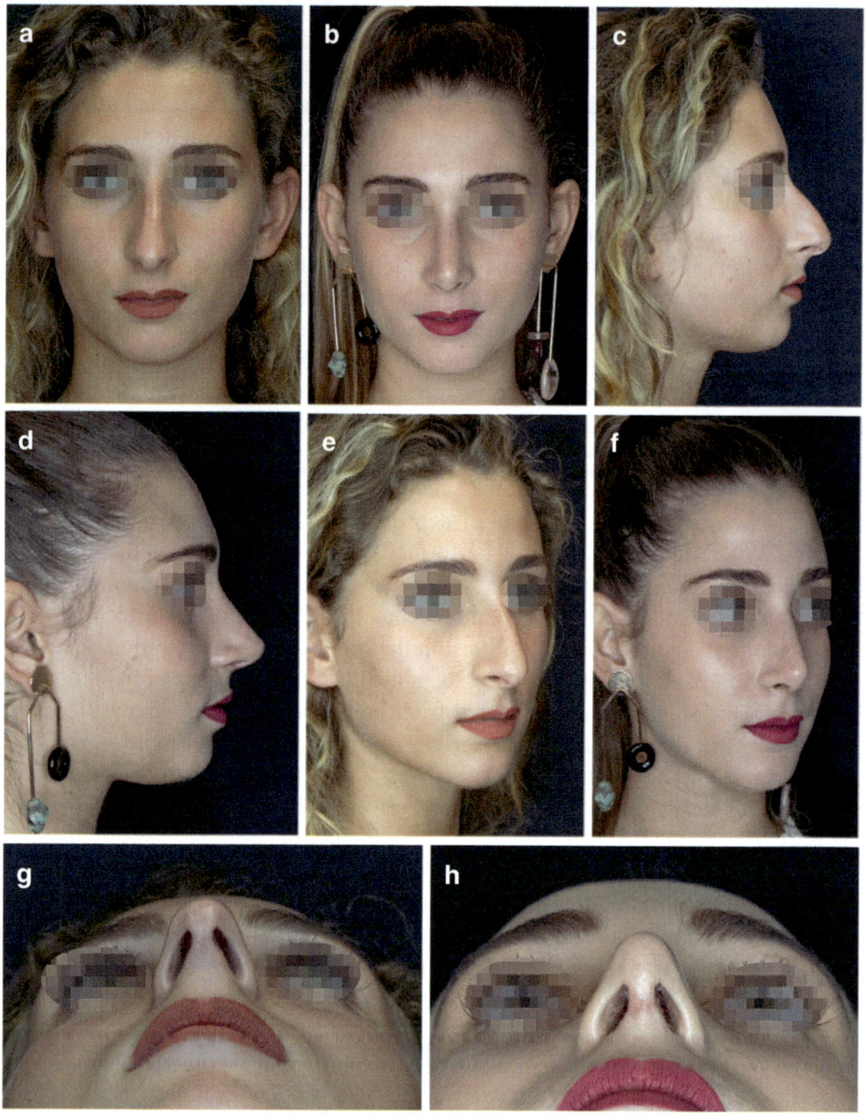

Fig. 9.18 Patient with a Mediterranean nose suffering from the hyperprojection of the nasal tip combined with ptosis. (**a**, **c**, **e**, **g**) Preoperative images; (**b**, **d**, **f**, **h**) corresponding post-op images

When discussing techniques that make use of grafts, we must consider the Peck graft, a shield graft or the columellar strut graft. The latter has already been described when we discussed the rotation of the nasal tip and, depending on the cartilage consistency and its thickness, can ensure a marked increase in projection [23, 24]. The Peck graft must be well shaped to avoid palpability or visibility of the graft through the skin. In the case of severe projection deficit, it can also be used in several layers

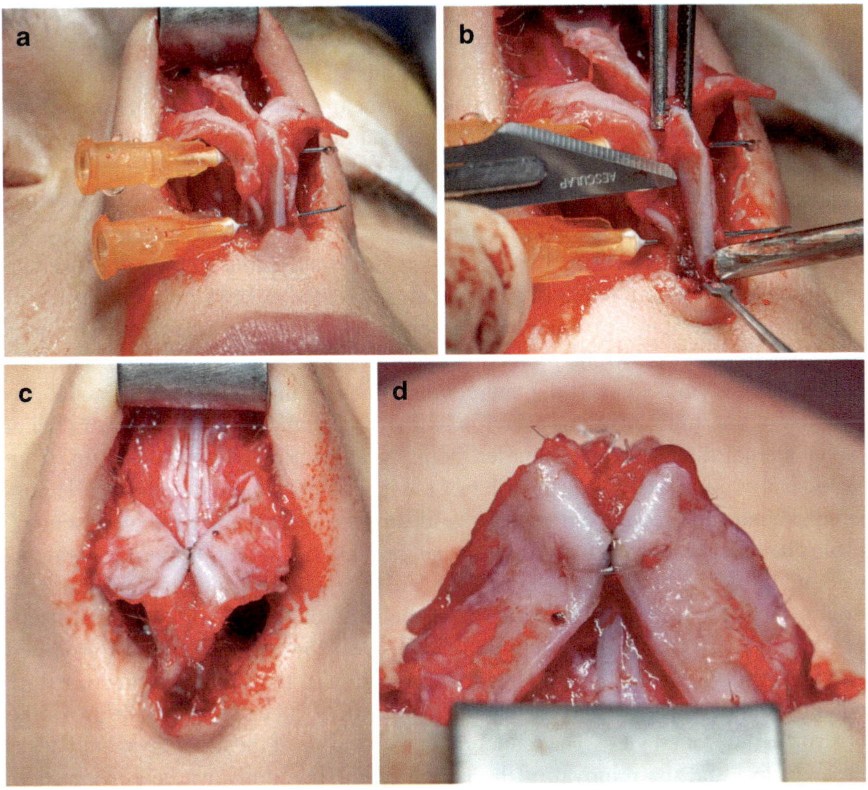

Fig. 9.19 Intraoperative images of the clinical case shown in Fig. 9.18. (**a**) Tongue-in-groove technique to reduce the projection of the alar cartilage; (**b**) Section of the excess caudal septum; (**c**) Shaping of the nasal tip by lateral crural steal and transdomal sutures to obtain a "diamond tip"; (**d**) Final intraoperative appearance of the nasal tip

and take a pyramidal shape (ziggurat graft) [34]. Finally, the shield graft is one of the most effective grafts for obtaining a good definition of the nasal tip in association with an increase in projection [35]. However, it is good to address the use of the shield and Peck grafts in patients with thick skin, as in the long term they could become visible and unsightly in patients with thin skin.

9.6 Modification of Nasal Tip Volume and Its Definition

The nasal tip in the Mediterranean nose is classically described as bulbous and in most cases patients request a decrease in its volume, along with an increase in definition. The first thing to understand when faced with a bulbous tip is whether its volume depends on an excess of cartilage or an excess of soft tissue, as the surgical approach is in fact very different and in some ways opposite. In the case of cartilaginous excess, this is usually caused by hypertrophy of the lateral crura of the alar cartilages. The cephalic resection of the alar cartilages is a classic maneuver in rhinoplasty that allows for the volume of the tip to be reduced, while also achieving a slight upward rotation of the nasal tip. Sometimes, it is not merely the volume of the lateral crura that determines the globularity of the tip, but also their consistency and curvature. Although both consistency and curvature can be reduced by the surgical maneuver of cephalic excision, it is often necessary to use additional surgical techniques to allow the curvature to be reduced. The most effective maneuver for "stretching" the lateral crus is the "lateral crural steal," which, by anteriorizing the lateral crus, it stretches it and straightens it. Inevitably, this technique causes an increase in the projection that is welcome in most cases of Mediterranean nose correction; however, it must be managed in some cases with other surgical techniques to reduce the increase of the projection caused by the lateral crural steal. This last technique also tends to evert the lateral crura, causing the correct craniocaudal orientation of the same. Also this eversion, with the cephalic border of the crura being more internal than the caudal border, helps to reduce the bulbous nasal tip. If an excessively caudalized inferior border of the lateral crura were to remain, it is possible to obtain an eversion of the same by means of a "lateral crura spanning suture." [36]. The latter can be performed with a single PDS 6.0 suture passed through corresponding points of the cephalic portion of the lateral crura and in the dorsal portion of the septum in order to bring the cephalic border closer to the septum itself, or it can be performed with a suture on each side. However, it must be considered that this type of suture could change the orientation of the axis of the lateral crura, which could become excessively cephalic, and lead to an excessive exposure of the nostrils in the frontal view. The reduction in the volume of the nasal tip should never be excessive and the removal of the lateral crura should always be conservative, leaving a thickness of 4–5 mm of the crus. In fact, if the support were reduced excessively, there could be a collapse of the external nasal valve that, in addition to causing an aesthetic deficit, will be the cause of functional dissatisfaction for the patient. To prevent the latter occurring, it is often necessary to reinforce the alar margin and the posterior portion of the alar itself. This is possible using different types of grafts, such as the alar batten graft, the alar strut graft and the alar extension graft [37]. The alar batten graft must be placed in a precise pocket that must reach the margin of the pyriform aperture and not be too thick to avoid it becoming visible and palpable through the skin. The alar strut graft, in addition to supporting the nasal ala, can play an important role in straightening it. Finally, the alar extension graft consists in an extension of the ala that can also be made with the previously excised portion of cephalic cartilage. The cartilage can be extended caudally if a frontal exposure of the nostrils is to be corrected, or posteriorly to prevent the collapse of the external nasal valve and ensure better triangularization of the tip. Definition of the nasal tip can be achieved with classic transdomal and interdomal sutures. The more the transdomal suture is applied cephalically at the level of the dome, greater divergence of the caudal portion of the dome and more accurate tip definition is achieved. The transdomal suture should equalize the domes, yet leave an angle of divergence between them of approximately 60°, so that two defined light points result below the skin.

On the other hand, when the bulbousity of the tip is caused by thick skin, a major cartilage excision should not be used. The more cartilage that is removed in these cases, the more shapeless and ill-defined the nasal tip will appear, as if it were a mass of soft tissue. To define a thick-skinned tip, we must triangulate the cartilage structure below the skin and, if appropriate, use grafts to stretch the skin and cause it to relax. Peck grafts, including overlapping grafts, or shield grafts can be used [34, 35]. On the contrary, if the skin is thin, these grafts should be avoided as much as possible, because over time they could become visible and palpable under the skin, creating an unnatural and unsightly effect.

The correct management of Pitanguy's ligament plays a particularly important role in defining the supratip region and avoiding the formation of a pollybeak deformity [21, 22]. Some surgeons extol its function in regulating the rotation and projection of the nasal tip. In my experience, this ligament should be isolated at the beginning of an open rhinoplasty and its repositioning at the end of the operation will be what allows for the supratip region to be defined. After the marginal incisions and the transcolumellar incision, the skin is detached from the caudal border of the medial crura, the domes and the lateral crura on a strictly subperichondrial plane, taking care not to dissect the connection between the subcutaneous tissue of the supratip region and the existing connective tissue between the domes and the medial crura. Next, the medial crura is detached and Pitanguy's ligament is isolated along with the transverse ligament and intercrural fibers until it rejoins the subcutaneous tissue in the supratip region. In this way, we obtain a sort of connective tissue cord that contains Pitanguy's ligament and that—at the end of the operation, when repositioned appropriately and anchored in the area of the columellar incision—will exert internal traction on the subcutaneous tissue of the supratip region, ensuring the pleasant definition of the latter and an adjustable supratip break depending on the tension applied with the suture. Figures 9.20 and 9.21 illustrate a clinical case in which tip definition was achieved by implementing the concepts outlined in this section.

9.7 Malposition or Malformation of the Lateral Crura

When dealing with a bulbous tip, consider that the problem is not always an excess of cartilage or the excessive curvature of the lateral crura. Sometimes, the latter can be malpositioned. In these cases, it is crucial that we ascertain the anatomical problem because surgical zeal in the resection of the crura can lead to serious aesthetic and functional sequelae. The correct orientation of the lateral crura should be oblique-horizontal, leaving an angle equal to or greater than 45° from the midline [38]. As most surgeons do not normally use a goniometer in the operating room, the lateral canthus is a useful reference, as the lateral crus should be directed towards it. When the crus is directed medially to the lateral canthus or even towards the medial canthus, the orientation is defined as cephalic and the crus is cephalically or vertically malpositioned. Aesthetically, this deformity results in a bulbous and unsightly tip with the "bracket deformity." In addition to the aesthetic deficit, this malposition can also cause functional problems. In fact, since all the cartilage is directed cephalically, the caudal

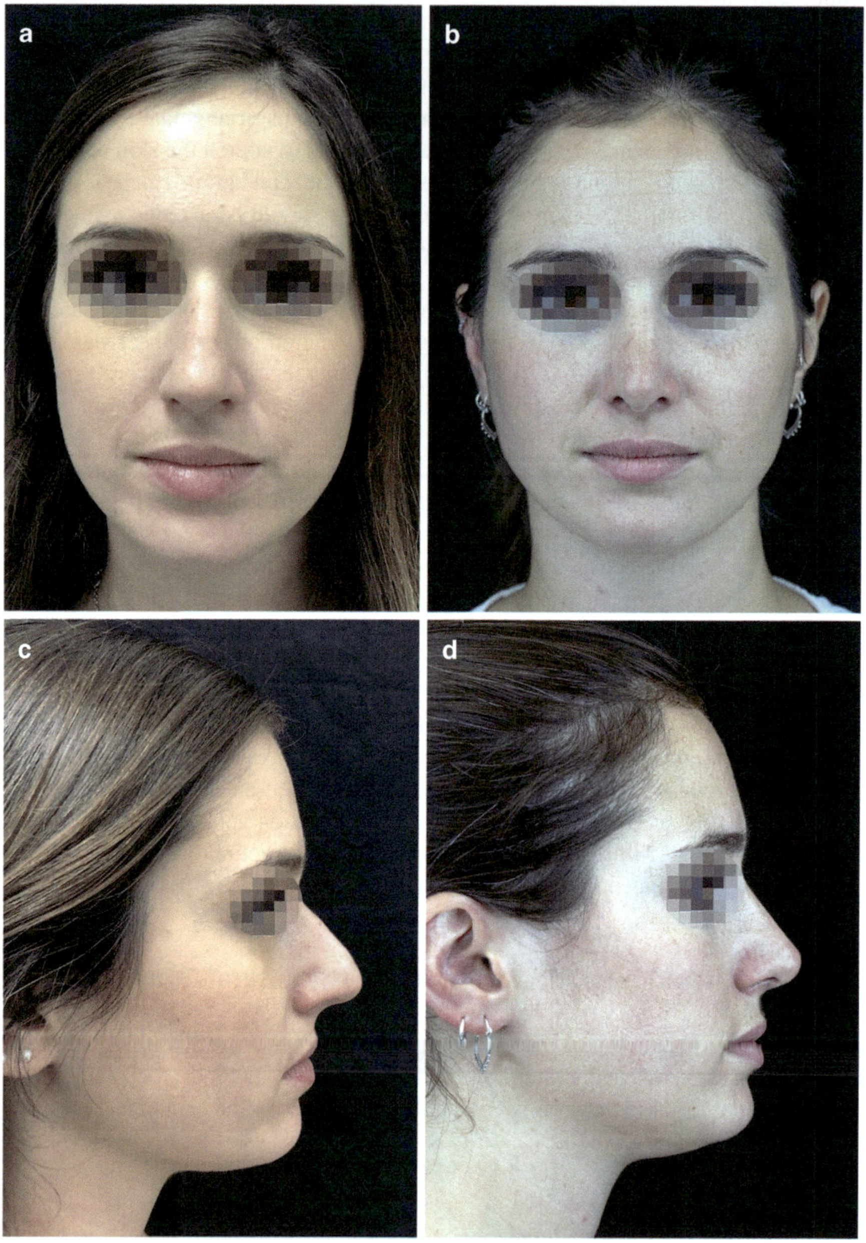

Fig. 9.20 Patient with globular tip and high dorsum. Note that despite having reduced the size of the tip and reduced the height of the dorsum, the nose continues to have a natural, "Mediterranean" appearance. (**a**, **c**, **e**, **g**) Preoperative images; (**b**, **d**, **f**, **h**) Corresponding post-op images

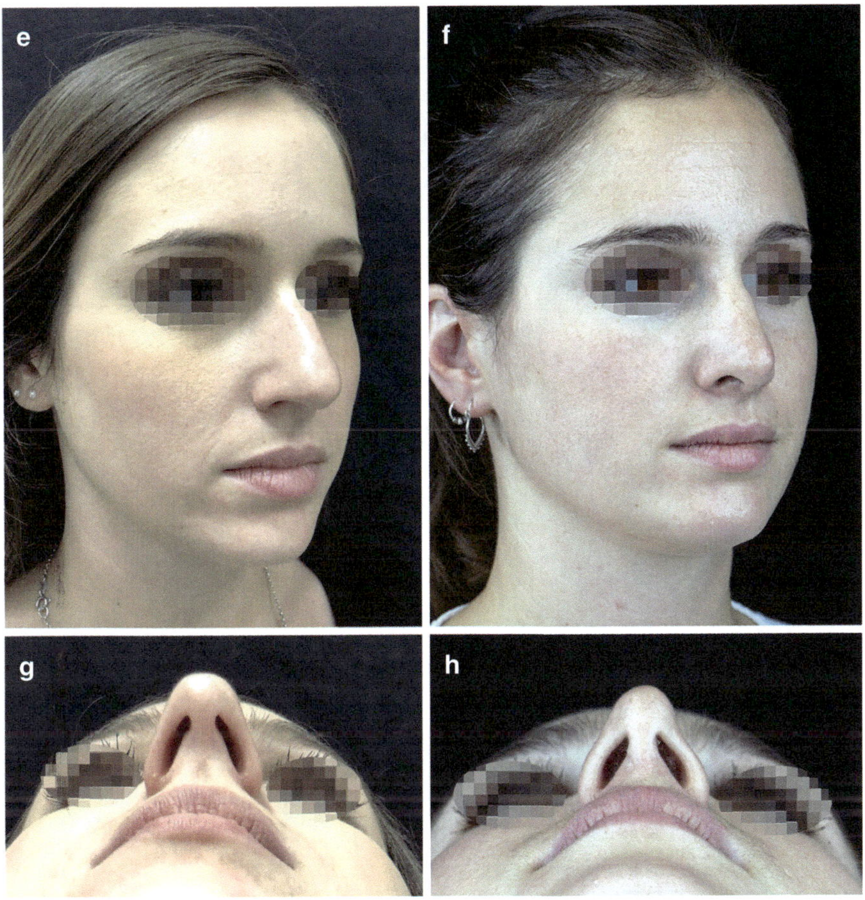

Fig. 9.20 (continued)

portion of the alae remains composed exclusively of soft tissue and some sesamoid cartilage. This often results in the pinching of the external nasal valve and failure to provide cartilage support for this region, especially during forced inspiration. The goal of all the surgical techniques described to correct the cephalic malpositioning of the lateral crura is to change its orientation. In the classic repositioning technique, the lateral crus is freed from the underlying vestibular skin and its orientation is changed [39, 40]. It can be fixed in its new position by transfixed sutures in the vestibular skin. If the length of the crus is adequate, it may only require repositioning, without the need for structural reinforcement with grafts. If, on the other hand, we need to intervene more decisively to reposition the alar and straighten a convex lateral crus, we can resort to the lateral crural strut graft, as described by Gunter in 1997 [41]. This graft, preferably taken from the septum, must be very long—about 20–25 mm—thin, and about 3 mm wide, and should extend from the domal region to the pocket made in the direction of the lateral canthus to the pyriform aperture. Another technique for

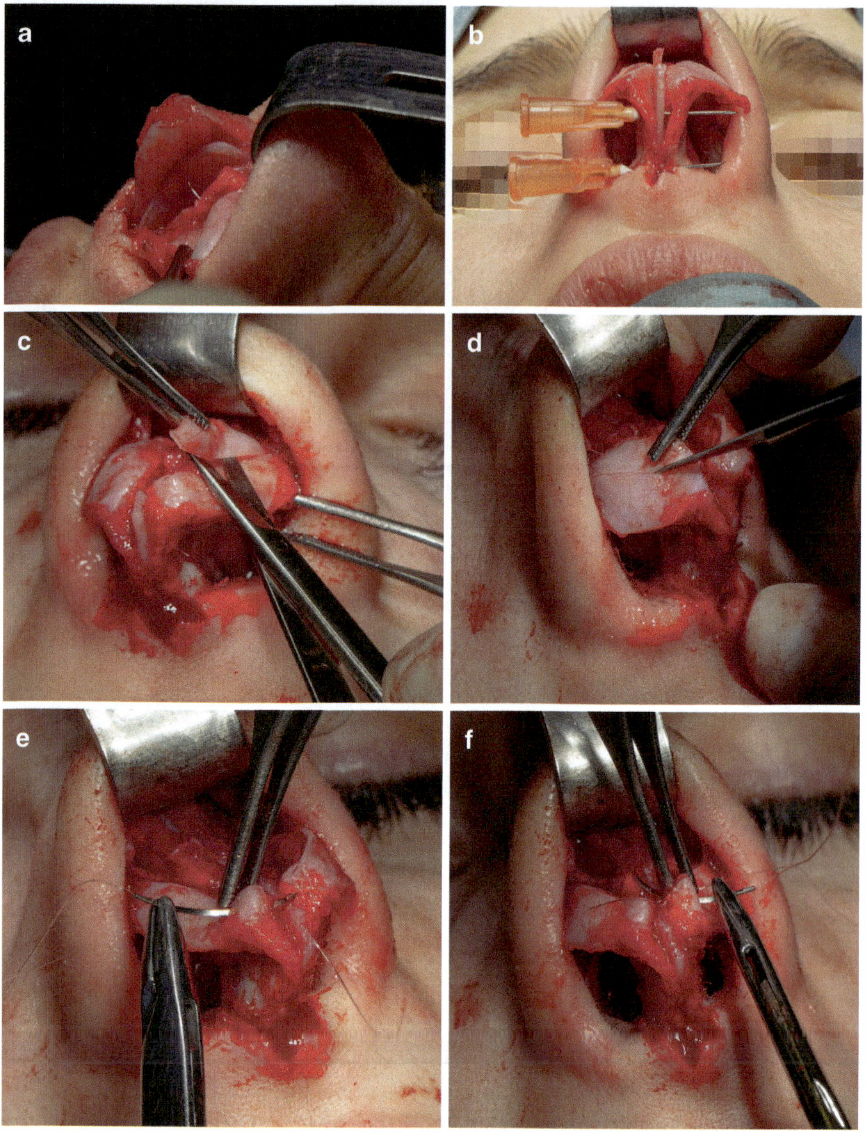

Fig. 9.21 Intraoperative images of the clinical case shown in Fig. 9.20. (**a**) Septal extension graft to define the rotation and projection of the tip. In this case the tip has been deprojected; (**b**) "Tongue-in-groove" on septal extension graft; (**c**) Left lateral crus cephalic resection; (**d**) Right lateral crus cephalic resection; (**e**) Right lateral crural steal; (**f**) Left lateral crural steal; (**g**) Interdomal suture; (**h**) Final appearance of the tip with reinforcement of the posterior portion by a lateral crural extension graft posteriorly with cartilage obtained from the cephalic excision of the same crus. (**i**) Helicopter view of the final structure of the tip. (**j**) Creation of Pitanguy's ligament to give definition to the supratip region

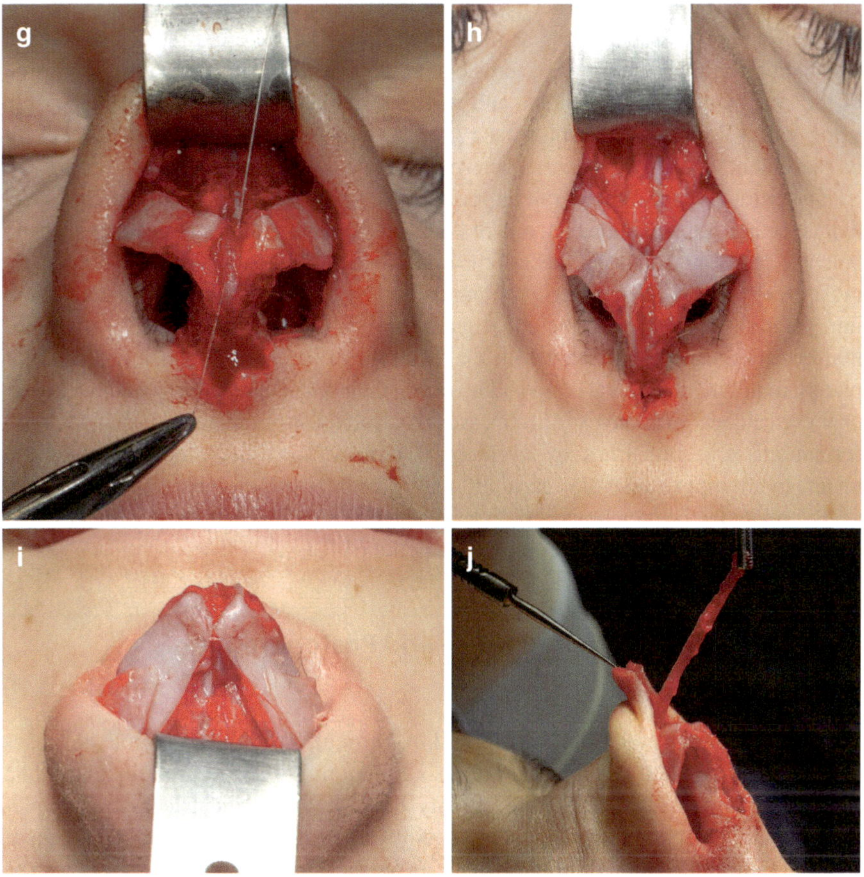

Fig. 9.21 (continued)

modifying the cephalic direction of the lateral crura was described in 2006 by Boccieri [42] and represents a modification of Kridel's lateral crural overlay [17]. This technique, known as the lateral crural stairstep technique, involves a stepped incision in the posterior portion of the lateral crura. The vestibular skin is removed and the lateral crura are spatially repositioned by connecting the cephalic portion of the anterior fragment with the caudal portion of the posterior fragment. Recently, other innovative techniques have also been proposed for the correction of this malposition. Kovacevic [43] proposed a repositioning of the lateral crura by using a turn-in flap of the lower portion of the alar cartilage, while Goksel [44] described an oblique turnover flap of the cephalic portion of the lateral crus on the caudal portion. Another solution may be to create a posterior lateral crural extension graft. In this case, it is possible to proceed with a classic cephalic excision of the alar cartilage according to what should be the correct axis of the lateral crus. In the case of cephalic malposition, this involves a section of a large part of the crus cephalically aligned with this axis. However, the same large portion of crus that has been removed can be used to reconstitute the entire lateral crus along the correct axis, as if it were a lower lateral crura replacement graft. The fixation of this portion of the crus can be done with the residual anterior portion of the crus using PDS 6.0 sutures and with transfixed sutures on the vestibular skin using Vicryl Rapide 5.0. We must take great care in creating the posterior pocket for its placement, because this pocket determines the correct orientation of the crus.

The crura can present several malformations. Apart from the asymmetrical aspect that is the norm in deviated tips, one of the most frequent malformations that needs to be corrected is the concave aspect of the crura. In addition to the aesthetic problem, in most cases there is a functional problem caused by the protrusion of the lateral crura into the nasal vestibule and the consequent stenosis of the external nasal valve. This malformation can be corrected with the "Barrel roll technique," which entails completely removing the lateral crura and inverting their original position so that what was concave can become convex [45]. In cases of severe post-traumatic or iatrogenic malformations, it is sometimes inconvenient, in terms of operative time and achievable result, to attempt to give alar cartilage with present, dysmorphic residues a correct shape and it may be more appropriate to completely reconstruct the alar with auricular concha cartilage according to Pedroza's technique [46].

9.8 Skin Thickness and Intra- and Postoperative Skin Management

The Mediterranean nose often has thick skin, particularly in the tip region, but cases of patients with notably thin skin are also common. Discerning the thickness and quality of the skin is an absolute priority because the surgical technique implemented and postoperative management will have to change depending on these characteristics. The skin cannot be seen as an inert coating and is sometimes the factor that most determines the end result. Thin skin allows for more accurate results in defining the nasal tip, but it also presents the problem posed by small underlying cartilage defects, which can become evident when postoperative swelling has resolved. The best way to avoid future problems in patients with thin skin is to be maniacally precise until complete symmetry of the tip cartilage is achieved. Onlay grafts, such as Peck and shield grafts, should be avoided as much as possible, because they would definitely become visible and unsightly over time. The possibility of using "soft" subcutaneous regularization grafts above the cartilage structure of the tip could be extremely useful in order to reduce irregularities and to achieve a more uniform result. Tissue that can be used for this purpose may be the retroauricular or temporalis fascia, the auricular perichondrium, or even heterologous resorbable membranes of porcine or equine pericardium. Recently, fluid cartilage or cartilaginous gel has also been introduced [47, 48]. This can be obtained by "scratching" a fragment of removed septal cartilage with a 15 blade and obtaining a kind of gel that can be placed directly on the tip cartilage before the columellar suture or introduced from the marginal incision with a syringe. It can be extremely useful in smoothing and evening out the cartilage structure. The same function can be performed by crushed cartilage (Figs. 9.22 and 9.23).

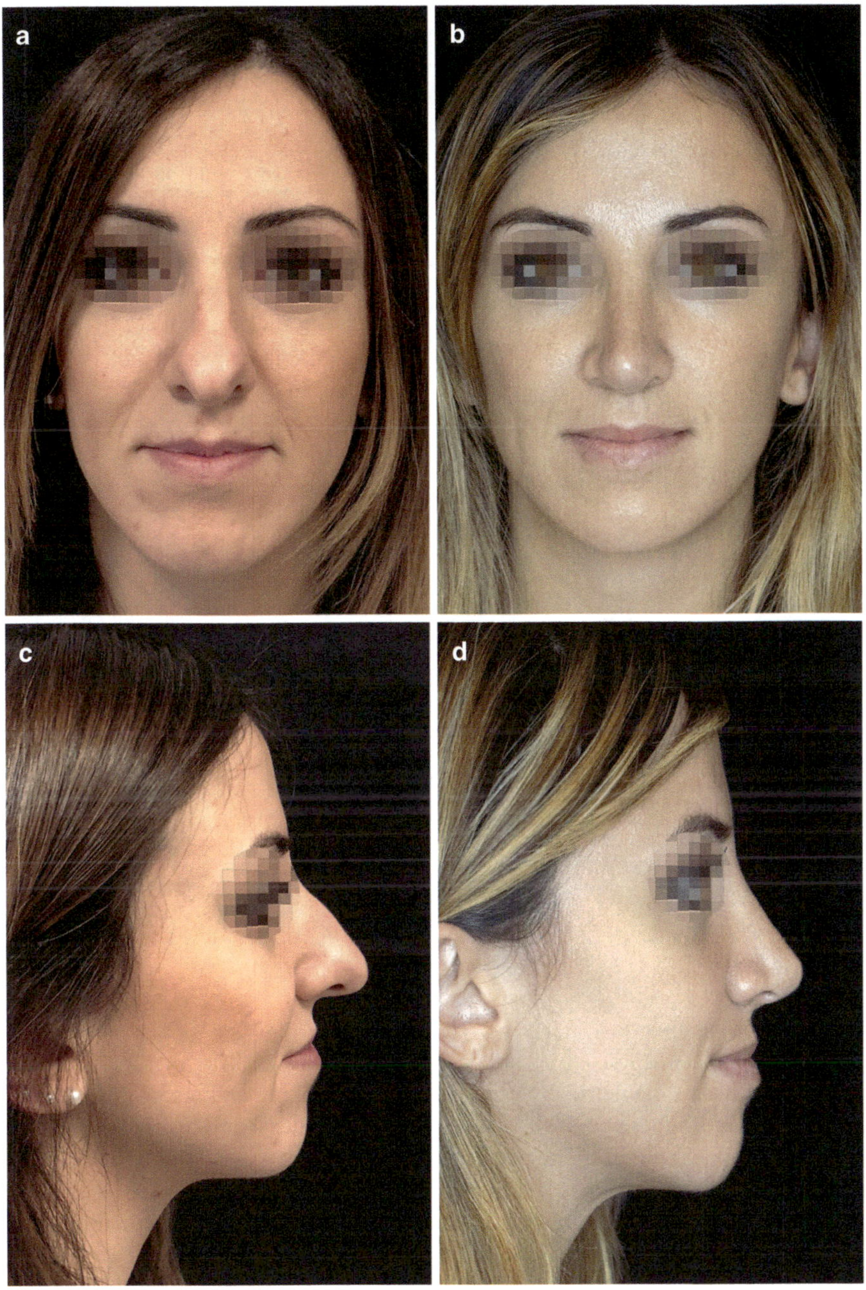

Fig. 9.22 Patient with cephalic malposition of the lateral crura. (**a**, **c**, **e**, **g**) Preoperative images; (**b**, **d**, **f**, **h**) Corresponding post-op images

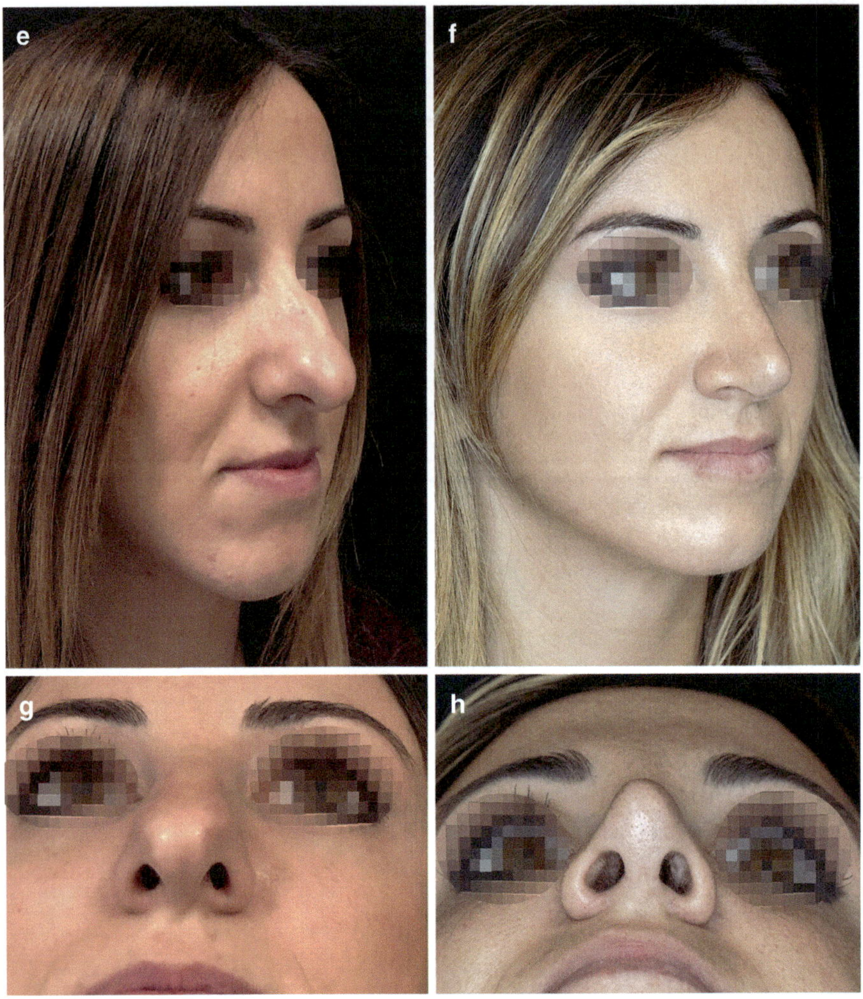

Fig. 9.22 (continued)

We must take a diametrically opposed way of thinking and acting for patients with thick skin. In these cases, it is necessary to consider that the skin needs to be stretched to appear thinner. The first requirement in these cases is to ensure strong support for the nasal tip. This can be provided by resorting to grafts, such as a strong columellar strut graft or, even better, a septal extension graft. The tongue-in-groove technique, when indicated, also provides strong support to the nasal tip. The defatting proposed by some surgeons to thin the skin on the tip, in my personal experience has proven to be not merely dangerous, but inadequate in resolving the issue, because over time the skin returned to its original thickness [49]. The definition and triangularization of the cartilaginous structure of the tip, which is required to "push" the skin from the inside and give a defined appearance to the tip, can be provided by

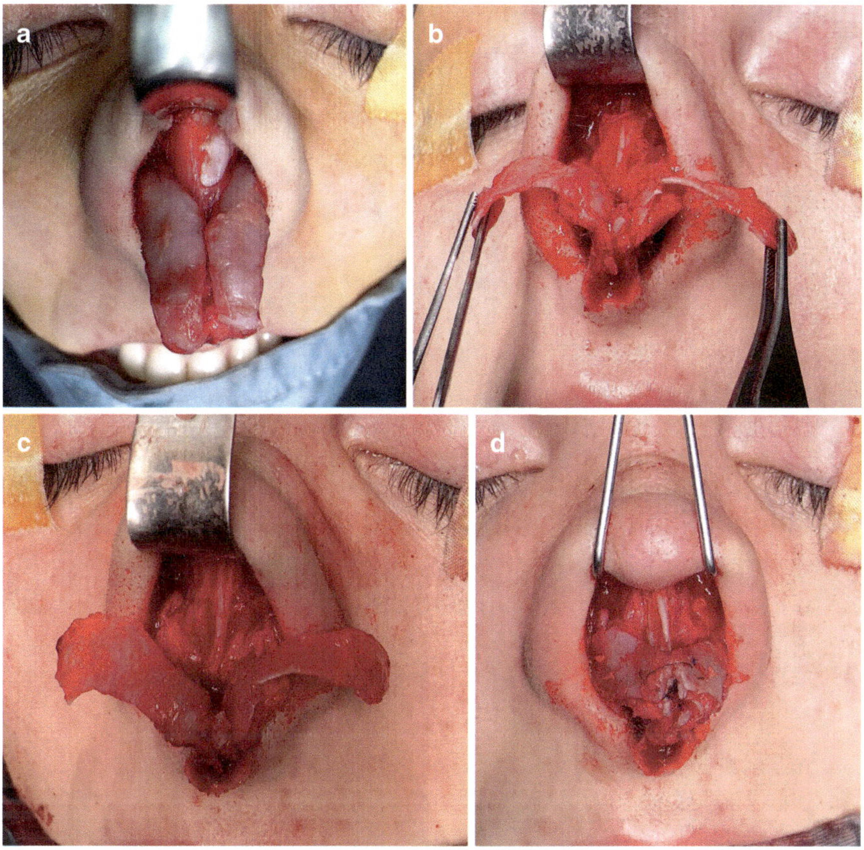

Fig. 9.23 Intraoperative images of the clinical case shown in Fig. 9.22. (**a**) Clear cephalic malposition of lateral crura; (**b**, **c**) Lateral crura released from vestibular skin and free to be repositioned according to the correct direction; (**d**) Lateral crura repositioned caudally

using Peck grafts, even in an overlapping orientation, and shield grafts. The latter in particular is excellent in defining thick-skinned tips. Figures 9.24 and 9.25 show a clinical case in which the definition of the nasal tip in a patient with thick skin was achieved using the shield graft.

Postoperative care also needs to differ depending on whether your patient has thick or thin skin. The final result can be achieved much earlier in a patient with thin skin. During the postoperative period, it is sometimes necessary to resort to hyaluronic acid infiltrations to correct small skin irregularities. It is my personal experience that if these small corrections are carried out very early, within a few months after the rhinoplasty procedure, they can largely stabilize because fibrosis is induced in the region of the injection, which gradually replaces the hyaluronic acid while it is reabsorbed over the course of months. Consequently, the effect determined by the hyaluronic acid can persist over time. Some scientific studies support my personal experience, but further studies are required to confirm this [50, 51].

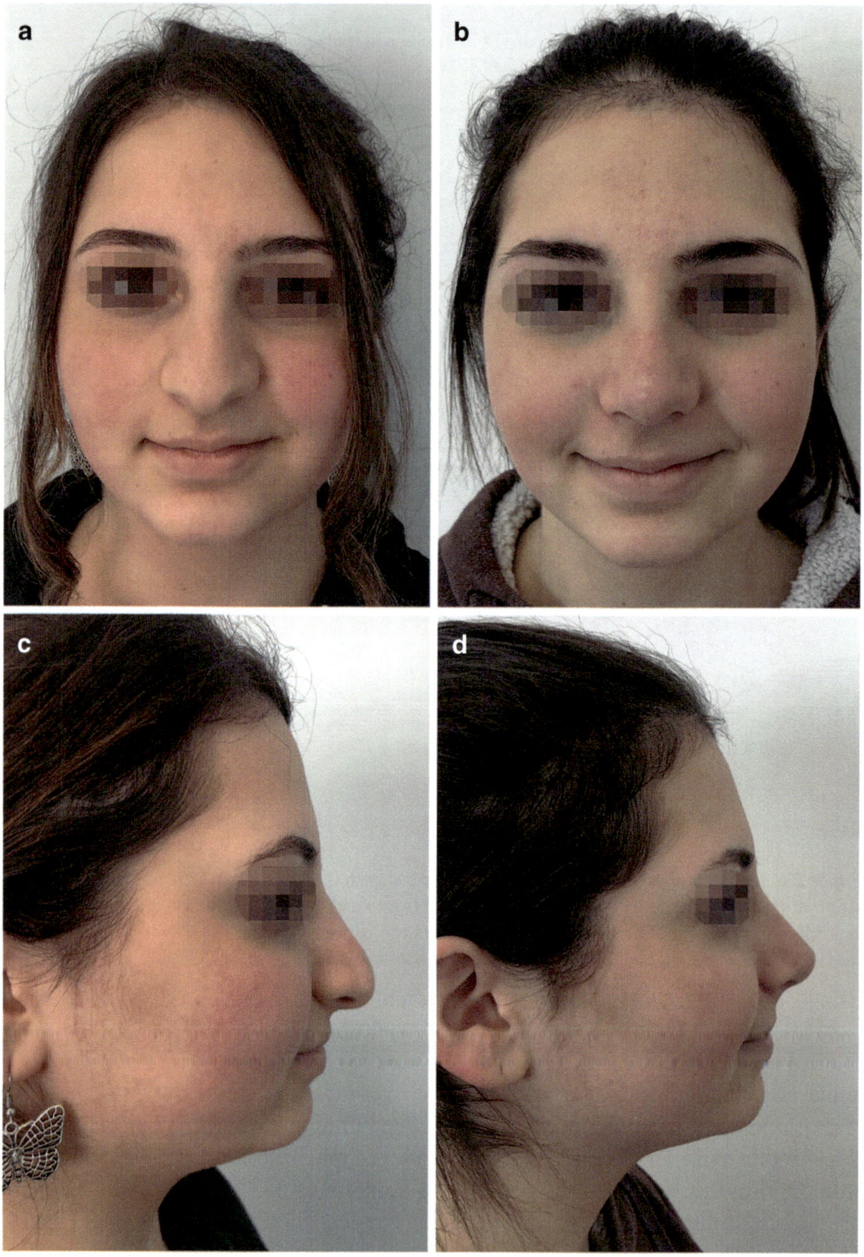

Fig. 9.24 Patient suffering from hyporotation and hypoprojection of the nasal tip combined with very thick skin. (**a**, **c**, **e**, **g**) Preoperative images; (**b**, **d**, **f**, **h**) Corresponding post-op images

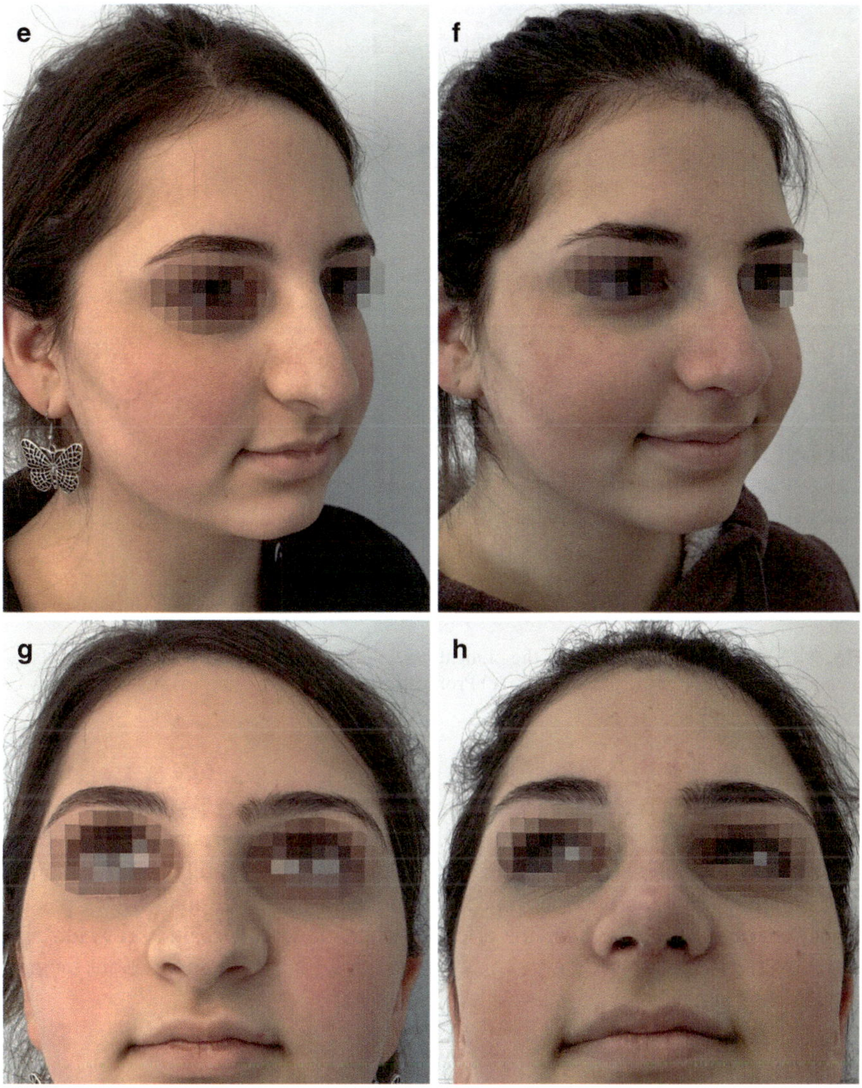

Fig. 9.24 (continued)

The pharmaceutical that is almost always required during the postoperative management period for thick skin following rhinoplasty is cortisone. Corticosteroids reduce fibroblast proliferation and the inflammatory response. This has the effect of reducing collagen and glycosaminoglycan synthesis and reducing tissue fibrosis, as well as having a direct collagenase-stimulating effect. There are numerous studies in the literature describing the correction of scar-based pollybeak deformities with triamcinolone injections. Kridel uses the injection of 1–2 mL of triamcinolone 10 mg/mL 2 weeks after surgery when needed and then every 4 weeks depending on

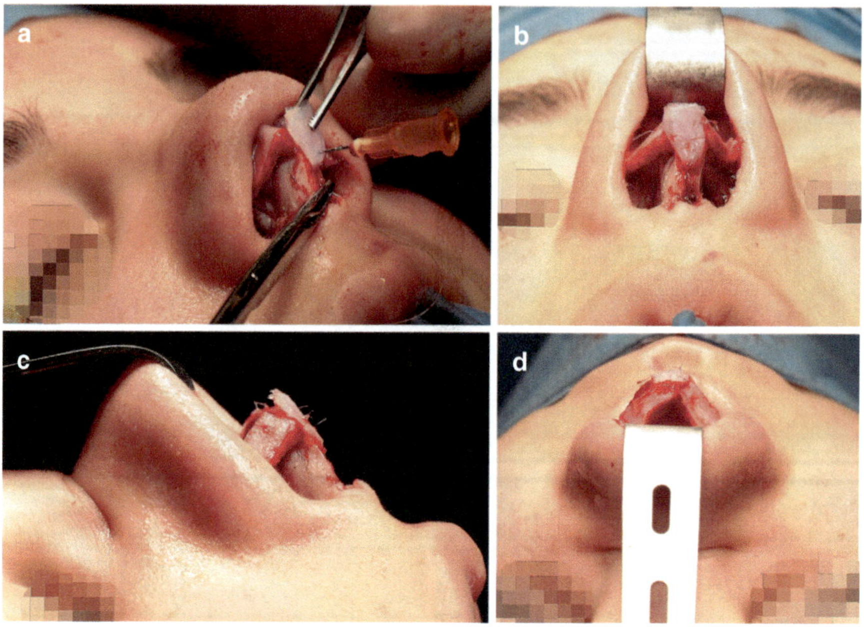

Fig. 9.25 Intraoperative images of the clinical case shown in Fig. 9.24. (**a**) Shield graft placement; (**b**) Axial view of the placed graft; (**c**) Profile view of the shield graft; (**d**) Helicopter view of the same graft

response [52]. Pastorek suggests earlier use, even intraoperatively or 1 week after surgery [52]. In my personal experience, the most frequent use is 40 mg/mL triamcinolone, but in a very small amount (0.05 or 0.1 mL) directly into the necessary spot. The first injection is usually given at 2 months and only rarely before 1 month. The important thing is never to repeat the injection before 2 months have passed from the previous one because the effect of triamcinolone lasts up to 6 weeks and could overlap, causing unsightly skin complications. Possible complications include depigmentation, telangiectasias, and skin necrosis.

9.9 Conclusions

In conclusion, the tip of the Mediterranean nose can present several malformations. Faced with these, it is essential to carry out a careful preoperative analysis in order to determine whether the tip is deviated, hypo or hyperprojected, hypo or hyperrotated, whether it is too voluminous, whether it has the right support, whether the lateral crura are in the right direction, and what type of skin it is covered by. Our surgical arsenal should include all surgical techniques to address different anatomical issues. Preoperative planning must always be accurate and must direct us towards the surgical technique to be used, but intraoperatively we can shift towards another technique if the anatomical condition requires it. Regardless of the techniques used, the main goal must remain in the surgeon's mind to achieve a natural, non-stereotypical result. "To change, without distorting" and avoid "surgical" results must always be the philosophy of the surgeon when performing rhinoplasty procedures.

References

1. Ripley WZ. The races of Europe: a sociological study. New York: D. Appleton and Co.; 1899.
2. Boccieri A. The surgical approach to the Mediterranean nose. Facial Plast Surg. 2010;26(2):119–30.
3. Palma P, Bignami M, Delù G, De Bernardi F, Castelnuovo P. Rhinoplasty for the Mediterranean nose. Facial Plast Surg. 2003;19(3):279–94.
4. Loyo M, Wang TD. Management of the deviated nasal dorsum. Facial Plast Surg. 2015;31(3):216–27.
5. Boccieri A. The crooked nose. Acta Otorhinolaryngol Ital. 2003;33(3):163–8.
6. Rudy S, Moubayed SP, Most SP. Midvault reconstruction in primary rhinoplasty. Facial Plast Surg. 2017;33(2):133–8.
7. Rohrich RJ, Hollier LH. Use of spreader grafts in external approach to rhinoplasty. Clin Plast Surg. 1996;23(2):255–62.
8. Byrd HS, Meade RA, Gonyon DL. Using the autospreader flap in primary rhinoplasty. Plast Reconstr Surg. 2007;119(6):1897–902.
9. Boccieri A, Pascali M. Septal crossbar graft for the correction of the crooked nose. Plast Reconstr Surg. 2003;111(2):629–38.
10. Gubisch W. Extracorporeal septoplasty for the markedly deviated septum. Arch Facial Plast Surg. 2005;7(4):218–26.
11. Rohrich RJ, Griffin JR. Correction of intrinsic nasal tip asymmetries in primary rhinoplasty. Plast Reconstr Surg. 2003;112(6):1699–712.
12. Gunter JP, Rohrich RJ. Management of the deviated nose. The importance of septal reconstruction. Clin Plast Surg. 1988;15(1):43–55.
13. Kridel RW, Konior RJ. Dome truncation for management of the overprojected nasal tip. Ann Plast Surg. 1990;24(5):385–96.
14. Kridel RWH, Konior RJ. Controlled nasal tip rotation via the lateral crural overlay technique. Arch Otolaryngol Head Neck Surg. 1991;117(4):411–5.
15. Manafi A, Rajaee A, Manafi A. Concomitant overlap steal tip-plasty: a versatile technique to simultaneously adjust the rotation, definition, projection, and symmetry of the nasal tip. Aesthet Surg J. 2016;36(2):147–55.
16. Pascali M, Boccieri A, Carinci F, Cervelli V. Treatment of the crooked nose. J Craniofac Surg. 2017;28(2):372 8.
17. Foda HMT, Kridel RWH. Lateral crural steal and lateral crural overlay. Arch Otolaryngol Neck Surg. 1999;125(12):1365.
18. Kridel RW, Scott BA, Foda HM. The tongue-in-groove technique in septorhinoplasty. A 10-year experience. Arch Facial Plast Surg. 2013;1(4):246–56; discussion 257–8.
19. Boccieri A, Sciuto S, Cervelli V, Pascali M. Dome division: a viable technique today? Facial Plast Surg. 2016;32(6):664–70.
20. Goldman IB. The importance of the mesial crura in nasal-tip reconstruction. Arch Otolaryngol—Head Neck Surg. 1957;65(2):143–7.
21. Pitanguy I. Surgical importance of a dermocartilaginous ligament in bulbous noses. Plast Reconstr Surg. 1965;36:247–53.
22. Daniel RK, Palhazi P. The nasal ligaments and tip support in rhinoplasty: an anatomical study. Aesthet Surg J. 2018;38(4):357–68.

23. Rohrich RJ, Kurkjian TJ, Hoxworth RE, Stephan PJ, Mojallal A. The effect of the columellar strut graft on nasal tip position in primary rhinoplasty. Plast Reconstr Surg. 2012;130(4):926–32.
24. Giacomini PG, Rubino S, Mocella S, Pascali M, Di Girolamo S. Approach to the correction of drooping tip: common problems and solutions. Acta Otorhinolaryngol Ital. 2017;37(4):295–302.
25. Byrd HS, Andochick S, Copit S. Septal extension grafts: a method of controlling tip projection shape. Plast Reconstr Surg. 1997;100:999–1010.
26. Park JH, Mangoba DCS, Mun SJ, et al. Lengthening the short nose in Asians. Key maneuvers and surgical results. Facial Plast Surg. 2013;15(6):439–47.
27. Kim K, Kim H-S. Secondary Asian rhinoplasty: lengthening the short nose. Aesthet Surg J. 2013;33:353–62.
28. Scattolin A, Galzignato P-F, Longari F, D'Ascanio L. Septal extension graft in "closed" revision rhinoplasty: a simplified technique. Am J Rhinol Allergy. 2017;31:260–4.
29. Toriumi DM. Discussion: control of nasal tip position: quantitative assessment of columellar strut versus caudal septal extension graft. Plast Reconstr Surg. 2019;144(5):781e–3e.
30. Sawh-Martinez R, Perkins K, Madari S, Steinbacher DM. Control of nasal tip position: quantitative assessment of columellar strut versus caudal septal extension graft. Plast Reconstr Surg. 2019;144:772e–80e.
31. Simons RL. Adjunctive measures in rhinoplasty. Otolaryngol Clin North Am. 1975;8:717–42.
32. Crumley RL, Lanser M. Quantitative analysis of nasal tip projection. Laryngoscope. 1988;98:202–8.
33. Soliemanzadeh P, Kridel RW. Nasal tip overprojection: algorithm of surgical deprojection techniques and introduction of medial crural overlay. Arch Facial Plast Surg. 2005;7:374–80.
34. Peck GC. The onlay graft for nasal tip projection. Plast Reconstr Surg. 1983;71:27–39.
35. Sheen JH. Tip graft: a 20-year retrospective. Plast Reconstr Surg. 1993;91:48–63.
36. Perkins SW, Sufyan AS. The alar-spanning suture: a useful tool in rhinoplasty. Arch Facial Plast Surg. 2011;13(6):421–4.
37. Gunter JP, Landecker A, Cochran CS. Frequently used grafts in rhinoplasty: nomenclature and analysis. Plast Reconstr Surg. 2006;118(1):14e–29e.
38. Toriumi DM. New concepts in nasal tip contouring. Arch Facial Plast Surg. 2006;8:156–85.
39. Mohebbi A, Azizi A, Tabatabaiee S. Repositioned lateral crural flap technique for cephalic malposition in rhinoplasty. Plast Surg. 2015;23(3):183–8.
40. Toriumi DM, Asher SA. Lateral crural repositioning for treatment of cephalic malposition. Facial Plast Surg Clin North Am. 2015;23(1):55–71.
41. Gunter JP, Friedman RM. Lateral crural strut graft: technique and clinical applications in rhinoplasty. Plast Reconstr Surg. 1997;99:943–52.
42. Boccieri A, Raimondi G. The lateral crural stairstep technique: a modification of the Kridel lateral crural overlay technique. Arch Facial Plast Surg. 2008;10:56–64.
43. Kovacevic M, et al. Management of the cephalically malpositioned lower lateral crus. Facial Plast Surg. 2017;33(5):491–8.
44. Göksel A, Vladykina E. Oblique turnover flap for repositioning and flattening of the lateral crura: a novel technique to manage cephalic malposition of lower lateral cartilage. Facial Plast Surg. 2017;33(5):483–90.
45. Boccieri A, Marianetti TM. Barrel roll technique for the correction of long and concave lateral crura. Arch Facial Plast Surg. 2010;12(6):415–21.
46. Pedroza F, Anjos GC, Patrocinio LG, Barreto JM, Cortes J, Quessep SH. Seagull wing graft: a technique for the replacement of lower lateral cartilages. Arch Facial Plast Surg. 2006;8(6):396–403.
47. Manafi A, Hamedi ZS, Rajabiani A, Rajaee A, Manafi F. Injectable cartilage shaving: an autologous and long lasting filler material for correction of minor contour deformities in rhinoplasty. World J Plast Surg. 2015;4:93–100.
48. Trivisonno A, Cohen SR, Magalon G, Magalon J, Steodimas A, Pascali M, Cervelli V, Toietta G, Colapietra A, Calcagni F, Orlandi A, Scioli MG, Gentile P. Fluid cartilage as new autolo-

gous biomaterial in the treatment of minor nose defects: clinical and microscopic difference amongst diced, crushed and fluid cartilage. Materials. 2019;31 (12:1062–70.
49. Nemati S, Banan R, Alizadeh A, Leili EK, Kerdari H. Ultrasonographic evaluation of long-term results of nasal tip defatting in rhinoplasty cases. Laryngoscope. 2013;123(9):2131–5.
50. Liapakis IE, Englader M, Vrentos NP, Derdas SP, Paschalis EI. Secondary rhinoplasty fixations with hyaluronic acid. J Cosmet Dermatol 2013; 12 (£): 235–239.
51. Mehta U, Fridirici Z. Advanced techniques in nonsurgical rhinoplasty. Facial Plast Surg Clin North Am. 2019;27(3):355–65.
52. Hanasono MM, Kridel RWH, Pastorek NJ, Glasgold MJ, Koch RJ. Correction of the soft tissue pollybeak using triamcinolone injection. Arch Facial Plast Surg. 2002;4(1):26–30.

Western Mediterranean Rhinoplasty

10

José Carlos Neves and Diego Arancibia Tagle

10.1 Introduction

In the last 20 years, there is a growing demand for facial plastic surgery, especially rhinoplasty, due to the big influence of social media and that young generations normalize the fact of undergoing a surgical procedure.

Due to migration and a growing number of ethnic groups in the big cities, the facial plastic surgeon increasingly will be confronted with patients with ethnic features who seek cosmetic surgery to improve self-esteem and aesthetic appearance [1]. Having said that, years ago many of these patients seek a Caucasian appearance, but now is more frequent that they want to preserve some of their ethnics features, so facial plastic surgeons will need to develop a clear understanding of facial aesthetics in the context of race, ethnicity, and culture. This insight is imperative to surgical planning and ultimately patient satisfaction in rhinoplasty [2].

Each of this groups present different characteristics which need a unique approach to solve their "problems."

The ethnic rhinoplasty (commonly used to refer to rhinoplasty in the non-Caucasian population) includes patients of African, East Asian (e.g., Korean, Chinese, Japanese, and Filipino), Middle Eastern (e.g., Persian/Iranian, and Arab), and Hispanic (e.g., Castilian or Mexican American) descent. As such, the term ethnic rhinoplasty is not a single entity, but rather a generic term with many inherent complexities [3].

The Mediterranean nose doesn't fit any of the groups described previously, because of their mix origins (Romans, Greeks, Spanish, Jews, Turks, Phoenicians,

J. C. Neves (✉)
MyFace Clinics and Academy, Lisbon, Portugal

D. A. Tagle
Hospital Son Espases, Palma de Mallorca, Spain

P. G. Giacomini (ed.), *Mediterranean Rhinoplasty*,
https://doi.org/10.1007/978-3-031-05551-5_10

and Egyptians), giving birth to a sharply defined race whose characteristics are still present today [4].

If we search on the literature, Daniel proposed a classification regarding the Hispanic nose, consisting of three nasal types: Castilian, Mexican American, and mestizo, and this was reinforced by Higuera and colleagues, who similarly identified three archetypes of Hispanic noses [5, 6].

The most similar archetype to the Mediterranean nose could be the Castilian profile that has a variable skin thickness that is thinner than the African American population. The radix is generally in a high to normal position with prominent nasal bones, and there is a high arched osseocartilaginous dorsum. Although the tip projection is similar to the Caucasian population, the tip width may appear slightly wide, and there is variability in the width of the base [2].

Boccieri [4] described a Mediterranean race. These include typical traits like dark coloring of the eyes and skin, black hair, a low-medium brow, strongly marked lineaments, and a prominent nose. The nose tends to be convex in profile with some thickness of the upper third in frontal view. The tip is often ptotic and the skin somewhat thick.

Apart from its particular anatomic features, however, the Mediterranean face is particularly expressive due to its marked lineaments and deep, penetrating gaze. An overly prominent conformation of the nose can therefore attract attention and impair this particular expressiveness by clashing with what can be regarded as the Mediterranean aesthetic canons.

The purpose of this chapter is to describe and analyze our casuistic, the surgical approach and management of the dorsum and tip, that will help us to obtain the best result possible in these kind of noses.

10.2 Casuistic Analysis

We analyze 1 (from June 2020 till May 2021) year of primary rhinoplasty in Western Mediterranean patients. We operated 161 patients, 112 females (69.6%) and 49 males (30.4%). The most common complaints were nasal dorsal humps (145 pts, 90.0%), ptotic tips (137 pts, 85.1%), tip asymmetries (67 pts, 41.6%), deviated pyramids (56 pts, 34.8%), and nasal trauma consequences (23 pts, 14.3%).

A tension nose with a droopy tip, most of them showing some degree of asymmetry, is the typical global diagnosis among the patient we do surgery in.

Regarding the approach, a closed approach was used in 2.1% of the patients (42 patients), while the open approach was the most frequent one, in 119 patients that represents 73.9%.

The actual intense discussion about the philosophy adopted to reduce the dorsal hump is something that we analyze also in our statistic. Since 2007 that the main author is performing conservative reduction of the nasal dorsal humps using foundation techniques, push-down or let-down (the preferred one), when the proper indication is made. We did preservation surgery in 110 patients (68.3%), 69 of which (62.7%) applying the Tetris concept, an intermediate strip approach, and 41 patients

(37.3%) were operated with a Modified Septal and Pyramid Adjustment and Replacement (SPAR, developed by Wilson Dewes based on the low strip approach championed by Cottle). The remaining 51 patients (31.7%) had no indication for preservation techniques, and we did a direct resection of the nasal dorsum, always structuring and rebuilding the pyramid framework.

10.3 Tension Nose

The tension nose concept has been described by many authors, each one of them with a minimal variant. Johnson et al. used the term "tension nose deformity" to "connote a high nasal dorsum, with stretching of the skin and soft tissue of the nose over a highly arched and narrow nasal vault" with "anterior and sometimes inferior displacement of the nasal tip cartilages" [7]. Gunter et al. describe the "excessive septum" in their description of the overprojected nose [8].

The "tension nose deformity" essentially combine the definitions mentioned before, includes any excessive external septum (dorsally or caudally) that stretches adjacent soft tissue [9].

To solve this kind of deformity we have two options, the first being a dorsal preservation approach or the classic joseph respective technique [10, 11].

10.3.1 Preservation

Conservative dorsal rhinoplasty, until recently called the push-down rhinoplasty, has been written about extensively. Since the end of the nineteenth century, some works have shown how to reduce a projected dorsum without impairing the surface anatomy of the nasal pyramid [12].

Even though the concept of dorsal preservation was already more than one-half of a century old, it was Cottle [13, 14] who popularized the "push-down technique" in 1946, combining several steps described by other surgeons. The principle of the technique was to preserve the continuity of the nasal dorsum by impacting the bony and cartilaginous hump around the keystone point.

The fundament goal of the conservative dorsal rhinoplasty is to preserve both the keystone area (K-area) and the continuity of the cartilaginous vault. This conservative approach avoids nasal valve collapse, with its adverse effects on respiration and the dorsal esthetic lines [15].

The main concept of the preservation techniques is to preserve the dorsum by addressing the middle wall, "the septum" and the lateral walls, the "nasal pyramid." The later can be addressed by a push or let-down technique.

Recently, Ferreira et al. [16] suggested a classification for the dorsal preservation approach, dividing it into two groups: Type I. Foundation Techniques, with dorsal impaction; Type II. Surface Techniques, with dorsal modulation.

Following this idea, in most of our cases, we perform a Foundation Technique (the Segmental Preservation Rhinoplasty) using the Tetris concept or the low strip approach, which is a modification of the SPAR [17]. It is also a Surface Technique that remodels the dorsal profile and lateral walls by sculpting with powered instruments (our preference) or rasps, and, in some cases, remodeling the cartilaginous vault with sutures or grafts, namely, spreader grafts.

In this chapter, we will describe the Segmental Preservation.

10.3.1.1 Lateral Wall

The pushdown technique mainly consists in a septal slice resection followed by lateral and transverse osteotomies, with subsequent impaction of the bony vault downward into the pyriform aperture (Fig. 10.1).

The let-down technique shares the septal resection but is followed by resecting a portion of the ascending frontal process of the maxilla. Then, the nasal pyramid is moved downward into the frontal process of the maxilla (Fig. 10.1) [15].

The let-down technique is our preference for approaching the lateral nasal wall because it gives us better mobilization of the pyramid and avoids bone impaction into the nasal cavity.

To create the flattening of the dorsal profile, the lateral walls must show some plasticity. To achieve that goal, the lateral articulation between the upper lateral cartilage (ULC) and the nasal bones in its posterior cephalic border can be released so that the "Lateral Wall Split Maneuver movement is facilitated. Goksel and Saban [18] also described this maneuver as the ballerina maneuver. After the lateral bony wedge is removed, we dissect the inner surface of the lateral in a subperiosteal

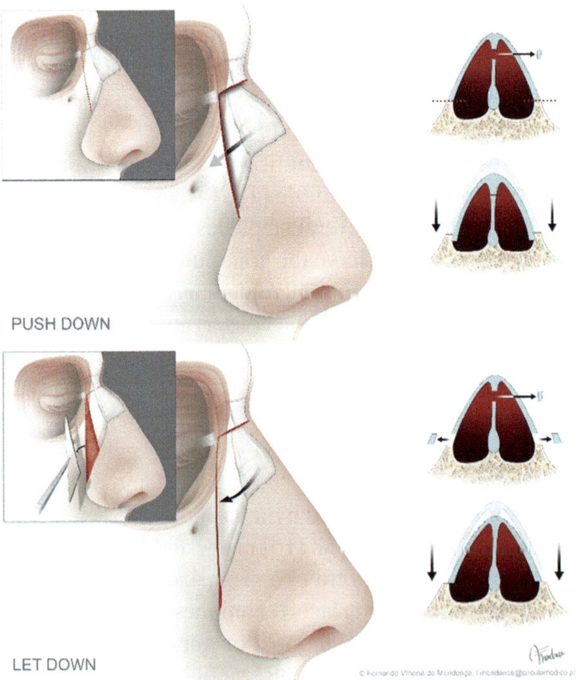

Fig. 10.1 Artist's sketch of push-down technique and the let-down technique

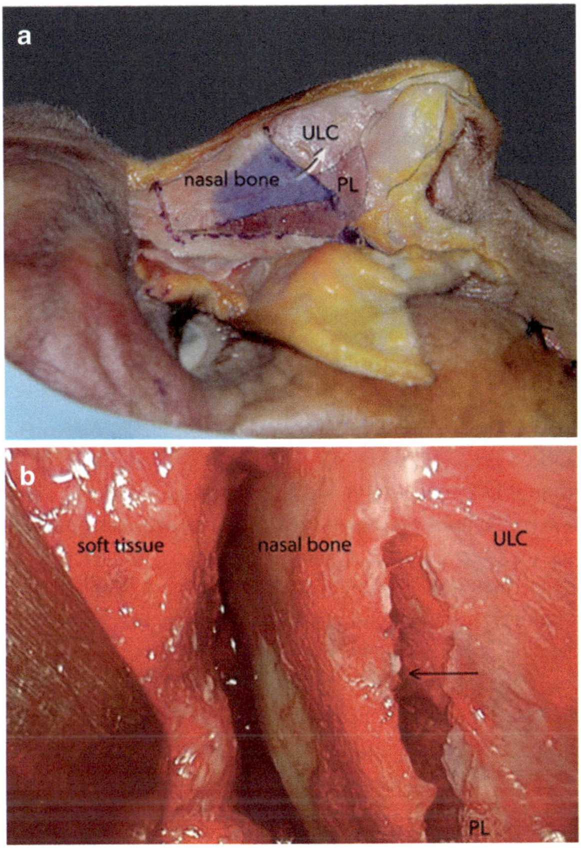

Fig. 10.2 The lateral articulation of the ULCs and pyriform ligament (PL) with the lateral bony wall must be released (**a**—light blue area) to facilitate the lateral wall "front splits maneuver" (**b**—arrow)

plane, to protect ULC and soft tissues. The pyriform ligaments are also liberated. This dissection will allow for an anterior and caudal sliding movement of the middle third of the lateral wall (Fig. 10.2) [15].

10.3.1.2 Middle Wall

Conceptually, in preservation techniques, the septum can be addressed lower in its base, keeping the attachment with the cartilaginous vault intact bringing all the structure down as a unit, and it can be addressed higher at the junction with the ULCs, pushing down exclusively the cartilaginous vault. It can also be addressed splitting the septum in a strategical medial position, bringing the ULCs and the remained attached septum down. Each one of these approaches has its pros and cons [12].

The main author has developed one modification of the let-down technique with a septal intermediate resection, the split preservation rhinoplasty [15] that showed the real advantage of the intermediate resection in stabilizing the rhinion position by putting a suture from our free anterior dorsal septal cartilaginous flap to the basal posterior stabile septum. In fact, this is a critical stitch for predictably keeping the

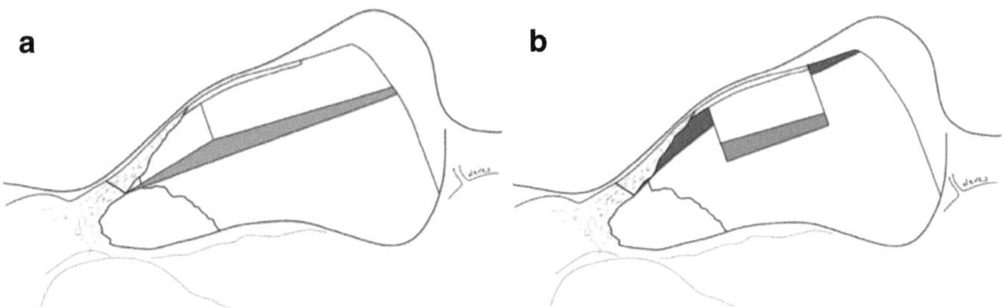

Fig. 10.3 The intermediate septal approach. (**a**) The intermediate split, where a fragment of septum is removed from the caudal border of the septum till the perpendicular plate at the level of the transverse osteotomy. (**b**) The segmental Tetris concept, where three segments are created with the key player being the Tetris block. The common gray area in both images is exactly at the same position

rhinion in the desired position with great accuracy. The "Tetris concept" is an evolution of the split preservation technique, with some advantages, which include suturing the free anterior septum (the Tetris block) in two vectors, craniocaudal and posteroanterior, conferring more stability to the pyramid in two axes and preserving a natural caudal septal strut, which allows us to control the supratip area and keep the caudal border and its relationship with the anterior nasal spine stable. As a general concept, these two techniques share the most relevant factor, the design of an intermediate fragment of cartilage below the rhinion to be anchored and consequently creating stability to the final dorsal profile (Fig. 10.3).

For more details of the surgical technique, we invite you to read the original articles "The Split Preservation Rhinoplasty, The Vitruvian Man Split Maneuver" and "The Segmental Preservation Rhinoplasty, The Split Tetris concept." [19]

The Tetris concept is a modified intermediate septal resection consisting of the following steps (Fig. 10.4). A 5–8 mm rectangular piece of septal cartilage will be designed below the cartilaginous hump in between the most prominent point of the hump (at or slightly caudal to the rhinion) and the caudal border of the ULC (the W point). The block is defined by two lines perpendicular and one horizontal to the dorsum (Fig. 10.5a). We prefer the block (quadrangular or rectangular) figure compared with a triangular shape, for instance. This is because it is designed to achieve a more stable structure, and once we have stabilized a vertical and a horizontal vector, we can avoid tilting of the free pyramid in the coronal and sagittal planes.

Two new shapes will be designed; one below the rectangular block and another below the bony hump. The shape below the block must have the height that we intend to decrease the dorsal projection. The shape of the excised area will usually be trapezoidal because the reduction will be bigger under the most projected point of the hump and less in the more caudal region. Below the bony hump, we draw a triangular excision area with its vertex at the level of the transverse osteotomies. The marked areas will be excised, which creates the space for the descending dorsum (Fig. 10.5b). Using a 15 blade, the caudal, posterior, and cephalic borders of the rectangular block are cut. It is essential to free the cartilaginous hump. When pushed

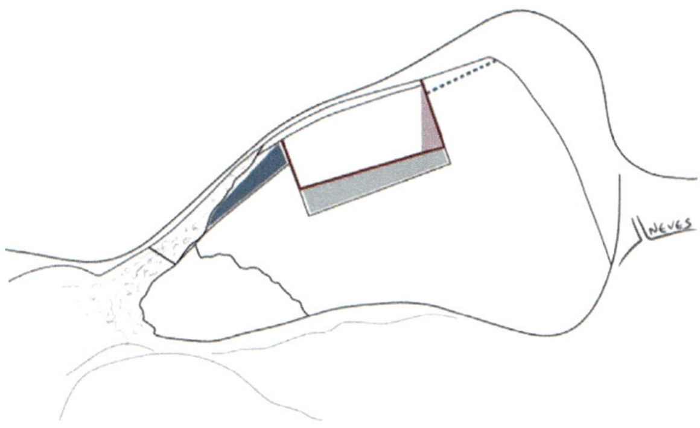

Fig. 10.4 The Tetris concept. A 5- to 8-mm height block is designed in between the WASA and the dorsal hump most prominent point (red line); a trapezoid figure is drawn bellow the block, it represents the amount of the hump to be reduced (gray trapezoid); a triangular figure is drawn below the bone pyramid, from the block till the lateral wall transverse osteotomy level to facilitate the push-down movement (blue triangle); to avoid overlapping the caudal aspect of the Tetris block with the natural caudal septal strut, we trim a triangular portion of the block cartilage (purple triangle); to adjust the new dorsal profile level a trimming of the anterior border of the caudal septal strut must be performed (blue dots)

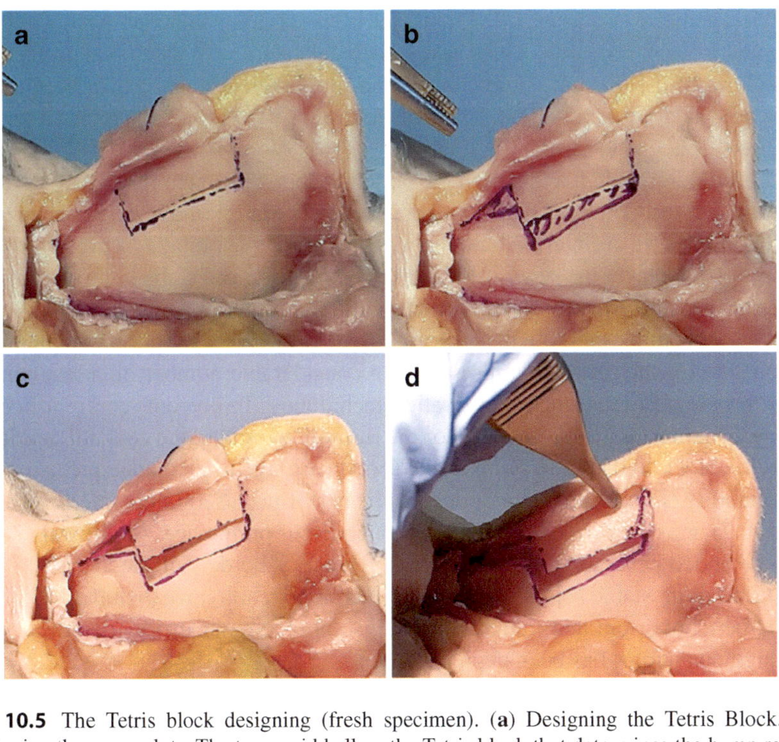

Fig. 10.5 The Tetris block designing (fresh specimen). (**a**) Designing the Tetris Block. (**b**) Designing the space slots. The trapezoid bellow the Tetris block that determines the hump reduction, and the triangular below the bony pyramid. (**c**) The Tetris block and the pyramid are free and can be repositioned. (**d**) A triangle to be resected was marked in the caudal border of the Tetris block to avoid overlapping with the natural caudal strut

down, the block overlaps with the stable septal cartilage, and we create a saddle nose below the UCL caudal border. Next, the triangular segment below the bony hump is removed using scissors. The cut always starts at a tangent to the undersurface of the bony vault to avoid an excess resection that can lead to a radix step. We initially remove a small triangular piece, and then perform the push down maneuver and analyze how much we have deprojected. If not enough, we go in again and remove another triangular slice until reaching the desired level. In some cases, we only remove cartilage, whereas in other cases we have to remove a small piece of bone, for which scissors are often necessary as well. Rarely, we use a baby rongeur, which we try to avoid, because it can create a bigger space than is needed and the radix step will appear as a consequence (Fig. 10.5c).

Now, the hump can be reduced and the cartilage block overlaps the stable basal septal cartilage; and because we have isolated the Tetris block we press it down, and by a rotational movement, posterior and caudal, we can create the side splits effect, thereby eliminating any residual dorsal hump. We are ready to remove the trapezoid slot, and thus create the space for our Tetris block. The rotational movement of the block, downwards and caudal, creates an overlap of a small portion of cartilage of its caudal border with the caudal septum strut we have left intact. Thus, we trim the caudal border of the block so that it fits the slot created perfectly (Fig. 10.5d). This movement brings the pieces down into their spaces in a perfect match resembling the Tetris game, so we have called it the Tetris preservation concept. At this point in the operation, the surgeon decides how satisfied they are with the dorsal profile line. Sometimes, if the dorsum is too convex or a more concave shape is desired then a Tetris split is done at this time. The first suture of 5-0 PDS is placed between the posterior aspect of the caudal border of the Tetris block to the caudal septal strut, which stretches and helps to flatten the dorsum. This movement resembles what we performed in the Cottle push down technique, and because of this here we can see a mini-Cottle, using an intermediate approach, with the advantage of preserving the stability of the rest of the septum. After performing this suture, the hump is reduced. Nevertheless, immediately we observe a small relapse of the hump that will slightly increase with time, the so-called spring effect (Fig. 10.6c). This phenomenon is responsible for the residual hump seen in a considerable number of cases, being a major problem of the dorsal preservation techniques. To prevent recurrent humps, we use a rhinion suture. At the level of the rhinion, we suture the cephalic border of the Tetris block to the underlying stable septal cartilage to guarantee precision and predictability (Fig. 10.6d). This suture can be performed as a simple interrupted one (Fig. 10.7) or as a figure-of-eight stitch, which is our preference. Additional sutures must be added between the caudal and the posterior borders of the Tetris block to the surrounding stable septal cartilage. To increase stability, we include the contralateral perichondrium and mucosa. With this approach, our incidence of recurrent cartilaginous humps has been negligible.

At this point, the dorsum has been brought down to its ideal position, except at the level of the caudal septal strut, which was previously preserved. In fact, one can often end up with a slight polybeak appearance. The anterior border of this natural strut must be addressed, and most often it is trimmed to achieve the desired dorsal

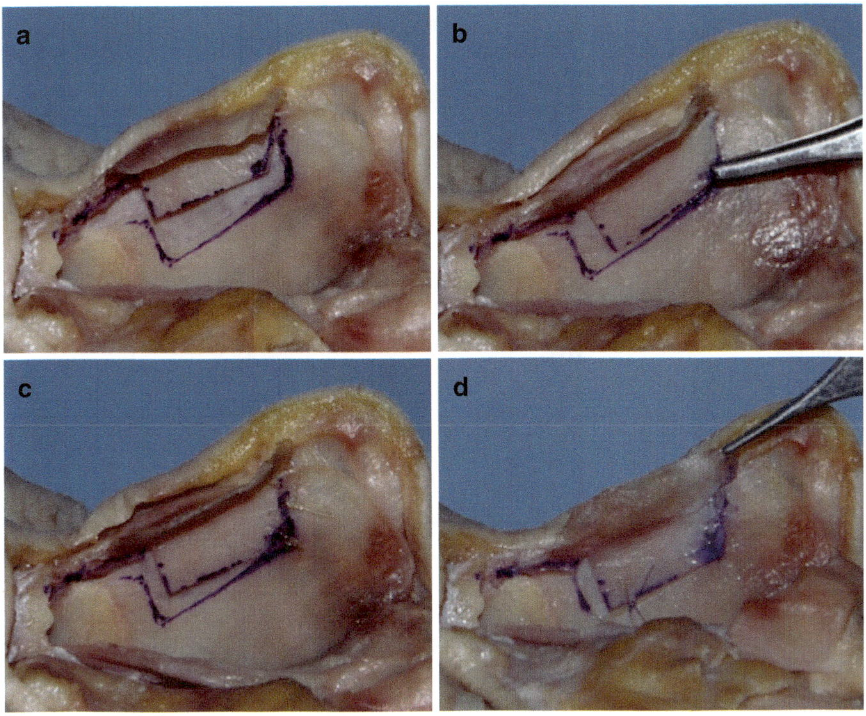

Fig. 10.6 The Tetris concept (fresh specimen). (**a**) The space slots are prepared to allow the push-down movement. (**b**) Adjusting the Tetris block, the profile is checked. (**c**) Two PDS 5-0 sutures have stabilized the caudal border of the block; the stabilization of this border of the block is paramount to avoid pyramid lateralization. Note the spring effect bellow the rhinion, a gap is created in the cephalic aspect of the space slot below the rhinion. (**d**) The 5-0 PDS suture was placed below the rhinion. The stabilization of the dorsum in a predictable final nasal dorsum position is probably the greatest achievement of this technique

height (Fig. 10.8b). Alternatively, it can be left partially at its maximum height to act like a strut to the tip or to support the stabilization of a septal extension graft (Fig. 10.8d). In deviated noses, one can suture the overlapped cartilages side by side without resecting the trapezoid piece. The rectangular block is sutured on the opposite side to the deviation so it can compensate.

In a nasal dorsal hump, the cartilaginous component tends to be convex. Even after hump reduction, a curved line can persist that creates a small hump in between the rhinion and the supratip region; in some cases, it is essential to flatten this cartilaginous curve. One or two additional vertical cuts are made into the septal block converting it from a single entity into two or three new blocks that will be brought caudally into rotational movement. The creation of multiple pieces allows the dorsum to flex, which resembles the spreading of fingers. This movement brings the pieces down into their spaces in a perfect match resembling the popular game and thus the name—the split Tetris preservation rhinoplasty. The more the block pieces are moved apart, the more concave the profile becomes [12].

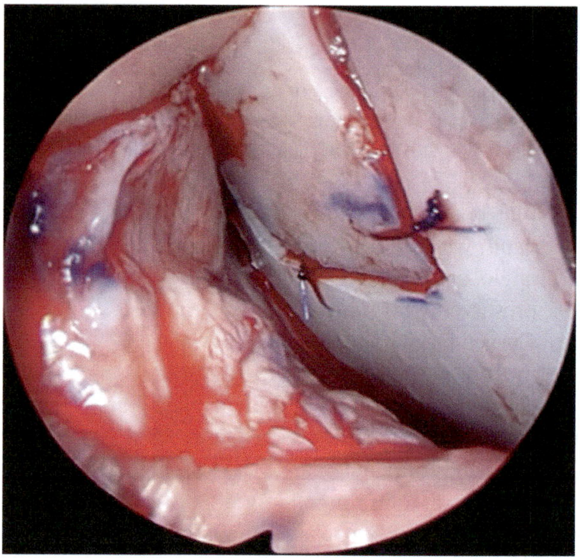

Fig. 10.7 The Tetris block. Intraoperative picture showing the two most important block sutures. Additional sutures will be added to complete stabilization. (Note that the stabilization of the two borders that are perpendicular promotes an affective stability to the pyramid, eventually like no other dorsal preservation technique)

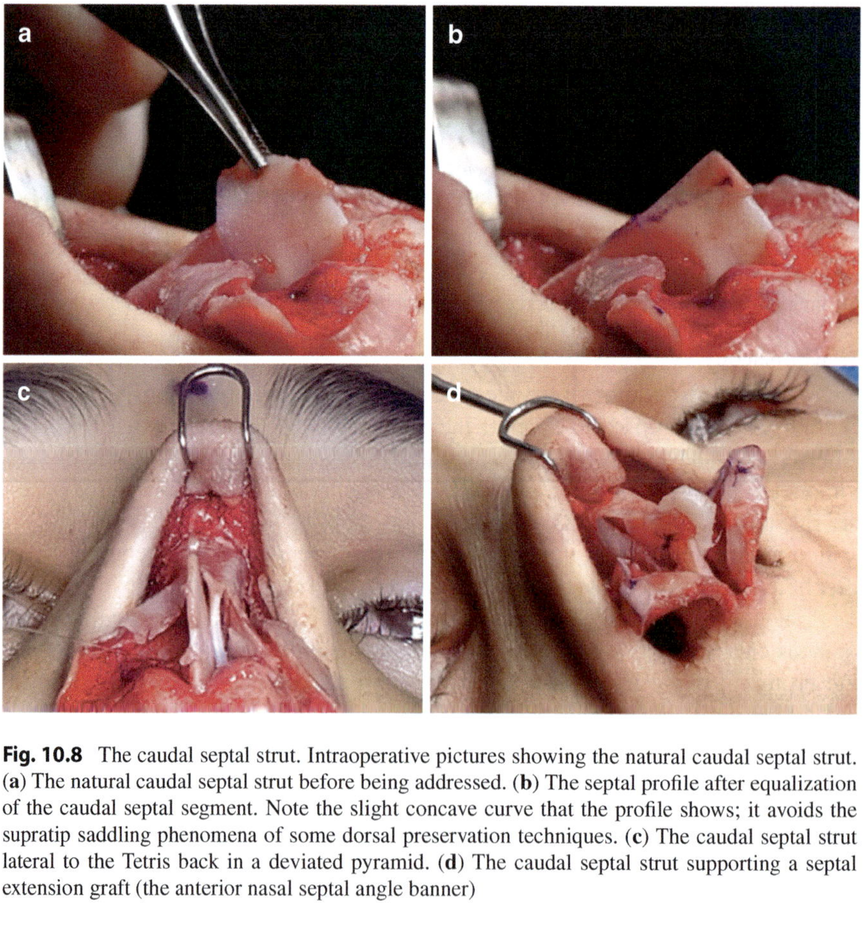

Fig. 10.8 The caudal septal strut. Intraoperative pictures showing the natural caudal septal strut. (**a**) The natural caudal septal strut before being addressed. (**b**) The septal profile after equalization of the caudal septal segment. Note the slight concave curve that the profile shows; it avoids the supratip saddling phenomena of some dorsal preservation techniques. (**c**) The caudal septal strut lateral to the Tetris back in a deviated pyramid. (**d**) The caudal septal strut supporting a septal extension graft (the anterior nasal septal angle banner)

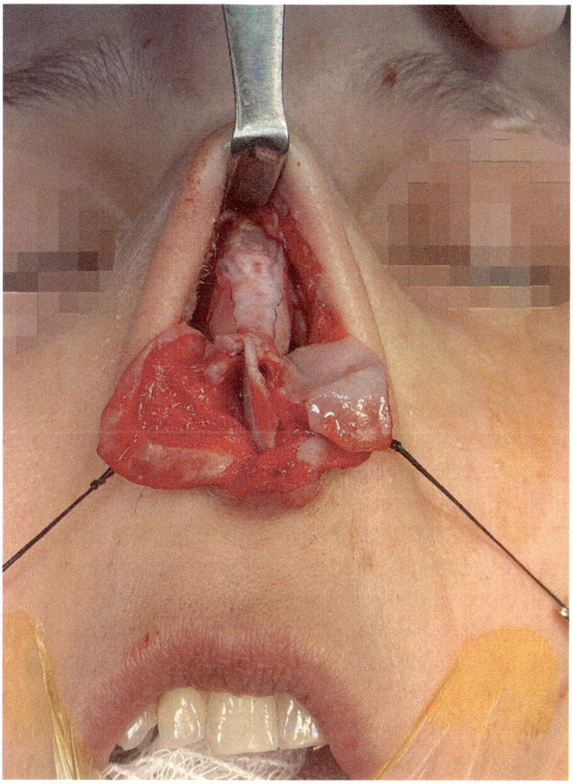

Fig. 10.9 A burr was used to sculpt the bony vault; A continuous suture was placed to reduce the cartilaginous vault width

Surface Technique

After defining the new position of the dorsum, it is time to refine the shape. In most cases, we use burrs (following the "precision rhinoplasty" concept developed by Emre Ilhan) but rasps or piezo can also be used. The advantages of using burrs is their capacity to achieve smoother bony surfaces by including the capacity of reshaping the cartilaginous framework (Fig. 10.9).

We analyze the profile dorsal line and, if needed, as in the S-shape dorsal lines, we sculpt it. The lateral wall is also specifically addressed in irregularities, broad bony pyramids, and palpable transitions in the let-down osteotomies. Eventually, in the case of broader noses, a paramedian green stick osteotomy, using a Piezo, is performed.

With respect to the cartilaginous vault, in some cases the width needs to be reduced, and we use sutures to achieve this (Fig. 10.9), while in others, irregularities need to be addressed with grafts being a possible solution such as the placement of a spreader graft in a depressed ULC, mainly seen in crooked noses, where we use the modified SPAR.

10.3.2 Resection

When the nose does not have the ideal characteristics for a preservation approach, we prepare the resection of the hump and a consequent reconstruction of the new dorsal profile.

The cartilaginous vault is preferentially dissected in a supra-perichondral plane, preserving the continuity of the perichondrium with the pyriform densification found at the perichondrium periosteum fusion, part of the pyriform attachment, to keep the LKA stability and achieve a softer transition and a beautiful and stable eyebrow-tip aesthetic line. The approaches that look to preserve or resect the dorsum aim for the same objective but in an opposite manner. In the first one, the keystone area and the eyebrow tip line is preserved and the LKA is released to allow the flattening movement of the dorsum, whilst in the second, the keystone area is sacrificed (the stability of the upper third depends mainly of a stable LKA). The dissection proceeds in a sub-periosteal plane. The periosteum is incised immediately after the pyriform aperture (Fig. 10.10).

The ULCs are separated from the quadrangular cartilage, creating three independent cartilages. Laterally the ULCs are separated from the inner surface of the bony pyramid up to the level of the new dorsum. It is important to keep the rest of the LKA intact, as mentioned. At this point, we may decide to keep the perichondrium attached to the ULC or to elevate and preserve it to be sutured as a blanked over the rebuilt middle third (Fig. 10.11). The excess of cartilaginous septum is removed with straight scissors or a scalpel (Fig. 10.12). The excessive osseous hump is removed with an accurate ultrasonic device, or with a 3 mm osteotome, defining the fracture lines on each side of the hump to be removed (we always avoid using a wide Ruby osteatome). In smaller humps (even if it can be used in all humps), sculpting the bone is also an option (with powered devices or rasps). An open roof is created without sacrificing the ULCs.

Even in dorsal resections, we like to try and preserve the ULCs and spare the septal cartilage by tailoring spread flaps. The ULCs with perichondrium show an

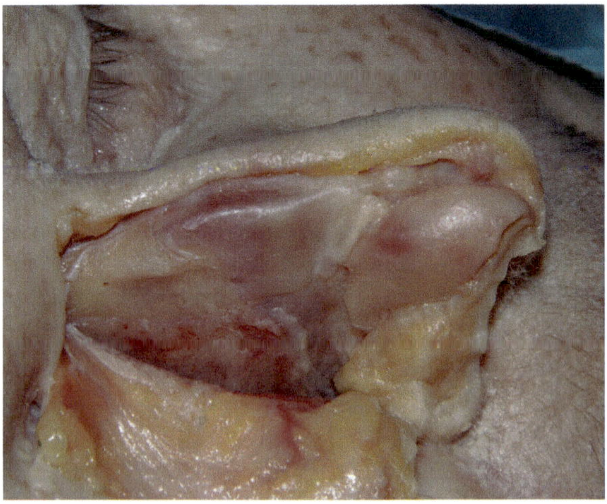

Fig. 10.10 Supra-perichondral and sub-periostal dissection in a cadaveric human specimen

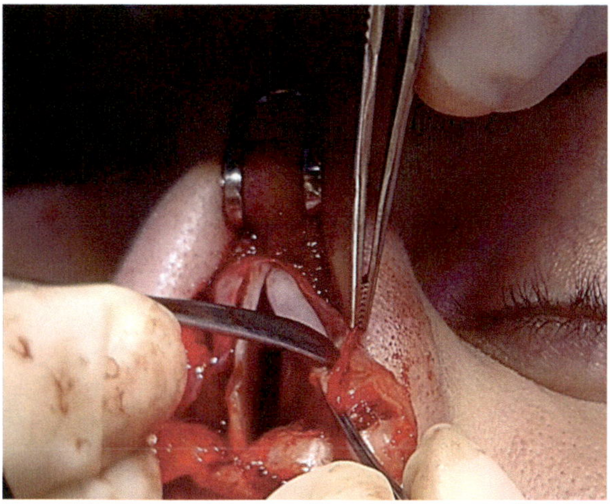

Fig. 10.11 The ULC perichondrium is elevated

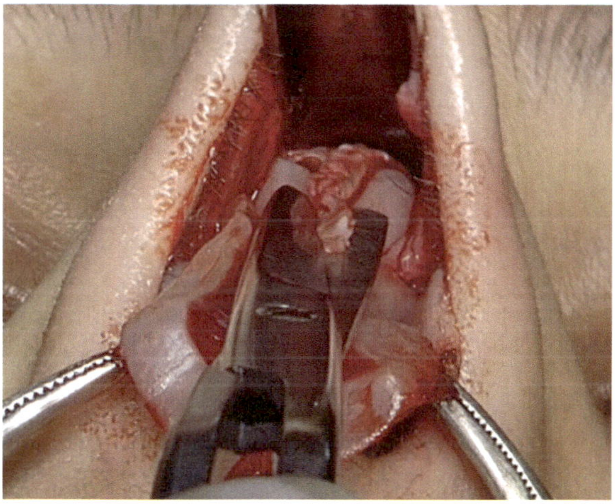

Fig. 10.12 The excess of the cartilaginous septum is removed with a straight scissors

interesting resilience to sutures and a useful tension when rebuilding a stable and elastic middle third. Proceeding with spreader flaps (Fig. 10.13) or grafts (Figs. 10.14 and 10.15), the first 5.0 PDS suture is placed with the ULC under tension towards caudal, to get stabilization, definition, and symmetry. The new mid third should be wider at the rhinion area when compared to the W point. When following this principle, the spreaders must shape as well as placing the sutures at the spreader flaps.

The osteotomies must mobilize the bone to a proper position with a predictable stability closing the open roof. Regarding dissection, our preference is to elevate the periosteum in a wide approach exposing the nasofacial groove. This allows direct vision when performing the lateral wall osteotomies and the ideal exposure to sculp the basal width of the nose, as described by Emre Ilhan in his "precision rhinoplasty" concept. We commonly shape the lateral wall with a burr to smooth any irregularities. The nasofacial groove is also shaped. An oblique osteotomy is

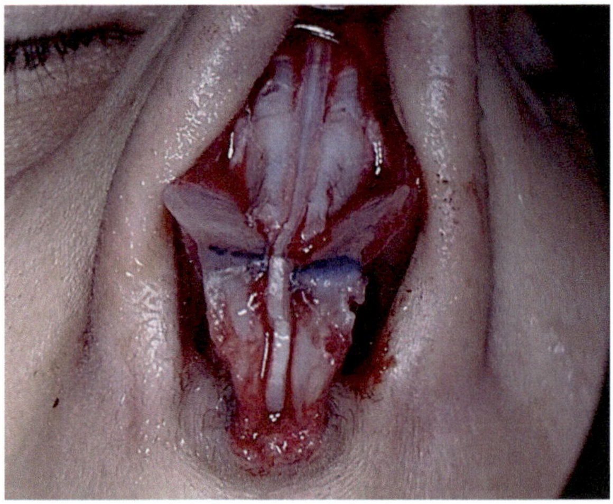

Fig. 10.13 Spreader flaps

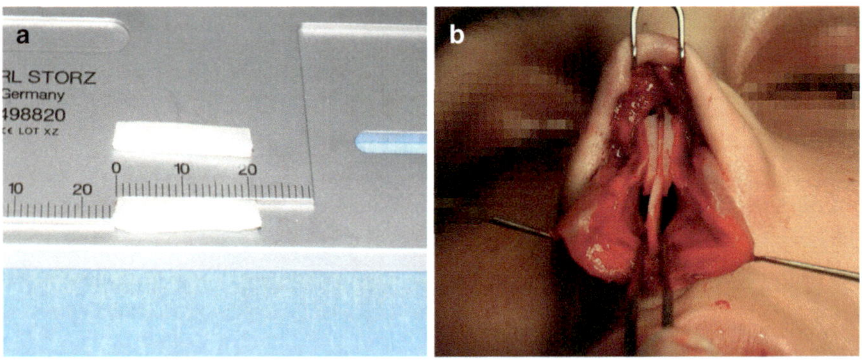

Fig. 10.14 (**a**) Designing the spreader grafts. (**b**) Spreader grafts in closed approach

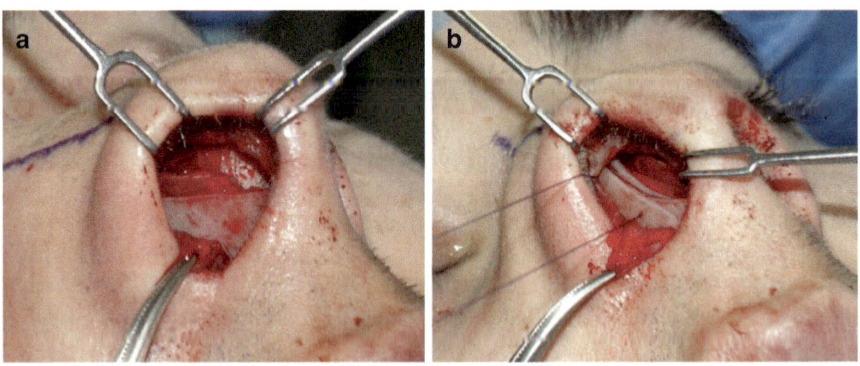

Fig. 10.15 (**a**, **b**) Placing the spreader grafts in a closed approach rhinoplasty

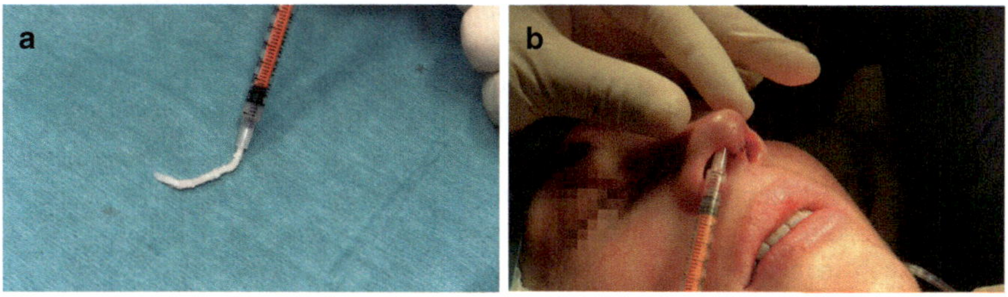

Fig. 10.16 (**a**) Cartilage gel. (**b**) Gel being placed at the nasal tip

designed following the eyebrow tip line. Then a low lateral osteotomy is placed with an ultrasonic device (or eventually with a 3 mm osteotome). A green stick fracture is created uniting the two previous osteotomies.

With the osteotomies performed and the cartilaginous vault rebuilt, it is time for refinements. The burr can be used to smooth the angles of bones and cartilages; some additional sutures may be necessary, and some camouflage considered such as cartilage gel, bony dust, fascia, or periosteum (Fig. 10.16).

10.4 Nasal Tip Surgery

10.4.1 Tip Dynamics and Support Mechanism

The nasal tip is probably the richest chapter in rhinoplasty procedures book. Its anatomical variations, compound anatomy, its relationship with the middle third of the nose and lip, and how these tissues behave post-surgically as well as many other factors that are involved in creating a pleasing and functional tip are responsible for that.

Jack Sheen was one of the main contributors to this subject, since the mid-70s, and has helped us understand this complex anatomy. It was he who described the ideal tip shape as two equilateral geodesic triangles with a common base formed by a line connecting both domes, among other characteristics [20].

Toriumi, in 2006, [21] introduced the concept of nasal tip contour as a series of surface highlights and shadows created by underlying anatomical high and low points. He described that a favorable nasal tip contour has a horizontal orientation with a shadow in the supratip area that continues into the supra-alar regions. There is a smooth transition between different subunits without a clear line of demarcation. The nasal tip will have highlights and shadows in specific areas depending on the underlying tip structure that we should preserve or modify, depending on each case, which will give a natural and pleasing non-operated look.

In 2012, Çakir [22–24] introduced the concept of polygons for analyzing the aesthetic lines and volumes of the nose, based on drawings and sculptures that he developed throughout his career as a rhinoplasty surgeon. These geometric distributions of the fundamental structure of the nose will have an important effect on the nasal external appearance, achieving a combination of shadows and highlights, with very good aesthetic results.

Apart from these authors, plenty of articles have been published by many surgeons regarding the management of special areas of the tip.

Understanding the domal segment was the main focus on developing tip plasty techniques. The Lateral Crura (LC) was mainly seen as a structure to be reduced cephalically, sometimes dramatically, in order to rotate, reduce volume, and refine the tip. Such maneuvers have the tendency of creating unsatisfactory outcomes, such as ala retractions, pinched tips, supratip fullness, irregularities, and external valve impairment. It is clear today that the LC work represents a fundamental and delicate step in tip plasty.

In an aesthetic tip, the caudal margin of the lateral crus lies close to the same level as the cephalic margin [25]. In addition, the caudal margin of the dome should be positioned above the cephalic margin of the dome [21].

The inversion of the caudal border promotes a reduction of the alar rim support which leads to a break of continuous light from the tip to the alar lobule, creating an unattractive appearance of an isolated tip. Functionally, the external valve can be compromised.

10.4.2 Lateral Crura Control

- ***Defining the Lower Lateral Cartilage New Architecture***

  The tip position is determined, and the rest of the process will follow this tridimensional decision. We design the length and width of the LC, considering the desired dome position. This point will work as the anterior vertex of the elliptical vestibular ring. We stand at the head of the patient and create traction of the two LLC with two forceps to achieve better symmetry. The new caudal and cephalic domal point are marked; and since, we are creating tension forward in the LC, we lateralize the new domes (a generous LCS), on some occasions up to 10 mm. Having defined the domal points, we mark the new domes. A cephalic line, from the Intermediate Crus (IC) to the LC is marked taking into consideration that: the domes should have 4–5 mm, the intermediate segment of the LC should have 7–9 mm, which means that aggressive reductions must be avoided in order to prevent lobular pinching, alar retraction, asymmetries and irregularities, hyperrotation and loss of tip support, and an eventual valve collapse (Figs. 10.17 and 10.18).

  The circumstantial cephalic excess will be trimmed or occasionally used to create a turn- in flap. When indicated, the reduction of the LC in the short axis permits rotation and adjustment of the ideal Short Axis Angle [26].
- ***Cephalic Oblique Dome Suture***

  The domal creation suture is determinant for the final result.

  The main goal is to evert the caudal margin of the LC and elevate the caudal point of the new dome position [27]. The suture will be placed in the cephalic third of the LC and IC. The entry point is 1–2 mm below the new domal line at

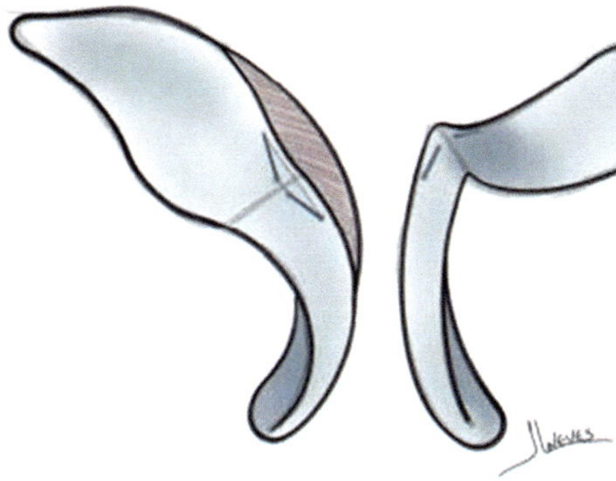

Fig. 10.17 Cephalic oblique domal suture: The suture will be placed in the cephalic third of the LC and IC. Two oblique lines will be designed lateral and medial to the new dome with the entry point 1–2 mm below the new domal line starting from medial to lateral. Then the suture runs over the surface around 4–5 mm oblique to the long axis towards the LC cephalic margin till it reenters as close as possible to the cartilage's cephalic border; it crosses the IC at the same level. The knot is placed in the medial surface of the IC

the junction of the medial third with the intermediate third of the medial surface of the IC. It will exit at the same level in the outer surface of the LC. The suture now runs at the surface around 4–5 mm oblique to the long axis towards the LC cephalic margin till it reenters as close as possible to the cartilage's cephalic border. It crosses the IC at the same level. The knot is placed in the medial surface of the IC (Fig. 10.17). When the knot is tight, the cephalic margins of the LC and IC become closer and leave the rest of the dome completely free. We can observe the elevation of the caudal border of the LC medial segment and the creation of a smooth concavity at the surface. The domal caudal point is also elevated.

If needed, we add one or two hemitransdomal sutures, as described by Dosanjh et al. [28] to increase this effect, and, due to the LCS we increased the intrinsic tension of the LC with consequent stretching of the four cartilaginous segments. Nevertheless, and, because we have performed a generous lateral steal, the domes fall slightly lateral and posterior, which makes it obligatory to reposition it in the proper previously defined dome position.

10.4.2.1 7X Lateral Crura Suture

As already described, the two lateral segments (the lateral segment of the LC and the AC segment) are often not directly addressed during tip plasty. When facing favorable anatomy (LC axis, intrinsic curvatures, LC-AC joint position), performing maneuvers in the anterior segments is usually sufficient. However, on some occasions less favorable anatomy may represent a real challenge, in controlling LC bulging and symmetry, controlling the supra-alar region and protecting the inner nasal valve. It is valid for most patients in cosmetic surgery that present overly wide nasal tips, and very often with asymmetries. As already described, the LC malposition concept led to the development of LC transposition techniques, usually with the

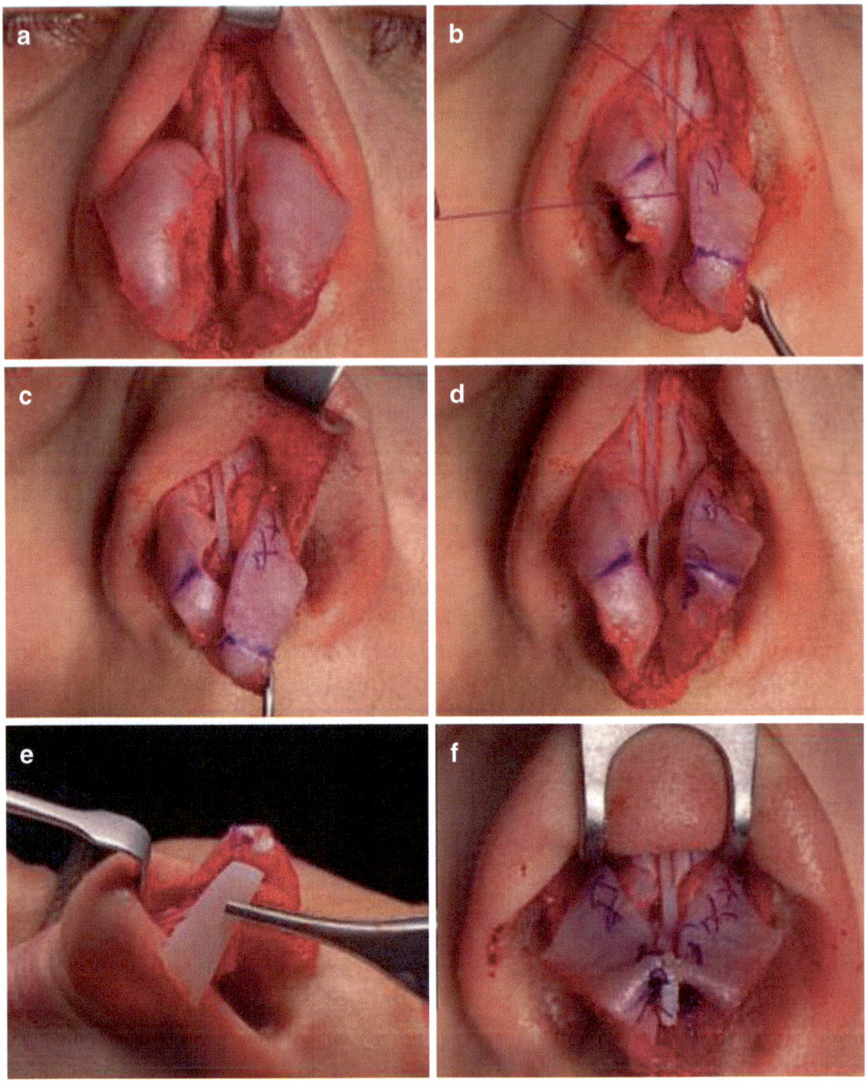

Fig. 10.18 Surgical sequence: (**a**) The Bulbous tip, LC crura with convex long axis and cephalic convexity of the short axis. (**b**) The new LLC anatomy was designed. LCS and turn-in flap (right crus); the 7 creation of the suture at the LC. (**c**) The 7X suture finalized with X appearance on the LC surface. (**d**) Left dome after the cephalic oblique suture. (**e**) Defining the ANSA banner orientation. (**f**) interdomal—ANSA banner suture stabilizing the tip. Note this suture follows the domal suture path. The LC is flat with the correct short axis orientation, the new LC medial segment is slightly concave meeting the dome, the LC caudal margins are everted and the caudal domal points are diverging

support of grafts (struts and battens), which are in fact powerful and effective maneuvers. However, we prefer to see the problem as an undesired LC surface or/ and LC-AC junction anatomy and an unfavorable vestibular ring curvature (wide ellipse) and try to correct the defect with conservative measures remodeling the cartilage surfaces and stretching the lateral component of the ring (narrowing the ellipse) bringing it to a more caudal position (correcting alar malposition), before considering more aggressive ones.

In convex LC surface, remodeling the dome region with sutures may lead to undesired side effects. Mispositioned domal sutures (mainly if no tension on the cartilage is created) may bring the two lateral segments medially and eventually posteriorly and collapse the LC-AC junction. It leads to obvious functional and aesthetic consequences. It is imperative then to also correct the anatomy of this region. By promoting the LCS (lateral crura steal) and LCT (lateral crura tensioning) we solve a great number of these issues but in marked convexities we may need to address the lateral segments structure, once the cephalic oblique domal sutures (or other domal suture) are not expected to correct these segments' anatomy. This is the same with severe concavities or irregular surfaces.

We have already mentioned the effectiveness of Grubber's sutures to correct convex cartilage surfaces. The long arms of the suture will be placed over the convex surface so it can become flat or concave, while the short arms will stay over the concave surface. We must avoid creating any relevant distortion with the suture short arms that in fact can increase concavity. We used this concept to develop our suture, the 7X suture (Fig. 10.19).

The horizontal mattress suture may present two problems. (1) The two suture passages in the concave surface will increase the concavity, that is why we should reduce their length as much as possible, and then create two short arms. In bulbous tips, where the two axis are convex, by placing a Gruber's suture to flatten the long axis we can increase the outer surface convexity of the short axis. (2) When a larger cartilage surface needs to be controlled, the use of a longer suture can distort the anatomy. As an example, in a bulbous tip, with convexity in both axis, when placing a larger mattress suture over the long axis it is difficult to determine the strength of the suture to get a flat surface, sometimes ending up with a non-desirable concave surface in between the two suture entrances of the longer arms. We can perform several mattress sutures (isolated or continuous [29]) but we may still encounter some of these problems. At the short axis, we can see an impairment of the convexity since the short arms act at the concave surface (Fig. 10.19a, b).

One solution to solve this suture weakness is by splitting the distance into three or four segments and crossing the sutures so no distortion will be created in any axis. Since we aim to have a strong and flat LC, we often perform the turn-in flap maneuver before we run the 7X suture. The goal of the turn-in flap (apart from opposing convexity against convexity or concavity against concavity helping to flatten the cartilage) is to have a thicker unit of cartilage to support the forces of the suture better, and mainly at the intermediate segment.

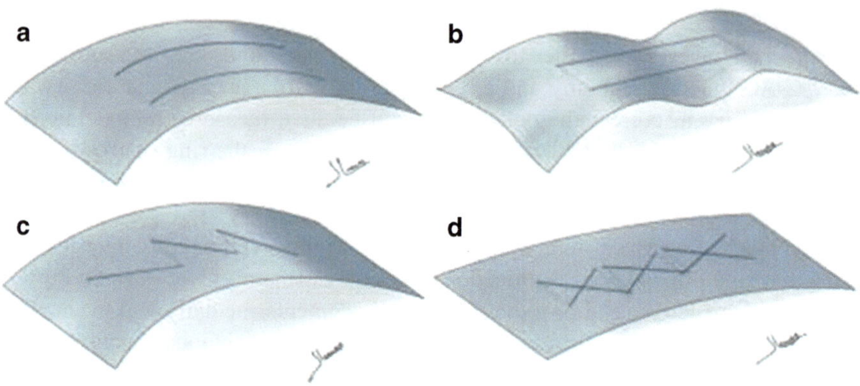

Fig. 10.19 (**a–d**) Based on the horizontal mattress suture and how it affects cartilage surfaces (Gruber), we developed the 7X suture. In overly convex LC a strategy to get a flat surface must be decided. In larger distances, the horizontal mattress suture does not accurately control the curvatures, and sometimes creates a concavity in between the sutures long axis entrances and forms or increases the convexity of the short axis. To avoid this, we split the forces into 3 or 4 points. The first passage creates a figure of 7, the second one an X, can deliver a flat surface with great accuracy

The entry point of the suture will be at the inner surface of the LC intermediate segment. The LC anterior segment is defined by the domal sutures, as already described. It runs slightly oblique to the long axis towards lateral for 3–5 mm over the outer surface. The suture again goes to the inner surface of the LC. We pass the suture to the outer surface around 1–2 mm (not bigger to avoid short axis distortions) from the previous exit in a perpendicular fashion regarding the same axis. These two suture lines, the outer oblique and inner perpendicular, form a seven-figure. We repeat this movement till we achieve the desired level of the LC lateral. On some occasions we include the first AC. Around three to four figures of seven's are created (Fig. 10.19c).

We start the way back repeating the same concept. The outer oblique suture lines will cross and create an X-figure. The inner perpendicular suture lines will remain parallel to themselves. By placing this suture, we can create a flat segment of the cartilage regarding the long axis with great accuracy without compromising the short one. The X shape in fact flattens both axis. In cases of concave LC, the X will be seen at the inner surface and the two parallel lines at the outer surface.

In cases of irregular surfaces (convex, concave), the concept must be adapted. The same when both axis are compromised. It is a very flexible suture that can be used in several circumstances (Fig. 10.18).

We use the 7X sutures in more delicate conditions of the LC, specifically in overly wide tips and considerable irregular LC surfaces (Image 4), where the rest of the maneuvers do not work properly. In the vast majority of cases, we anticipate the need of this step; however, we can decide to perform the suture at any stage of the surgery.

10.4.3 Midline Structuring

When we talk about midline structuring, we immediately think about giving the best and most stable support to the tip, so that we can obtain a long-lasting functional and aesthetic result.

10.4.3.1 ANSA Banner

We will stabilize the tip on a SEG (septal extension graft) to bring the lateralized domes forward and create LC tension, but we prefer to use a partial SEG, the ANSA banner. Banner because conceptually it works as a long strip of cartilage bearing the whole tip structure in a projected position. The partial SEGs are historically being used for many purposes, and specifically the anterior septal angle extension graft [30–34]. To prevent postoperative progressive descent of the nasal tip and to construct a permanent nasal tip, Byrd et al. [31] proposed the construction of a rigid skeletal connection between the septum and nasal tip cartilages. They published a series of 20 patients who were at risk of losing the nasal tip projection. Nasal tip stiffness and thickening of the septum in the nasal valve area where the major drawbacks of the paired SEG. In the following years, many have published modifications of this SEG with very good results regarding the projection, but with the inability to solve the lack of tip mobility.

We use the ANSA banner to support the LCT and avoid frozen tips as much as possible. It is a trapezoid structure, 10–15 mm long and 3–5 mm at the anterior aspect and 5–8 mm at the posterior aspect, which makes it a low cartilage consumer. Shape and size can be adapted to the available donor cartilage always taking into consideration that the graft is strong enough to resist to forces of retrodisplacement, overrotation or deprojection, depending on the orientation we give it.

The banner orientation is probably the most important detail of the concept. Following simple engineering principles, a moment of a force (torque) is a measure of the tendency of the force to rotate the body upon which it acts, which is dependent on the distance and the force itself.

In other words, it is the tendency of an applied force to spin an object around an axis, a principle that represents what happens in the nasal tip. If the force is perpendicular to the distance, we achieve the highest moment of force, which makes the object rotate. But if the vector of the force acts at the same vector of the distance moment of force is 0 Nm, which means there will be no rotational movement (Fig. 10.20).

We follow that rule to place our extension graft avoiding future rotations (specifically over rotation of the tip secondary to the LCS and tensioning). This is exactly what we are looking for in our banner's central axis orientation. It must align with the force vector that is represented by the anterior to posterior traction that the LC provoke in their long axis. By placing these two axis together we are creating a moment of force of 0 Nm, meaning there is no rotational forces.

Practically, we create an angle with the anterior septal border of 130° (115°–145°) to facilitate calculating at the surgical table, 40° (25°–55°) with a perpendicular line to the anterior septal border in the sagittal plane. If we imagine the patient is

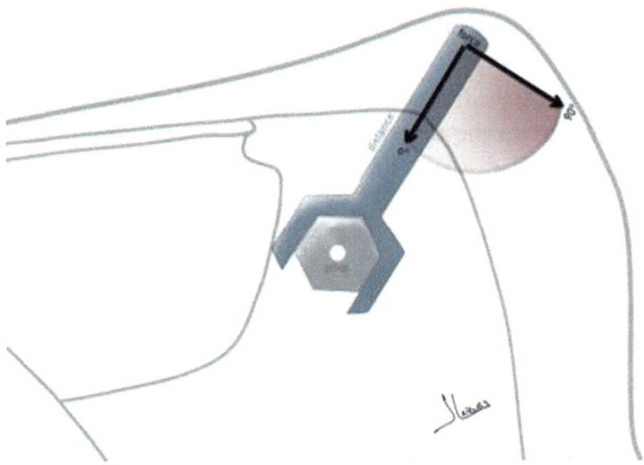

Fig. 10.20 The moment of a force. The moment of force depends on the distance and force applied. It represents the capacity to rotate an object around a pivotal point. If the force is perpendicular to the distance (90°), we achieve maximum rotation. If the force is performed in the same vector of distance (0°), the moment of the force is 0, and there is no movement. It is fundamental to choose the ANSA banner angle that must follow the LC long axis vector

standing still, the axis of the banner will be on the horizontal plane, as well as the horizontal (long) axis of the LC (Fig. 10.21).

Once have the correct angle, we are dependent now on the stabilization of the ANSA banner to the septum to avoid lineal retro (posterior) displacement. We use 5.0 PDS and make several passages, in a mattress suture fashion. To prevent long-term displacements, we finalize it with a 5.0 Prolene suture. The two cartilages will stand side by side. We need to analyze the best way to place the graft, including which side of the septum, in order to avoid the lateralization of the graft, which is also stabilized in the midline with the help of the mattress sutures. In our aesthetic concept, the ideal length of the extensor over the septal border is 4–5 mm but this is, of course, artist dependent. We usually suture it with a longer free arm (6 mm, 7 mm) so we can carve it for precise remodeling at the end of the process (Figs. 10.18e and 10.21).

Having the ANSA banner stabilized in the septum, it is now time to anchor the new tip, by performing an interdomal suture that includes the banner (Fig. 10.22). We will follow the same orientation of previously performed domes cephalic oblique suture. The six points sequence is as follows: (1) first through the graft at the level of the domes; (2) the first entry point of the domal suture, 1 mm from the domes from medial to outer surface; (3) the second point of the domal suture, 5 mm below, at the cephalic border of the LC; (4) through the extensor at the level of the previous passage; (5) the contralateral LC cephalic border, keeping the same level; (6) the domal point of the contralateral dome, from lateral to medial. The knot is tight in between the domes and the Ansa banner. An additional suture (circular or 8-figure) is passed including both domes for stabilization. With this approach, the domal caudal points diverge while the cephalic ones are in close contact in a

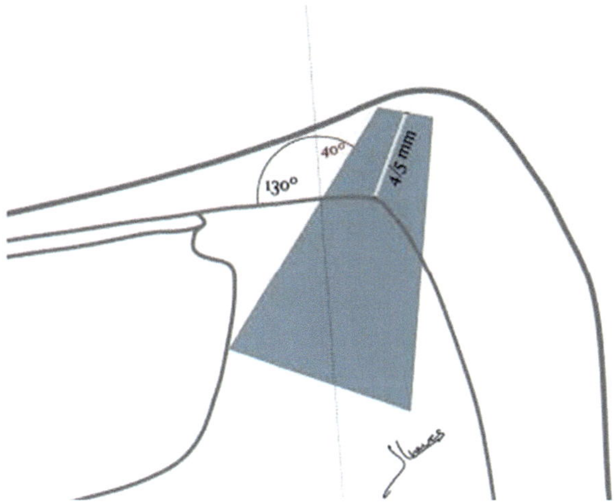

Fig. 10.21 The ANSA banner. Following the information given by the moment of force, we plan the ideal angle of the banner. Our preferred angle is 130° with the anterior border of the septum (or 40° if we consider a perpendicular line to the anterior border of the septum). The projection of the graft must be 4–5 mm on average, to achieve our aesthetic ideals

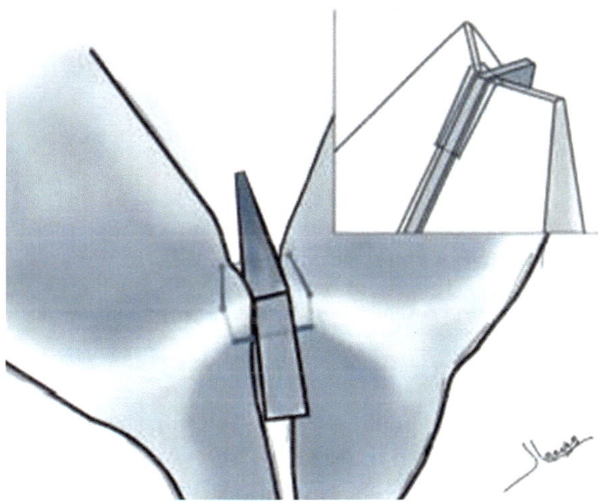

Fig. 10.22 Suturing the new domes to the ANSA banner. The suture follows the rule of the cephalic oblique domal suture in order to elevate the caudal margin of the LLC. This is an interdomal suture with the inclusion of the extension graft

symmetric and very stable fashion. The caudal border of the LC is everted. The lateral crura tension is then created.

10.4.3.2 Columellar Strut and Medial Crura Overlap

Having the domes ideal positioned with the proper shape and having the LC with the ideal short angle and the adequate long axis form and tension, we now need to address the MC and columella complex. Almost constantly, we use a columellar strut. It has a role in giving tip support but mainly avoiding columella retractions.

Anteriorly, we leave a gap between the anterior aspect of the ANSA banner and the strut to permit free columella movements (Fig. 10.23). It works as a functional joint, and this is the main reason we try to avoid "full" extensors and not to create frozen tips.

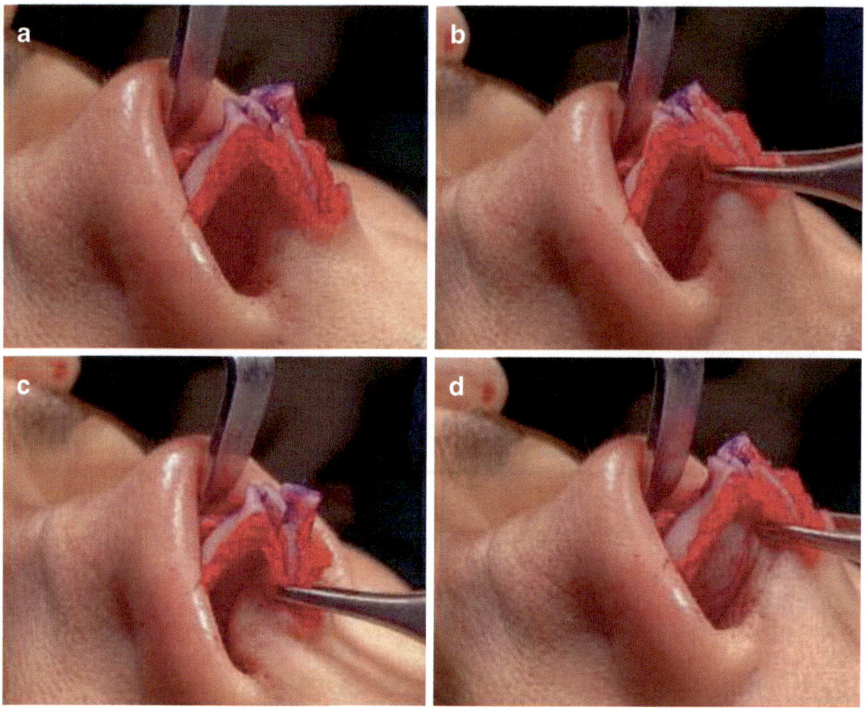

Fig. 10.23 ANSA banner and columellar strut. The two grafts are not connected. It permits the columella region to mobilize lateral and upwards avoiding the frozen tip. The banner supports the tip in pull-down movements (**c**). Pulling up (**b**) and lateralizing the columella (**a**–**d** Tip free movements)

This articulation allows lateral mobilization of the columella and posterior to anterior (projection) movements. The whole complex (LC tensioning, ANSA banner, columellar strut and medial SMAS repositioning) supports the tip in a stable tridimensional position, avoiding future tip ptosis. It seems to be the ideal scenario in tip surgery.

In ptotic tips, where typically the MC are foreshortened, the LCS elongates it creating the ideal balance with the LC, which in turn are shortened and tensioned. On some occasions, the MC become too long distorting the columella. If that happens, we create an overlap at the level of the columellar breakpoint.

10.4.3.3 Tip Medial SMAS and Vertical Scroll Ligament Repositioning

Even if this is not the topic of this chapter, just a quick note on soft tissues. The tip medial SMAS [35, 36] is transected at the level of the columella incision. The superficial SMAS often goes with the cutaneous flap, even if it can sometimes be

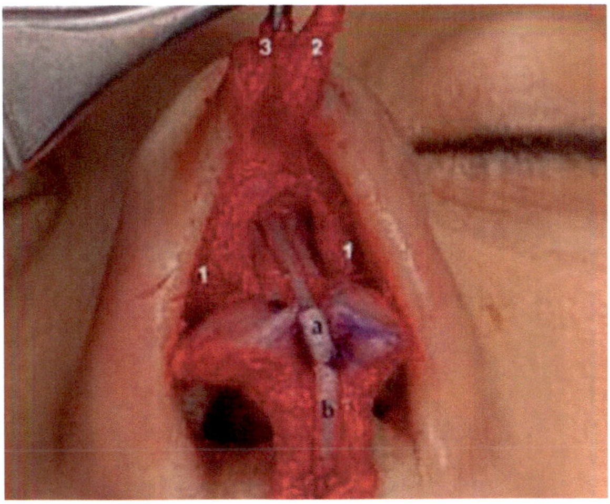

Fig. 10.24 Ligaments repositioning: The vertical scroll ligament (1) and Pitanguy ligament (2), the deep medial SMAS, are repositioned. The superficial medial SMAS goes with the columellar cutaneous flap. ANSA banner (a) and columella strut (b)

dissected separately. The deep medial SMAS (also known as the Pitanguy ligament) is dissected and kept attached to the supratip soft tissues. The vertical scroll ligament is isolated and preserved.

At the end of the surgery, the ligaments are repositioned. First, we recreate the scroll area. We suture the vertical scroll ligament in its proper place, in between the new cephalic border of the LC and the caudal border of the upper lateral cartilage with a 5.0 Vicryl. This is an additional maneuver to avoid cephalic migration of the LC. The deep SAMS ligament is then sutured to its origin. It will pass below the dome sutures immediately over the anterior septal angle in the midline (lateral to the ANSA banner), simulating the normal anatomy where the ligament runs in between the domal ligament and the caudal border of the septum. These three ligaments repositioning create a supratip and lateral crease definition, and work as stabilization net reducing dead space. At last, the superficial ligament will be repositioned with the skin flap at the columella incision level (Fig. 10.24).

10.5 Conclusion

Rhinoplasty is dynamic both on the operating table and in the history timeline. Some guidelines are important to be present in every surgeon armamentarium; however, it is essential to be able to adapt to any particular preferable strategy before and/or during surgery, and never only try to insist on one technical concept, which should never limit the quality of the result. We should adapt to the nose itself and the surgical requirements, and not the other way around.

This is why this chapter will never be completed.

10.6 Clinical Cases

Case 1

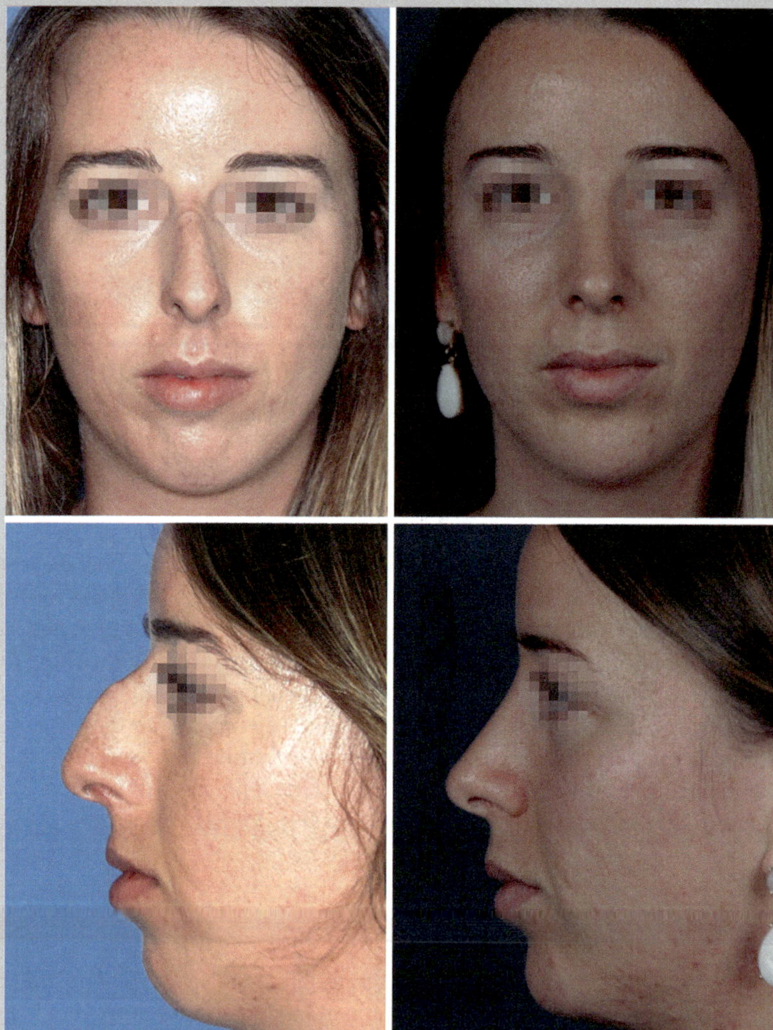

- *Closed approach*
- *Direct resection of the nasal hump; spreader grafts; oblique osteotomiesintermediate osteotomies; low basal osteotomies*
- *LLC cephalic trim; lateral crura steal; cephalic oblique domal sutures; interdormal sutures; columellar strut*

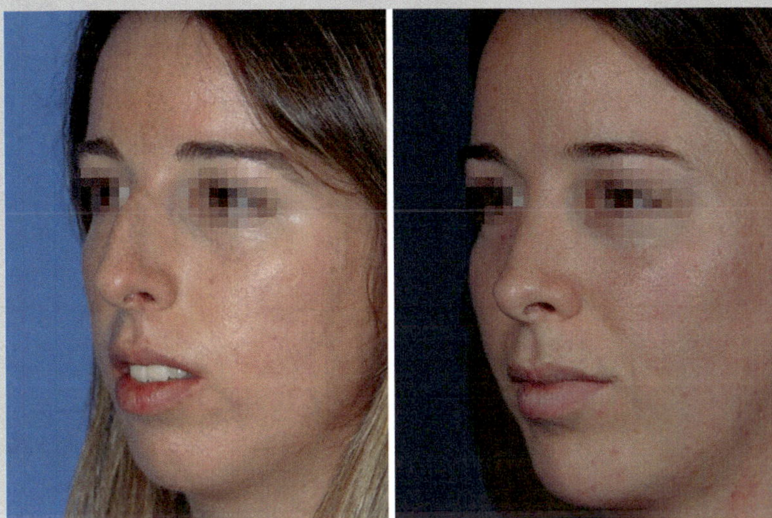

Case 2

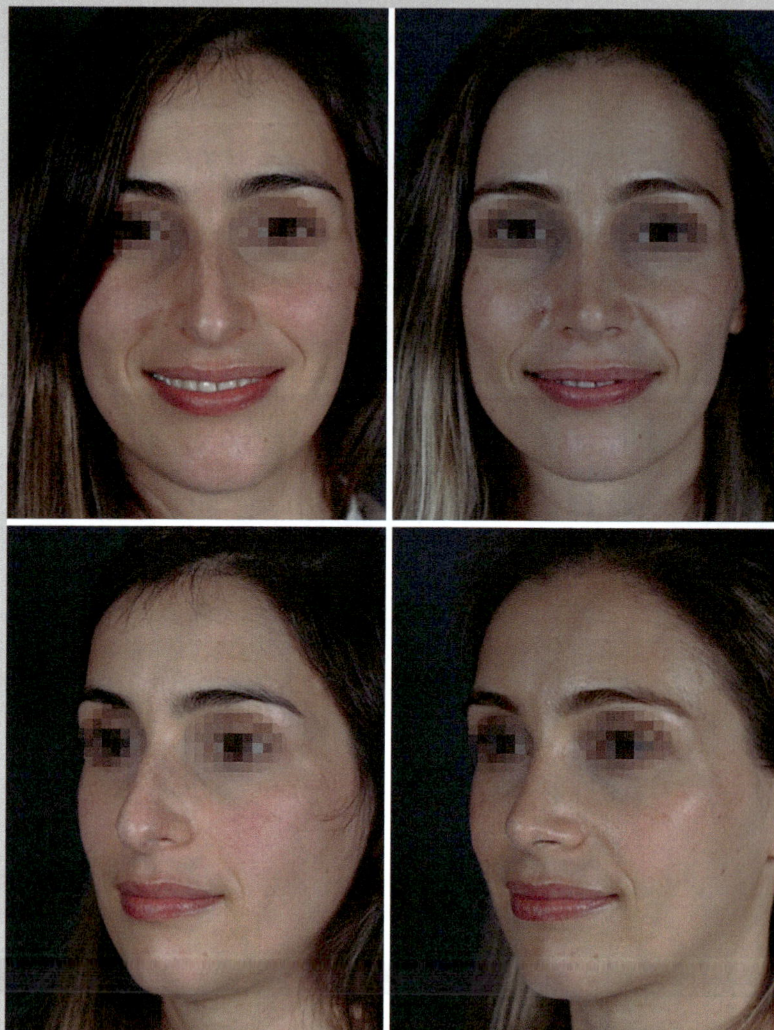

- *Open approach*
- *Segmental preservation approach, using the Tetris concept; Burrs were used to sculpt the dorsum*
- *LLC cephalic trim; lateral crura steal for lateral crura tensioning; cephalic oblique domal sutures; ANSA banner; interdomal sutures; columellar strut*

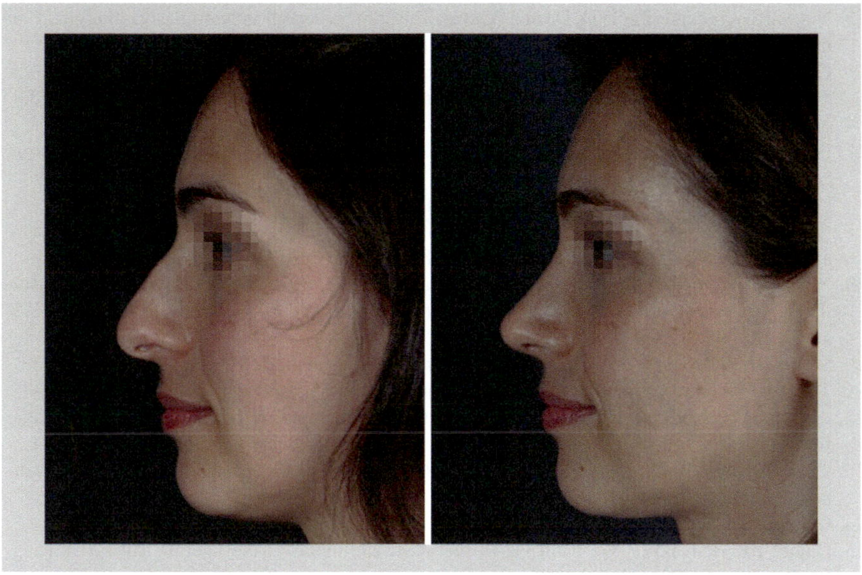

References

1. Fedok F, Nolst Trenité GJ, Becker DG, Gausas R. The ethnic nose. Facial Plast Surg. 2003;19(3).
2. Patel PN, Most SP. Concepts of facial aesthetics when considering ethnic rhinoplasty. Otolaryngol Clin North Am. 2020;53(2):195–208. https://doi.org/10.1016/j.otc.2019.12.001. Epub 2020 Jan 31. PMID: 32008729.
3. Rohrich RJ, Bolden K. Ethnic rhinoplasty. Clin Plast Surg. 2010;37(2):353–70.
4. Boccieri A. The surgical approach to the Mediterranean nose. Facial Plast Surg. 2010;26(2):119–30. https://doi.org/10.1055/s-0030-1253498. Epub 2010 May 4. PMID: 20446206.
5. Daniel RK. Hispanic rhinoplasty in the United States, with emphasis on the Mexican American nose. Plast Reconstr Surg. 2003;112(1):244–56. [discussion: 257–8].
6. Higuera S, Hatef DA, Stal S. Rhinoplasty in the Hispanic patient. Semin Plast Surg. 2009;23(3):207–14.
7. Johnson CM, Godin MS. The tension nose: open structure rhinoplasty approach. Plast Reconstr Surg. 1995;95(1):43–51.
8. Lee MR, Geissler P, Cochran S, Gunter JP, Rohrich RJ. Decreasing nasal tip projection in rhinoplasty. Plast Reconstr Surg. 2014;134(1):41e–9e.
9. Weinstock MS, Stupak HD. Bony/cartilaginous mismatch: a radiologic investigation into the cause of tension nose deformity. Plast Reconstr Surg. 2018;141(2):312–21. https://doi.org/10.1097/PRS.0000000000004059. PMID: 29019863.
10. Joseph J. The classic reprint: nasal reductions. Plast Reconstr Surg. 1971;47(1):79–83.
11. Joseph J. Beiträge zur Rhinoplastik. Berl Klin Wochenschrift. 1907;16:470–2.
12. Neves JC, Tagle DA, Dewes W, Ferraz M. A segmental approach in dorsal preservation rhinoplasty: the Tetris concept. Facial Plast Surg Clin North Am. 2021;29(1):85–99. https://doi.org/10.1016/j.fsc.2020.09.010. PMID: 33220847.
13. Cottle MH, Loring RM. Corrective surgery of the external nasal pyramid and the nasal septum for restoration of normal physiology. Ill Med J. 1946;90:119–35.
14. Cottle MH. Nasal roof repair and hump removal. AMA Arch Otolaryngol. 1954;60(4):408–14.

15. Neves JC, Arancibia Tagle D, Dewes W, et al. The split preservation rhinoplasty: "the Vitruvian man split maneuver". Eur J Plast Surg. 2020; https://doi.org/10.1007/s00238-019-01600-3.
16. Gonçalves Ferreira M, Toriumi DM. A practical classification system for dorsal preservation rhinoplasty techniques. Facial Plast Surg Aesthet Med. 2021;23(3):153–5. https://doi.org/10.1089/fpsam.2021.0030. Epub 2021 Apr 16. PMID: 33861635.
17. Ferraz MBJ, Zappelini CEM, Carvalho GM, Guimarães AC, Chone CT, Dewes W. Cirurgia conservadora do dorso nasal—a filosofia do reposicionamento e ajuste do septo piramidal (S.P.A.R.). Rev Bras Cir Cabeça Pescoço. 2013;42:124–30.
18. Goksel A, Saban Y. Open Piezo preservation rhinoplasty: a case report of the new rhinoplasty approach. Facial Plast Surg. 2019;35(1):113–8.
19. Neves JC, Arancibia-Tagle D, Dewes W, Ferraz M. The segmental preservation rhinoplasty: the Split Tetris concept. Facial Plast Surg. 2021;37(1):36–44. https://doi.org/10.1055/s-0040-1714672. Epub 2020 Sep 4. PMID: 32886949.
20. Sheen JH, Sheen AP. Aesthetic rhinoplasty. 2nd ed. St Louis: CV Mosby; 1987.
21. Toriumi DM. New concepts in nasal tip contouring. Arch Facial Plast Surg. 2006;8(3):156–85.
22. Çakir B, Oreroğlu AR, Doğan T, Akan M. A complete subperichondrial dissection technique for rhinoplasty with management of the nasal ligaments. Aesthet Surg J. 2012;32(5):64–74.
23. Çakir B, Doğan T, Öreroğlu AR, Daniel RK. Rhinoplasty: surface aesthetics and surgical techniques. Aesthet Surg J. 2013;33(3):363–75.
24. Çakır B. Aesthetic septorhinoplasty. Heidelberg: Springer; 2016.
25. Daniel RK, Palhazy P, Gerbault O, Kosins AM. Rhinoplasty: the lateral Crura-Alar Ring. Aesthet Surg J. 2014;34(4):526–37.
26. Neves JC, Tagle DA. Lateral Crura control in nasal tip plasty: cephalic oblique Domal suture, 7X suture and ANSA banner. Ann Plast Reconstr Surg. 2020;4(3):1059.
27. Kovacevic M, Wurm J. Cranial tip suture in nasal tip contouring. Facial Plast Surg. 2014;30(6):681–7.
28. Dosanjh AS, Hsu C, Gruber RP. The hemitransdomal suture for narrowing the nasal tip. Ann Plast Surg. 2010;64(6):708–12.
29. Neu BR. Suture correction of nasal tip cartilage concavities. Plast Reconstr Surg. 1996;98(6):971–9.
30. Davis RE. Lateral crural tensioning for refinement of the wide and under projected nasal tip: rethinking the lateral crural steal. Facial Plast Surg Clin North Am. 2015;23(1):23–53.
31. Byrd SH, Andochick S, Copit S, Walton GK. Septal extension grafts: a method of controlling tip projection shape. Plast Reconstr Surg. 1997;100(4):999–1010.
32. Ahmet S, Sema O, Ummahan O, Emin S. A simplified use of septal extension graft to control nasal tip location. Aesthet Plast Surg. 2007;31(5):506–11.
33. Richard H, Byrd H. Septal extension grafts revisited: 6-year experience in controlling nasal tip projection and shape. Plast Reconstr Surg. 2003;112(7):1929–35.
34. Kim JH, Song JW, Park SW, Oh WS, Lee JH. Effective septal extension graft for Asian rhinoplasty. Arch Plast Surg. 2014;41(1):3–11.
35. Saban Y, Amodeo CA, Hammou JC, Polselli R. An anatomical study of the nasal superficial musculoaponeurotic system. Surgical applications in rhinoplasty. Arch Facial Plast Surg. 2008;10(2):109–15.
36. Cobo R. Superiorly pediculated superficial musculoaponeurotic system ligament flap to control the supratip. JAMA Facial Plast Surg. 2018;20(6):513–4.

Southern Mediterranean Nose Correction

11

Samit Unadkat and Hesham Saleh

Ideal nasal proportions have long been described in the literature and have been based on European Caucasian populations. Whilst these measurements can prove to be a useful guide when first starting out in rhinoplasty surgery, a nose which is considered to be "ideal" is one that is harmonious with the patients pre-existing features, ethnicity and skin type. Rhinoplasty surgery should also aim to be aesthetically pleasing to the patient without compromising on nasal function [1]. Additionally, as the world's population becomes more globalized than ever before, rhinoplasty surgeons too have had to adapt their knowledge and skill-set to individualize their approach for each patient.

Within Europe too, there are recognized specific ethnic groups with distinctive anatomical differences: Anglo-Saxon, Germanic, Latin and Slavic [2]. Increasingly there is a greater appreciation that one cannot simply group all Caucasian noses together and that there are specific hallmarks and characteristics one needs to consider. Even within these four groups, variations exist further.

The Southern Mediterranean Latin nose does not fit the classical description of a "Roman nose". The Southern Mediterranean region is a vast and culturally diverse region, which influences not just from Central and Northern Europe but also from North Africa, the Middle East and Arabian Gulf [2]. Consequently, many of the historical rhinoplasty techniques described in texts geared for the Northern and Central European populations are not always applicable for Southern Mediterranean noses.

S. Unadkat
Department of Rhinology and Facial Plastic Surgery, Royal National ENT and University College Hospital, London, UK

H. Saleh (✉)
Department of Rhinology and Facial Plastic Surgery, Charing Cross Hospital and Imperial College, London, UK

P. G. Giacomini (ed.), *Mediterranean Rhinoplasty*,
https://doi.org/10.1007/978-3-031-05551-5_11

Broadly speaking, in the authors' experience, the distinct considerations for Southern Mediterranean noses are relatively heavy, thick skin and soft tissue envelope with weak underlying cartilage. Of course, exceptions to this rule exist, and thus each patient requires a tailor-made approach. Based on our experiences of the Southern Mediterranean diaspora, we outline our approach herein.

11.1 Preoperative Work-Up

Prior to embarking on any rhinoplasty surgery, it is first crucial to gauge the patient's wishes and expectations from surgery. This can only initially be ascertained from a detailed history and examination. It is at this stage that any functional concerns can be elicited too. Should there be gross septal abnormalities, then these may impact the preoperative surgical plan. A comprehensive past medical and surgical history is important to exclude any underlying systemic inflammatory conditions or conditions such as diabetes which may impact post-surgical healing. History of previous nasal trauma or surgery too will affect surgical planning and whether additional graft materials are required. Smoking and recreational drug use will affect the post-surgical healing and in patients with thicker skin, which can have profoundly adverse outcomes.

As mentioned previously, the Southern Mediterranean nose is a variable entity from typical Northern Mediterranean noses, the former with greater influences from the Middle East and Arabian Gulf and the latter with greater Anglo-Saxon and Germanic influences. These variations mean that patients must be appropriately counselled of what is realistically achievable from surgery. Hallmarks of the Southern Mediterranean nose include a prominent nasal dorsum, ptotic nasal tips, thicker nasal skin and in a large proportion of patients, weaker cartilaginous support than their Northern Mediterranean counterparts. Unlike their Middle Eastern and Eastern Mediterranean counterparts, in the authors' experience, the inter-alar width is not excessively wide, and thus surgical correction is infrequently warranted.

11.2 Surgical Considerations

11.2.1 Skin Quality

As is well-established, having thicker skin is a double-edged sword. Whilst any post-surgical irregularities are often well-camouflaged, nasal tip refinement is certainly more challenging. Care should be taken to not thin the skin excessively (if at all) as contour irregularities, and telangiectasias over time become more visible which are very difficult to correct. If defatting is required, care must be taken to entirely avoid the dermis. Instead, in the authors' experience, close involvement with a dermatologist who has an interest in rhinoplasty patients is of paramount importance. Heavy, oily skin which is not uncommon in Southern Mediterranean rhinoplasty patients may require pre or postoperative treatment with drugs such as isotretinoin, in order to control the production of the sebaceous glands and thin the skin-subcutaneous tissue envelope (SSTE) in a uniform fashion without compromising the underlying bony and cartilaginous structures of the nose [3]. As side effects are common and potentially serious, such medication should only be started by a dermatologist.

Additional intra-operative considerations for the skin include meticulous elevation of the SSTE in a supra-perichondrial and sub-periosteal plane. Some authors suggest postoperative draping of the nose for up to 3 months after surgery to reduce the post-surgical swelling, although this is not our routine practice.

One of the longer-term complications of thicker skin and over-resection of cartilage in cephalic margins of the lower lateral cartilages is the potential for soft tissue pollybeak formation. Here, there is excessive scar tissue in the new dead space in the supra-tip region. Unlike a more conventional cartilaginous pollybeak deformity which is often easily corrected with cartilage excision, soft tissue pollybeak deformities are harder to correct [4]. The authors therefore recommend postoperative Triamcinolone (Kenalog) injections 10 mg/mL as early as 3 weeks post op then repeated monthly for up to three doses.

11.2.2 Nasal Tip

Nasal tip definition in patients of Southern Mediterranean descent can be challenging. Frequently, the heavy skin means that using only conventional suture techniques classically employed in Northern European patients, the nasal tip can appear unchanged once the skin is redraped. It is the authors' experience that although infrequent, some of these patients can also develop recurrent nasal tip swelling after surgery. This is through a combination of scar tissue formation and oedema.

As tip ptosis is a frequent complaint in Southern Mediterranean rhinoplasty patients, one has to take into account techniques to help project and rotate the nose. Pollybeak deformities are well-recognised complications in this group of patients, particularly in more inexperienced hands. Thus, good projection of the nose will avoid this phenomenon. It is in the authors' experience that in order to maintain good long-term projection, the tongue in groove technique, popularized by Kridel in 1999 is a reliable method to help recreate the nasal tip support mechanisms [5]. Tissue contracture can be greater in patients with thicker skin, and so it is the authors' preference to marginally over-project the nose rather than under-project. The precise degree of projection will depend on a combination of patient preference and surgeon assessment. Many critics of the TIG technique report excessive nasal stiffness as a complication. In the authors' experience, this is a seldom, if ever, reported complaint from patients in the long-term. The reproducibility, marked improvement in nasal projection and long-term results mean that it remains our technique of choice in patients of Southern Mediterranean descent. In patients with insufficient caudal septal cartilage requiring nasal lengthening, or in secondary rhinoplasty surgery patients, a septal extension graft (SEG) is also highly effective when secured in a TIG fashion.

In cases where the TIG/SEG is insufficient to achieve the desired projection of the nasal tip, different manoeuvres have been described to further increase tip projection including suture techniques, such as a lateral crural steal, or cartilage grafting techniques, such as cap grafts. In the authors' experience, cartilage grafting techniques in Southern Mediterranean noses are more effective due to the reasons previously mentioned of heavy skin and reduced likelihood of pollybeak formation.

11.2.3 Dorsal Humps

Southern Mediterranean rhinoplasty patients present with variations of the nasal dorsum, reflecting the wide-ranging cross-cultural mix of differing ethnic groups. Whilst the nasal dorsum can be prominent with large humps, in many patients the dorsum can be straight. Should dorsal de-humping be necessary, the authors prefer structural rhinoplasty techniques. Where there are moderate nasal humps, en-bloc resection of the dorsal hump is preferred. By contrast, where dorsal humps are larger than 6 mm or if the patients have short nasal bones with weak upper lateral cartilages, our preference is for a split hump technique, taking care to reconstruct the mid-third, in order to prevent inverted V deformities. Figures 11.1, 11.2, 11.3, 11.4, 11.5, and 11.6 show examples of Southern Mediterranean patients with descriptions of encountered deformities and operative solutions.

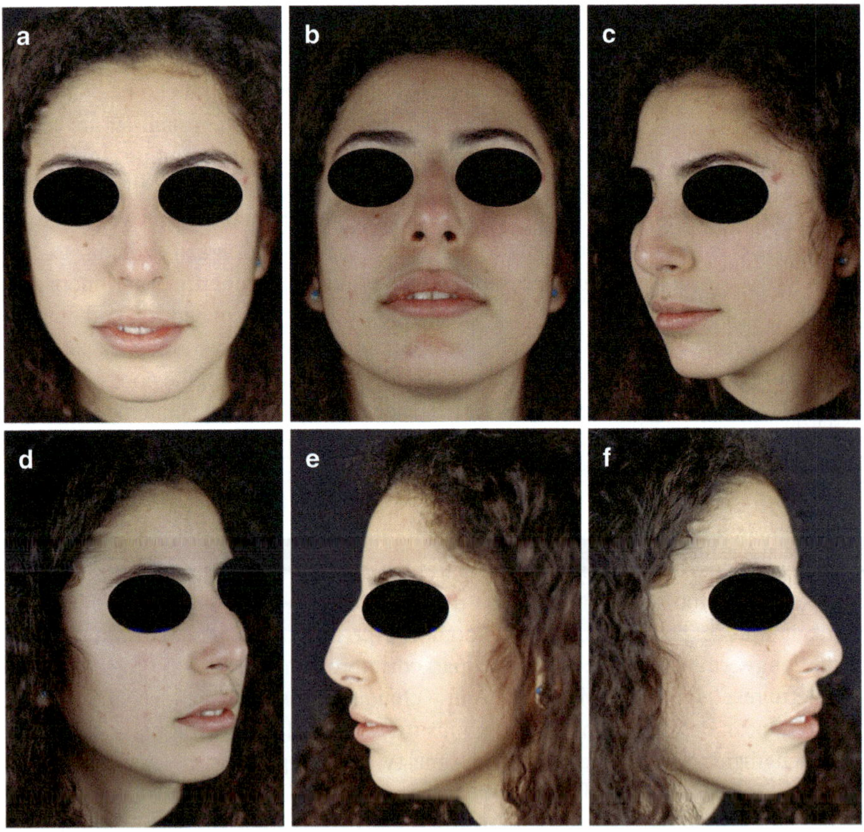

Fig. 11.1 Preoperative frontal (**a**), base (**b**), left oblique (**c**), right oblique (**d**), left lateral (**e**) and right lateral (**f**) views showing a 20-year-old patient with moderately thick skin, dorsal hump, moderately bulbous and under projected tip

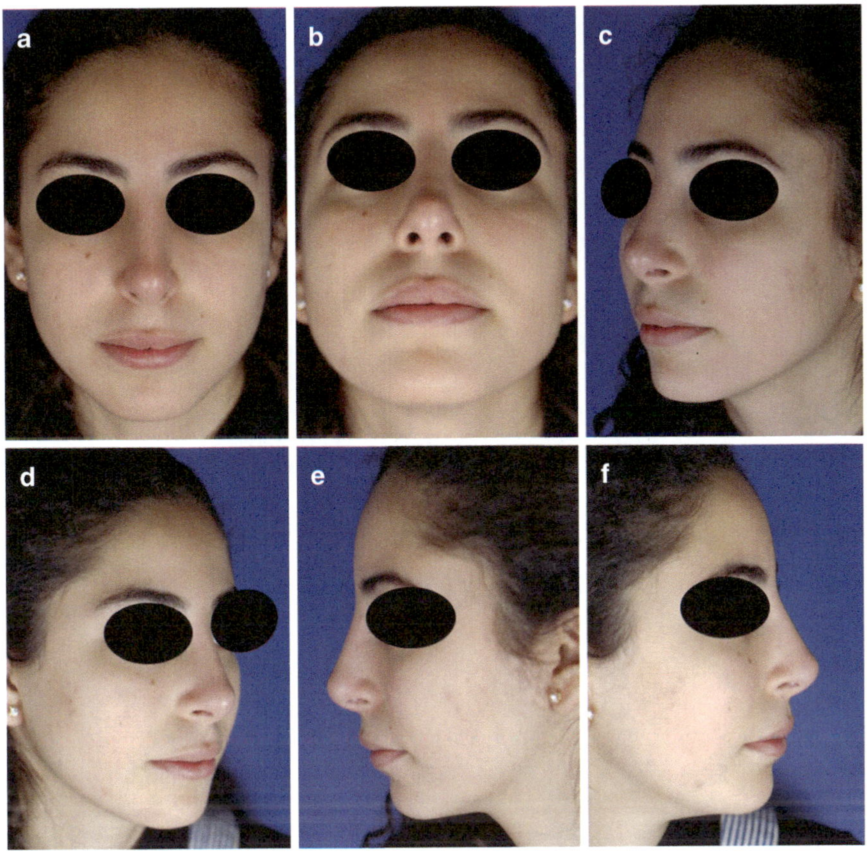

Fig. 11.2 Postoperative frontal (**a**), base (**b**), left oblique (**c**), right oblique (**d**), left lateral (**e**) and right lateral (**f**) photographs

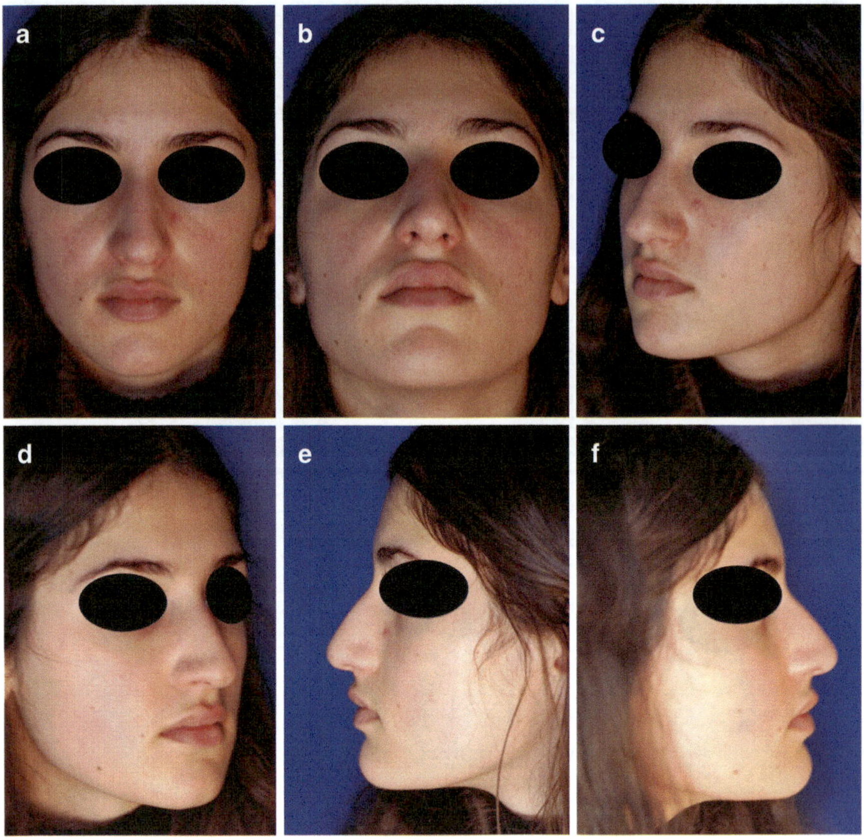

Fig. 11.3 Preoperative frontal (**a**), base (**b**), left oblique (**c**), right oblique (**d**), left lateral (**e**) and right lateral (**f**) views showing a 19-year-old patient with thin skin, small hump, down rotated bulbous tip with weak cartilage and strong depressor septae muscle

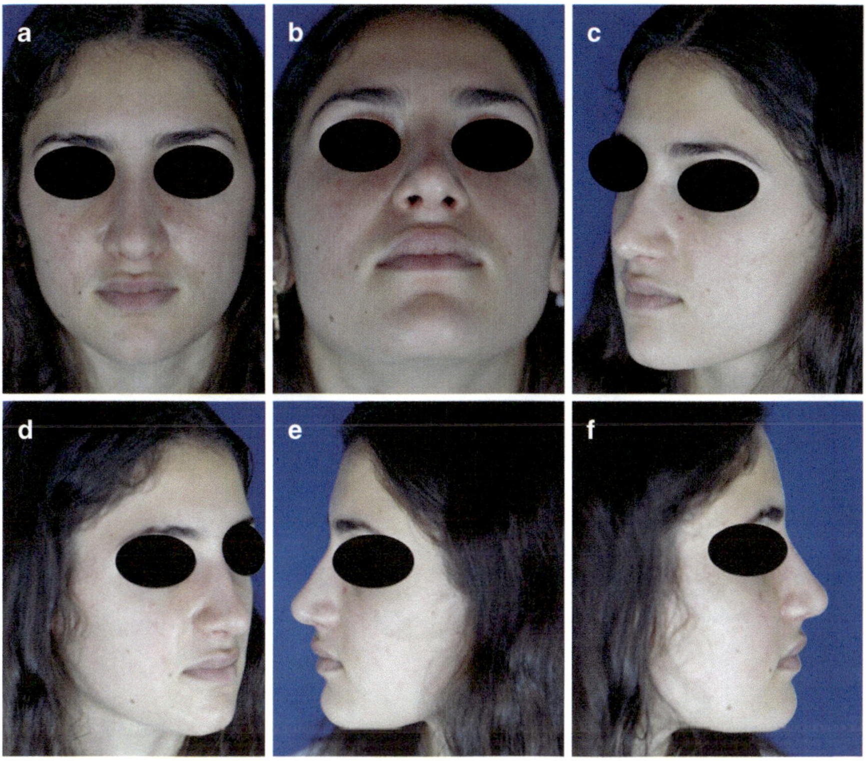

Fig. 11.4 Postoperative frontal (**a**), base (**b**), left oblique (**c**), right oblique (**d**), left lateral (**e**) and right lateral (**f**) photographs

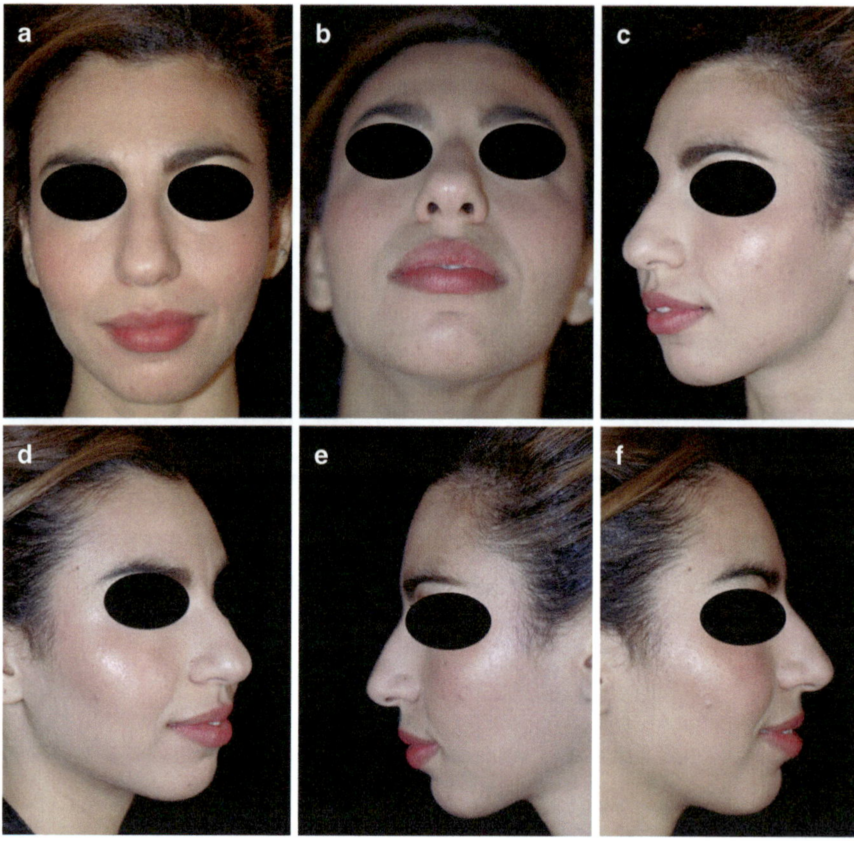

Fig. 11.5 Preoperative frontal (**a**), base (**b**), left oblique (**c**), right oblique (**d**), left lateral (**e**) and right lateral (**f**) views showing a 23-year-old patient with thick skin, large lower lateral cartilages and wide nasal dorsum

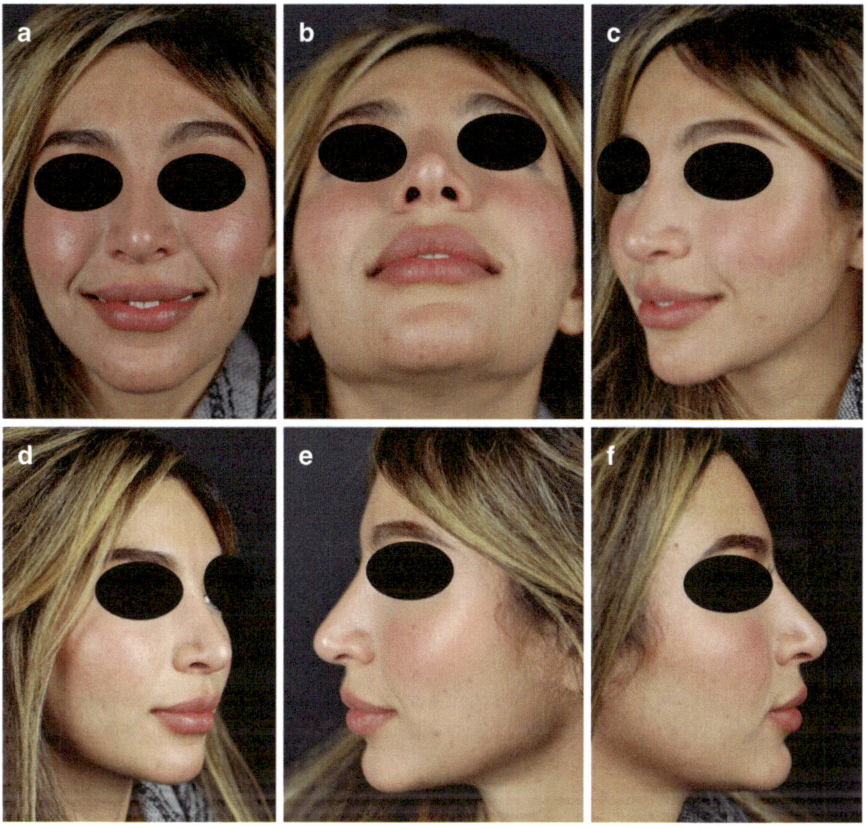

Fig. 11.6 Postoperative frontal (**a**), base (**b**), left oblique (**c**), right oblique (**d**), left lateral (**e**) and right lateral (**f**) photographs

11.3 Conclusions

Much of the classical descriptions of ideal nasal proportions are based on the art of Ancient Greece and of the Italian and European Renaissance [2]. The rhinoplasty techniques thus originally described were geared around these generalized proportions for a European Caucasian nose and do not take into account differing nasal archetypes. The Southern Mediterranean nose is very much a distinct entity from Northern Europe and even the Northern Mediterranean nose with influences from North Africa and the Middle East. Key concepts to remember include projection of the nasal tip, use of cartilage grafting and to consider involvement of a dermatologist if considering starting isotretinoin.

In conclusion, the patients presented herein are examples and the concepts described in the present chapter are generalized to the authors' experience of the Southern Mediterranean nose. There remains no substitute, however, for a thorough preoperative analysis, eliciting patient expectations and identifying the techniques that work in the surgeon's hands in order to produce aesthetically pleasing and balanced results.

References

1. Leong SC, White PS. A comparison of aesthetic proportions between the healthy Caucasian nose and the aesthetic ideal. J Plast Reconstr Aesthet Surg. 2006;59(3):248–52.
2. Palma P, Bignami M, Delù G, De Bernardi F, Castelnuovo P. Rhinoplasty for the Mediterranean nose. Facial Plast Surg. 2003;19(3):279–94.
3. Cobo R, Vitery L. Isotretinoin use in thick-skinned rhinoplasty patients. Facial Plast Surg. 2016;32(6):656–61.
4. Hanasono MM, Kridel RW, Pastorek NJ, Glasgold MJ, Koch RJ. Correction of the soft tissue pollybeak using triamcinolone injection. Arch Facial Plast Surg. 2002;4(1):26–30; discussion 31.
5. Kridel RW, Scott BA, Foda HM. The tongue-in-groove technique in septorhinoplasty. A 10-year experience. Arch Facial Plast Surg. 1999;1(4):246–56; discussion 257–8.

12 Eastern Mediterranean Nose Correction

Fazil Apaydin

12.1 Introduction

The Mediterrean Sea is at the heart of the ancient world. Throughout the centuries there were migrations all along these countries, while the sea route was the main way of transportation. Therefore, it is no surprise that one can meet similar faces in all regions of the Mediterranean Sea. Still, the southern part of the Mediterranean is closer to Ecuador so the color of the skin gets darker and the anatomical features of the face change as well. In the eastern part of the Mediterranean, the bigger countries are Turkey and Egypt. The smaller countries are Lebanon, Israel, and Syria. Having operated in all of these countries, I can say that the general features of the nose and face are identical in Turkey and Greece. However, in Egypt, Syria, and Lebanon most of the population are Arabic in origin.

We conducted a photogrammetric study in Turkish population and found that a crooked nose, obtuse nasofacial angle, and acute nasolabial angle were major problems for seeking rhinoplasty [1]. Similar results were reported for Arabic noses [2]. It has been mentioned that the Middle Eastern noses have thick skin, dorsal hump, overprojected radix, wide upper two-thirds, nasal deviation, poorly defined and underprojected tip, weak lower lateral cartilages, acute nasolabial angle, and nostril tip asymmetries [3–7]. I do confirm many of these findings except that in Turkey, the thick skin is rarer than the population in Egypt. Besides, the lower lateral cartilages are not weak in most patients. In my daily practice, dorsal hump, droopy, and wide tip are three main concerns of my patients. Crooked nose is less seen than these three complaints (Fig. 12.1).

F. Apaydin (✉)
Department of Otorhinolaryngology, Ege University Medical Faculty, İzmir, Turkey
e-mail: fazil.apaydin@ege.edu.tr

P. G. Giacomini (ed.), *Mediterranean Rhinoplasty*,
https://doi.org/10.1007/978-3-031-05551-5_12

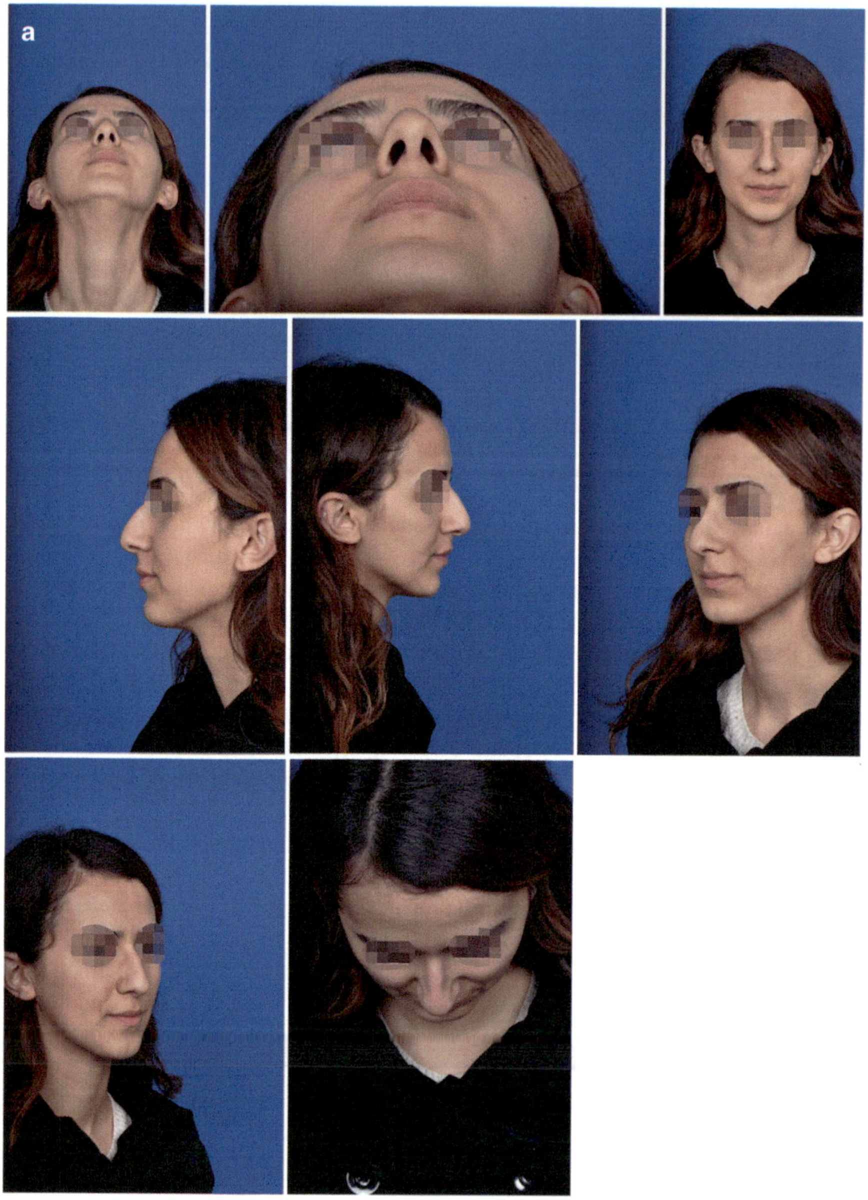

Fig. 12.1 A typical Turkish young woman seeking rhinoplasty with three most common complaints: dorsal hump, wide, and droopy tip. One can see the preoperative and 1-year postoperative pictures

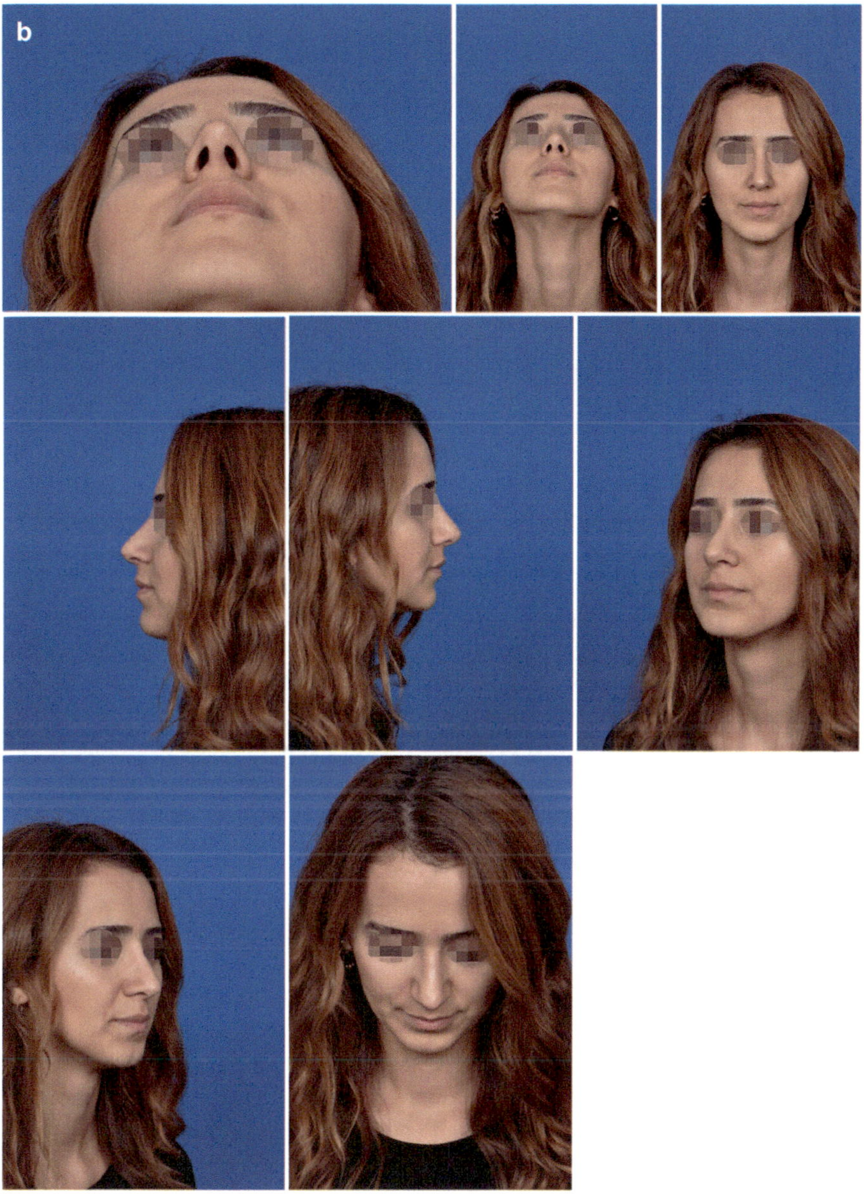

Fig. 12.1 (continued)

12.2 Preoperative Stage

The most important thing in rhinoplasty is to determine what the patient wants. All patients fill in a questionnaire composed of patient-reported outcome measure called SCHNOS (10-Item Standardized Cosmesis and Health Nasal Outcomes Survey) which was validated for Turkish [8] and a body dysmorphic disorder questionnaire [9]. The same questionnaire has been validated for Arabic [10] as well that makes it a unique tool as a multilingually validated patient-reported outcome measure. The answers in this questionnaire are detailed to learn more about what patient wants.

In my opinion, the best time to learn the demands of the patient is during imaging. At first, standard rhinoplasty pictures are taken in a studio with strobes placed at 45° with the patient's head. It consists of different views, namely, frontal, laterals, obliques, basal, frontal smiling, and lateral smiling, and three views by putting a ruler on one side of the head (frontal, lateral, basal). These pictures are transferred into a computer for imaging. The first facial analysis is performed during ENT examination, and the findings are discussed with the patient. The second time a facial analysis is realized while looking at the transferred pictures. The imaging is performed using frontal, lateral, and basal views (the ones including ruler) for operative planning. Then, an imaging session is realized with the patient where different scenarios are discussed to understand what the patient wants and show what can be done. The third facial analysis is done when the pictures are transferred into Rhinobase, a computer program designed specifically for rhinoplasty patients. In this program, it is possible to make an aesthetic and photometric analysis [11].

12.3 Surgery

12.3.1 Approach

I prefer to operate all patients under general anesthesia. In 80% of the cases, an external approach is used. The nasal septum is exposed by hemitransfixion incision if the rotation and projection of the tip is fine, otherwise the septum is approached from the midline through the external approach. An inverted-V incision and marginal incisions are made. The columellar flap is elevated using sharp curved scissors and the incision edges are cut perpendicular to the wound edges. Then, the caudal end of the medial crura and lateral crura is dissected free. Recently, the Pitanguy ligament is dissected and preserved while going between the medial crura and exposes the caudal margin of the nasal septum only if the rotation and projection of the tip will be changed [12] (Fig. 12.2). The middle third is dissected on a supraperichondrial plane. Then, the perichondrium of the middle third is cut in the midline and dissected laterally 3–4 mm. Then, the periosteum is dissected away creating a perichondrium-periosteal flap [13].

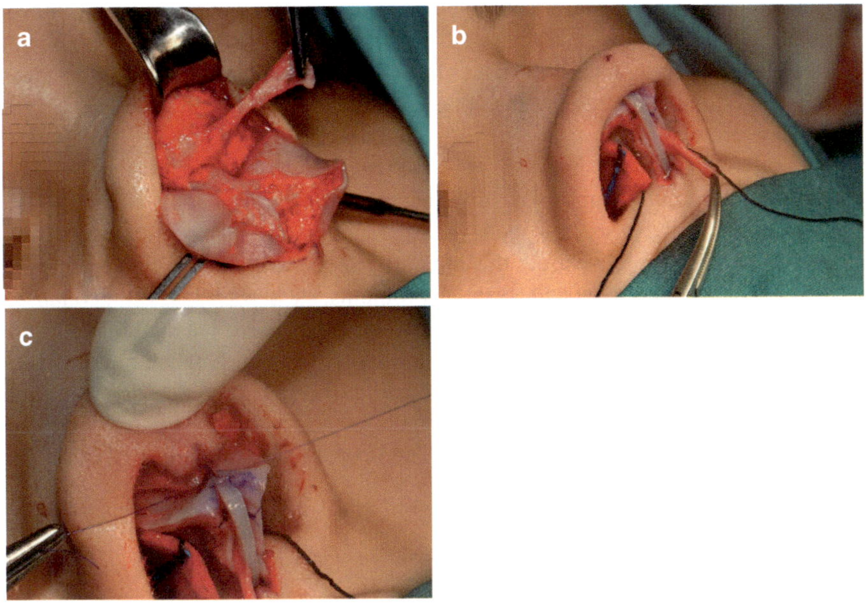

Fig. 12.2 Pitanguy ligament can be dissected during surgery (**a**) and sutured between the medial crura to obtain a nice supratip break (**b**, **c**)

12.3.2 Bony Skeleton

I have been using many instruments to reduce the bony hump such as Rubin osteotome, rasp, burrs, and piezo, which all work fine in my hands. I prefer to use Piezo more recently because of less risk of severing the soft tissues around and the ability to shape the bones under direct vision [14]. The most important thing is to keep the soft tissues under the bony hump, so it is less likely that a traditional open roof is seen.

I use 3-mm guarded osteotomes for lateral osteotomies because I do not like wide dissection of the bony skeleton to use Piezo. Because I do think that it can cause overmobilization of fractured segments, which can be more difficult to control. I prefer medial fading and lateral osteotomies except in crooked noses. In crooked noses, I like using paramedian and transverse osteotomies instead of fading medial osteotomy.

12.3.3 Middle Vault

There are many options to reduce the dorsal hump, and I have been using all of them:

1. En bloc hump removal.
2. Rasping the bony dorsum and en bloc removal.

3. Detaching the upper lateral cartilages from the nasal septum and then remove in pieces.
4. Detaching the upper lateral cartilages from the nasal septum and then resect only the septal hump and preserve the upper lateral cartilages.
5. Dorsum preservation.

Unfortunately, hump removal destroys the elegant natural anatomy of the middle and upper third of the nose. In Joseph type of reduction rhinoplasty, no special technique was reported to reconstruct this area after osseocartilaginous hump removal [15]. Some of the functional and aesthetic problems, such as middle vault collapse, inverted-V deformity, and internal nasal valve stenosis, have led surgeons to find solutions to these problems [16, 17]. The importance of rebuilding the middle vault after hump reduction has become popular within the last three decades by using spreader grafts and flaps [16–20].

The main reasons to use spreader grafts and/or spreader flaps in most of the cases are as follows [16, 20, 21]:

1. Reconstitute the anatomy of the middle vault.
2. Avoid middle vault collapse.
3. Restore, widen, or maintain the internal valves.
4. Recreate the brow-tip aesthetic lines.
5. Create a smooth transition at the key area.
6. Splint deviated dorsal segment of the nasal septum.

12.3.4 Spreader Flaps

Spreader flaps are my first choice in primary rhinoplasty to rebuild the middle vault. They were first used by Fomon et al. to overcome collapsed ala in 1950 [22]. After the upper lateral cartilages (ULCs) are dissected away from the nasal septum and the cartilaginous hump is resected, the medial portion of the upper lateral cartilages is folded inwards and sutured to the nasal septum (Fig. 12.3a, b). The major advantage over spreader grafts is that there is simply no need to use an additional graft obtained from anywhere else [18]. Besides when performed meticulously, it looks as if the dorsum is not touched at all. So in my mind this is a dorsum preservation technique as well.

When the ULCs are separated from the nasal septum, I use three techniques in reconstructing the middle vault [23]:

1. Suturing of the ULCs to the septum: In small and wide humps, this option is an elegant technique and the intact mucosa under dorsum acts as a soft tissue spreader.
2. Suturing of the ULCs over the septum: When there is a need to augment the middle third, this technique is useful.

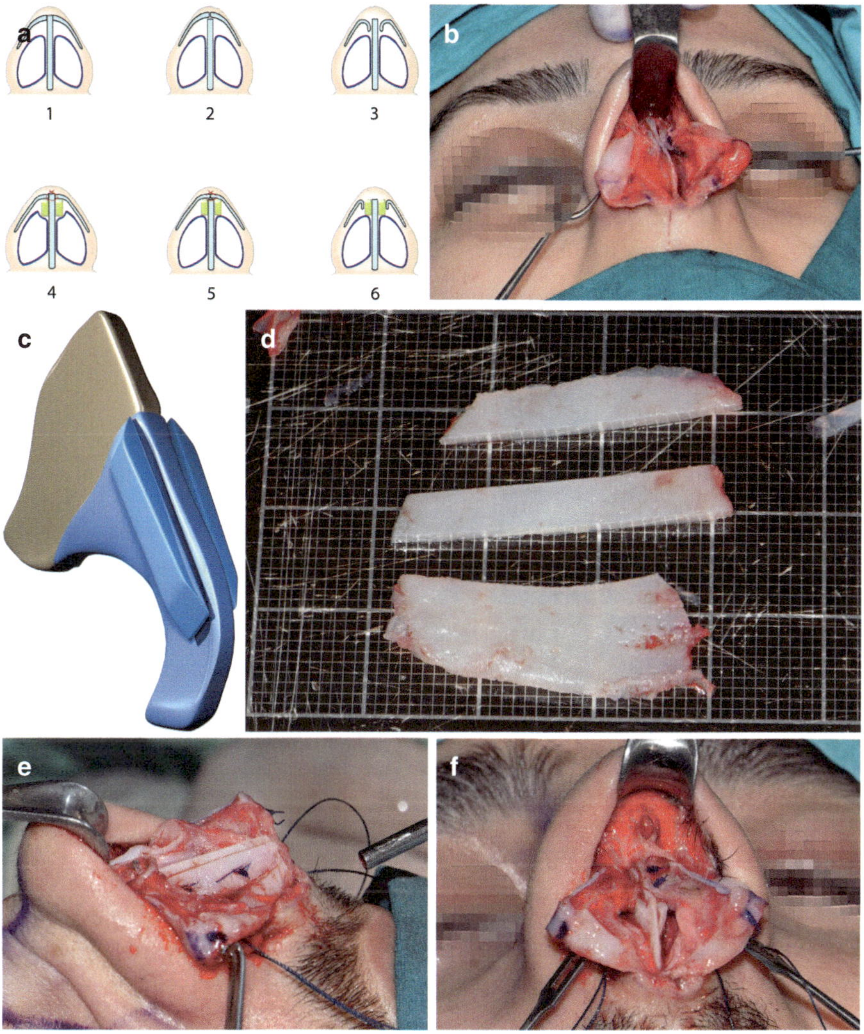

Fig. 12.3 In primary rhinoplasty, spreader flaps are easier to perform after septal hump removal. The upper lateral cartilages can be sutured to the nasal septum, above the septum or folded in and then sutured to septum (**a**, **b**). Spreader grafts are useful for middle vault reconstruction (**c**, **d**). Spreader grafts can be used together with spreader flaps (**e**, **f**)

3. Turn-in flaps: The medial portion of the ULC is folded inwards as much as required and then sutured to the nasal septum by two or three mattress sutures [13, 14, 19, 20]. In my daily practice, this technique is the one I mainly use.

If the perichondrium of the middle third is kept intact on the ULC, this creates a strong cartilage to fold inwards and small relieving incisions, especially at the key area may be needed for fine adjustments. However, if the perichondrium is dissected, the ULC is folded very easily, and the perichondrium is used as camouflage material.

12.3.5 Spreader Grafts

Spreader grafts are described to put between upper cartilages and nasal septum [16, 17] (Fig. 12.3c, d). They have been my workhorse after I started using external rhinoplasty for 21 years. I can easily say that through all these years, I am satisfied with their usage. They are carved from the harvested septal cartilage. In revision cases, or when multiple grafts are required, they can be obtained from the conchal or rib cartilage as well. In my hands, there are different ways to use spreader grafts [24]:

1. Traditional: Either rectangular in shape or beveled at the edges.
2. Modified:
   (a) One sided: They can be used on one side in crooked noses where there is a concave deformity of the dorsal segment [25, 26].
   (b) Asymmetric (thickness): In cases when there is significant asymmetry in the middle third, the spreader grafts can be carved in asymmetric thickness.
   (c) Two layers: When the cartilage is not thick enough, two layers of cartilage can be sutured to each other to obtain necessary thickness.
3. Splinting: In crooked noses, thicker and longer spreader grafts should be used to splint the dorsal deviations.
4. Reconstructive: In severe septal deviations, there are times that some part of the dorsal segment of the nasal septum.

In crooked nose and in some cases, I am much in favor of using a combined usage of spreader grafts and flaps [23] (Fig. 12.3e, f).

12.4 Dorsum Preservation

My philosophy in rhinoplasty is to keep control during all maneuvers in rhinoplasty. I am a structural rhinoplasty surgeon for the past 21 years. I am pretty happy with the results within all these years. However, recently the preservation techniques have been reintroduced with some refinements [26, 27]. Although the idea of preserving the dorsum looks appealing, during my first trials, I did not feel that I could keep control as much as I would like. Because to preserve the dorsum, the surgeon can be more aggressive with the osteotomies fully mobilizing the bony pyramid. In addition, detaching the upper lateral cartilages from the nasal bones can create problems we have never seen before. The third thing is that no secure way to keep the dorsal profile in place is easy. In selected cases such as high septal deviations, I like using Cottle type of dorsum preservation (Fig. 12.4). As mentioned before, spreader flaps act as if the dorsum is not touched at all, and the abovementioned three major problems do not exist at all. However, I should also add that in Turkey preservation techniques are popular among younger surgeons following the teachings of some prominent Turkish surgeons. On a final note, I will keep on using dorsum preservation techniques in selected cases.

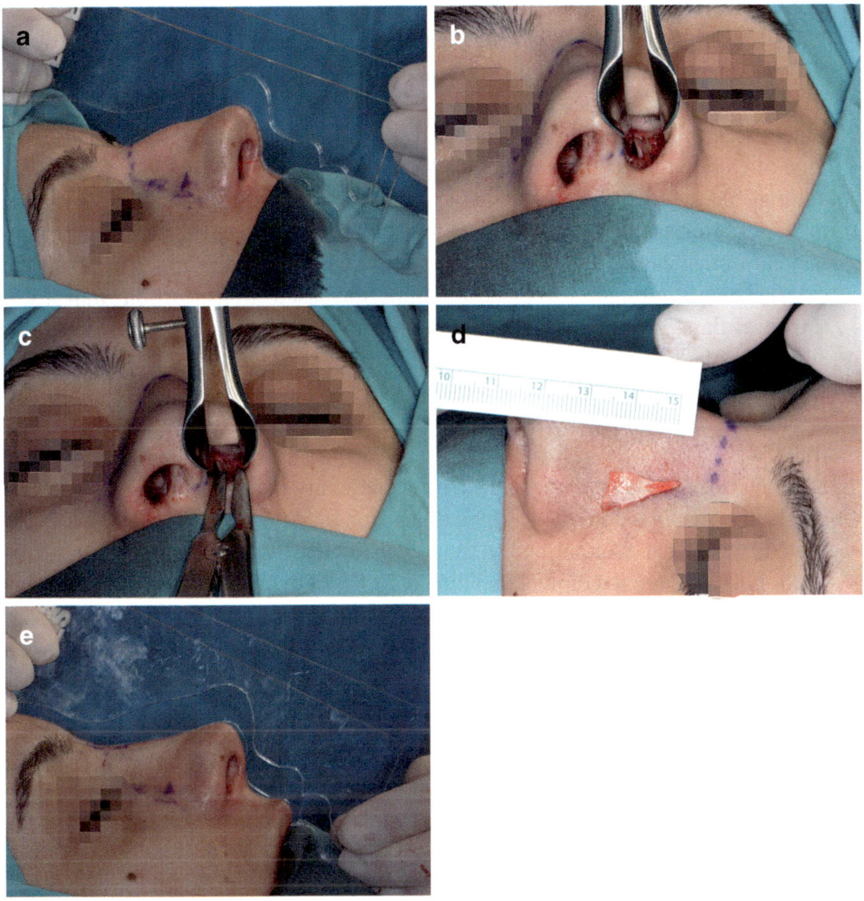

Fig. 12.4 Profile templates are used during surgery for precision profile plasty (**a**). These templates are created using the patient's preoperative picture and the requested profile obtained during imaging. In Cottle type of let-down rhinoplasty, a wedge resection is performed on both sides to preserve the dorsum by using a Beyer rongeur (**b**–**d**). At the end of surgery, it is checked if the targeted profile is obtained (**e**)

12.4.1 Tip

Tip bulbosity and droopiness are two major problems encountered in Eastern Mediterranean. The surgeon should be careful with the facial analysis to decipher the deformities causing these problems. The underlying reasons can be due to intrinsic forces, i.e., the shape, dimensions, resilience, and strength of the lower lateral cartilages. It can also be due to extrinsic forces such as overly developed caudal septum, anterior nasal spine, or deviated septum.

The lateral crura should be evaluated for shape, dimensions, strength, orientation, and axis. There are many options for lateral crural reshaping and/or restructuring:

1. Cephalic trim: This is a traditional way of decreasing the volume of the ala to make it aesthetically more pleasing and to shape the tip [15]. My preference for two decades is to leave 7 mm in females and 8 mm in males, both of which worked fine.
2. Lateral crural turn-in flap: Instead of resecting the cephalically trimmed cartilage, it can be turned in after dissecting the skin under the lateral crus and then sutured like a sandwich [28] (Fig. 12.5). It can be used in refining, reshaping, and restructuring the lateral crus. If the scroll can be kept intact, which in my hands in most cases, this flap serves as a unique technique supporting both the external and internal valves [29]. Superior-based transposition flap [30], turn-over flap [31], and sliding alar cartilage flap [32] have all been described for similar goals.
3. Lateral crural shortening: The lateral crus can be cut about 10 mm lateral to the dome and shortened by overlapping to decrease projection and increase rotation [33].
4. Lateral crural repositioning: In case of cephalically malpositioned lateral crura, this is a powerful technique to solve this problem. After the lateral crura are dissected free of the original bed, they are supported by lateral crural strut grafts and repositioned in a recipient bed directed toward to the lateral canthi [34]. This is a technically challenging technique and is not for novice surgeons. Honestly, I do not need to use this technique much because the lateral crural steal is powerful in changing the orientation of lateral crura and eliminate malposition. Another easier alternative that I like is to use alar battens [35] and/or articulated alar rim grafts [36].

12.5 Sutures

I like to apply a certain order with tip sutures. Before starting sutures, cephalic trim or lateral crural turn-in-flap is performed (Fig. 12.6a, b).

1. *Hemitransdomal suture:* This is the first suture I start with three things in mind: to reduce the dome width, to evert the lateral crus, and to obtain a straighter caudal border of the lateral crus [37]. It should not be sutured too tight, otherwise an exaggerated concavity can be seen lateral to the suture. If I want to use lateral crural technique, I decide at this stage on how much to steal (Fig. 12.6c–e).
2. *Domal suture:* This is a mattress suture I like using to obtain better symmetry on both sides with a dome definition [38, 39]. I prefer to put the suture at the upper half of the dome in order not to narrow the domal angle (Fig. 12.6c–e).
3. *Domal equalization suture:* This suture passes from the cephalic border of each dome to reduce the interdomal width and align the domes [39] (Fig. 12.6f, g).
4. *Septocolumellar suture:* The inner margins of the medial crura are sutured to the caudal septum to guarantee the tip projection and rotation [10]. Therefore, it is a key suture in my daily practice. When the intrinsic forces are overcome with the abovementioned sutures, there is not much stress on this suture. I usually suture

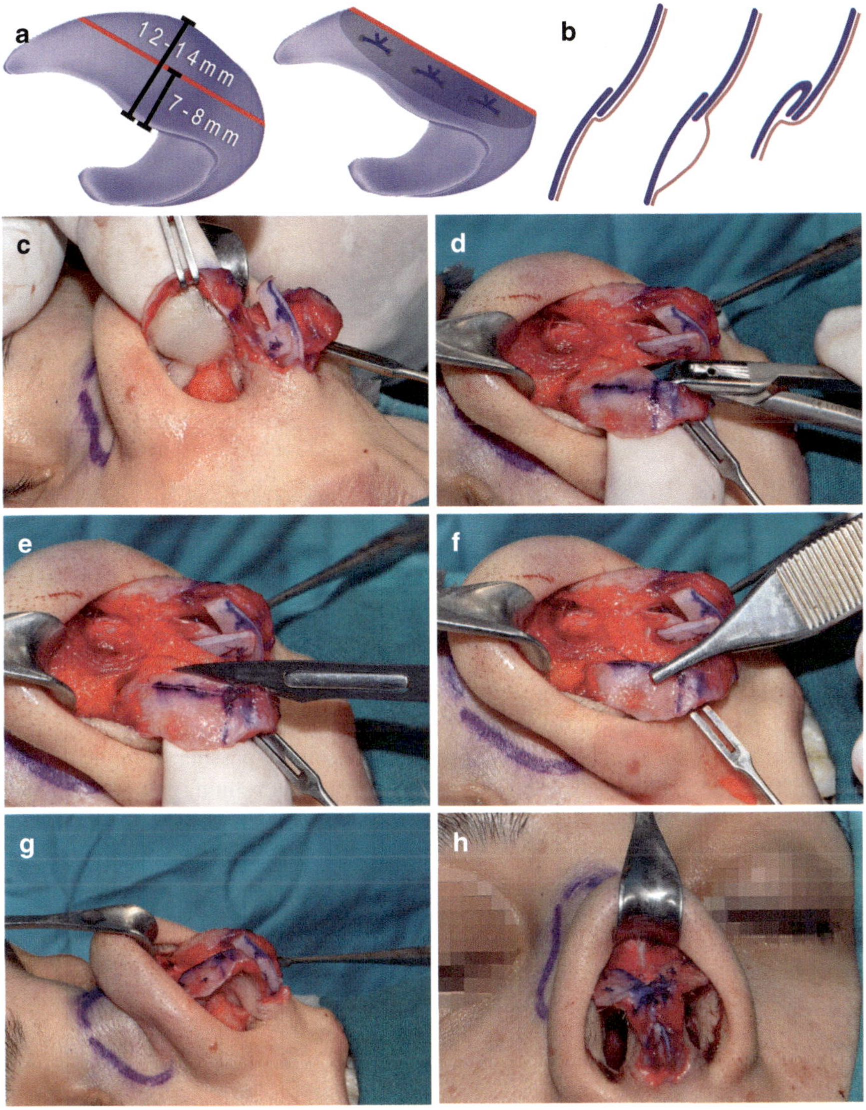

Fig. 12.5 Instead of cephalic trim, lateral crural turn-in flap is a powerful tool to reshape and support the lateral crura (**a**, **b**). After hydrolic dissection, the skin under the lateral crus is dissected (**c**, **d**). A linear partial incision is realized by leaving a 7 mm caudal portion (**e**). The cephalic portion is folded under the caudal portion and sutured by 5-0 PDS sutures like a sandwich (**f**). The dissected skin is reattached to the lateral crus (**g**). Tip plasty completed by sutures (**h**). In case of cephalically malpositioned lateral crura (**i**), lateral crura are dissected free and turn-in flap can be used to have a stronger and better shaped cartilage (**j**–**l**)

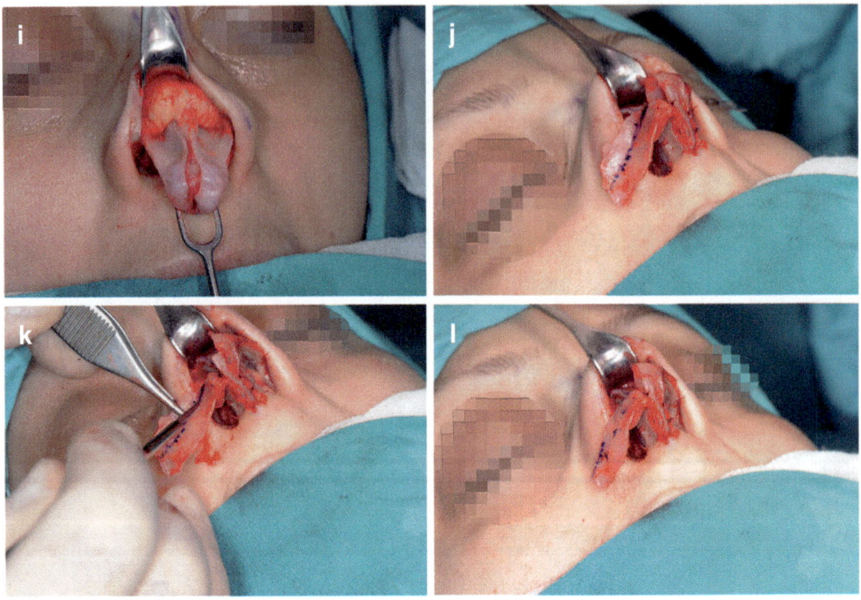

Fig. 12.5 (continued)

a long and strong boomerang-shape columellar strut between the medial crura by 5-0 PDS sutures (Fig. 12.6h, i).

5. *Transdomal suture:* This is a horizontal mattress suture passing from the domes to narrow and reorient the alar cartilage domes, thus refining the attitude and shape of the nasal tip and the lateral crura [40, 41] (Fig. 12.6j).
6. *Alar spanning suture:* This mattress suture starts at the caudal end of the middle vault and then passes from the cephalic margin of the lateral crura. The idea is to bring the cephalic margins closer to the nasal dorsum and rotate the axis of the lateral crus to a more favorable position [42] (Fig. 12.6k, l).

12.5.1 Grafts

I used to use tip grafts more in primary cases 15–20 years ago. Currently I am using them more in revision cases. They are at the surgeons's service to eliminate tip asymmetry, increase projection, change rotation, add structure, and reshape lateral crura. My favorite graft options are listed below.

1. Columellar strut: It is a rectangular or slightly curved graft sutured between the medial crura (Fig. 12.7a–e). It is used to:
   - Support the tip.
   - Spacer between the medial crura.
   - Control shape and profile configuration of the medial crura.

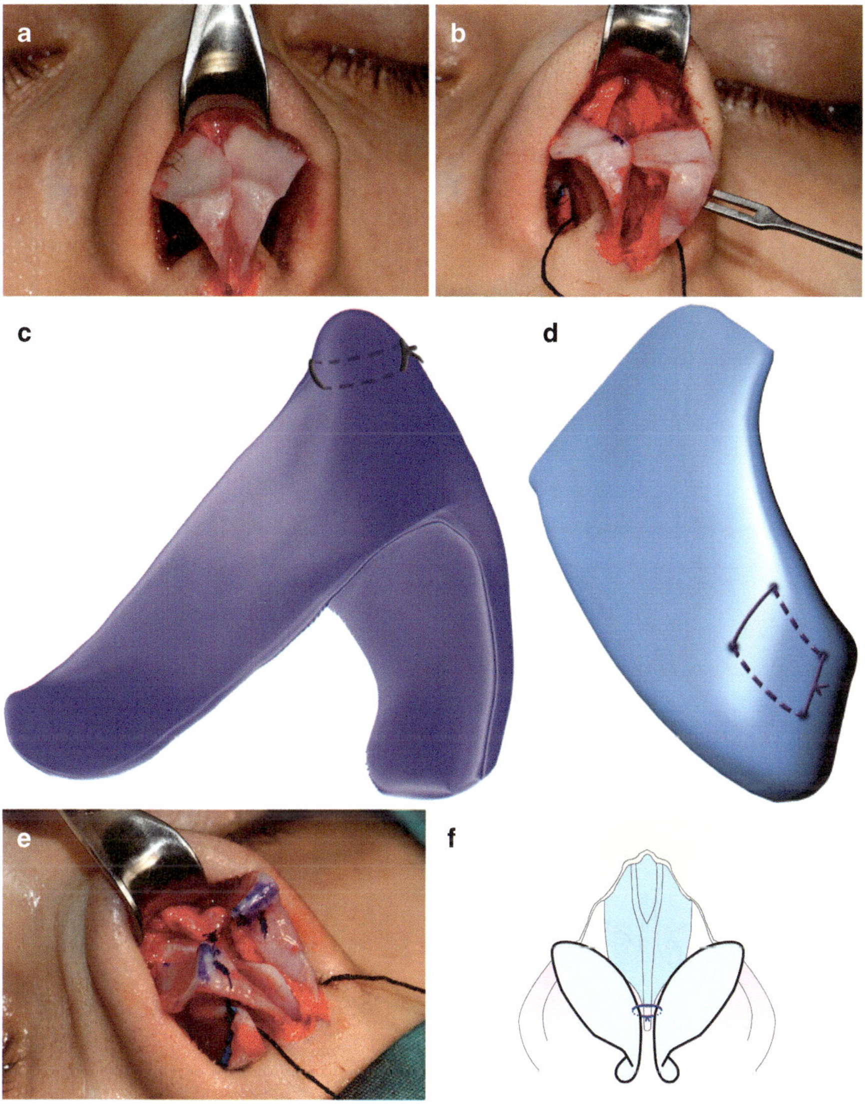

Fig. 12.6 Tip sutures are my favorite techniques to reshape the tip. In tip plasty, the first step is to perform cephalic trim or lateral crural turn-in flap (**a**, **b**). It is decided how much steal is needed such as 3–5 mm. The first suture is the hemitransdomal suture followed by high domal suture (**c**–**e**). The third suture is the dome equalizing suture (**f**, **g**). The fourth suture is two septocolumellar sutures, which is followed by adding a long columellar strut between the medial crura (**h**, **i**). Transdomal suture is helpful in fine tuning the interdomal distance (**j**). Alar spanning suture is used only when there is a need to approximate the cephalic margins to the upper lateral cartilages (**k**, **l**)

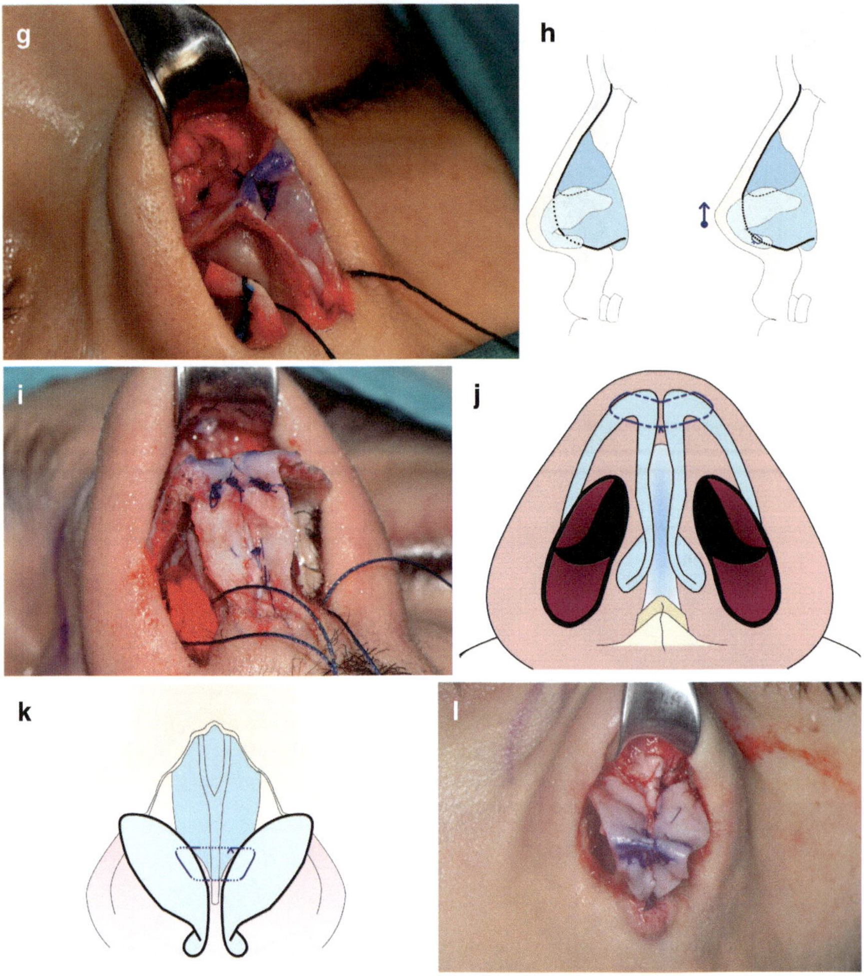

Fig. 12.6 (continued)

- Increase projection.
- Guarantee an angle of divergence.
- Correct medial crural anomalies.
  - Buckling.
  - Footplate flare.
  - Prominent double break angle.

In external rhinoplasty, it is routinely used to support the weakened tip cartilages in order not to lose projection and rotation [43]. When a bigger type of it is sutured to the caudal end of the septum either end-to-end or overlapping fashion, it is called caudal septal extension graft.

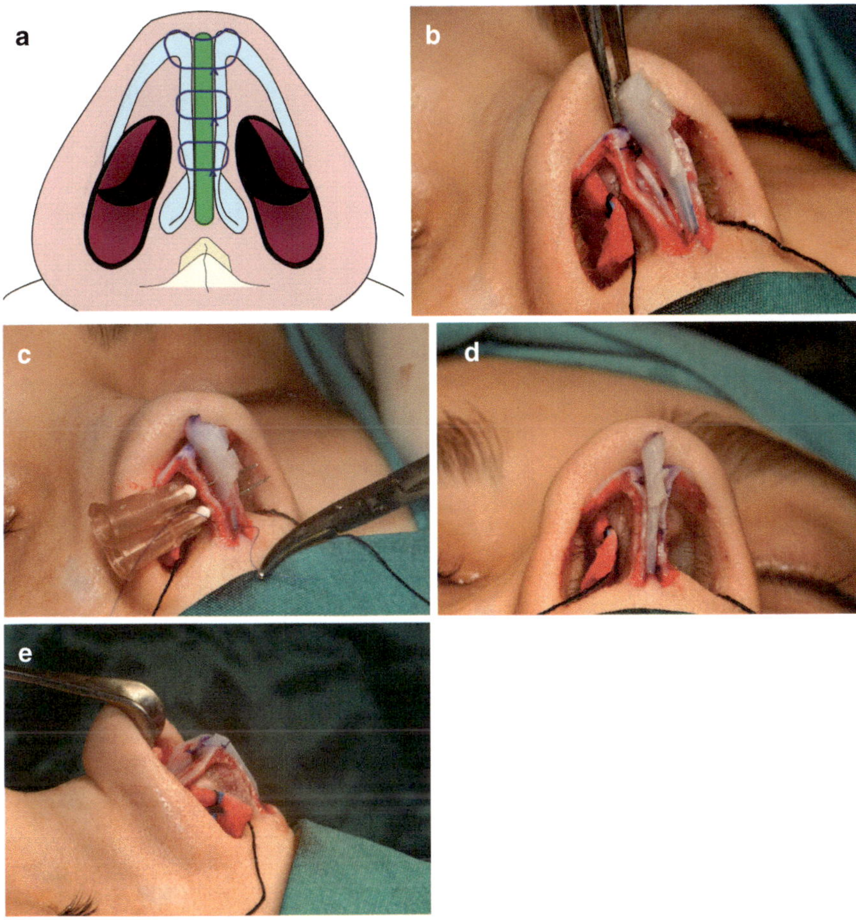

Fig. 12.7 Columellar strut is a useful graft sutured between the medial crura (**a**). I first finish the tip sutures. After performing two septocolumellar sutures, the medial crura look like an open book. A long, big, and slightly curved graft is fixed to the medial crura with 2 small needles (**b**, **c**). Then, 5-0 PDS sutures are out to keep the columellar strut in place and to give the final shape to the columella (**d**). The cartilage exceeding the medial crura margins is trimmed (**e**)

2. Shield graft: It is a piece of graft in the form of a shield to obtain better tip definition, to eliminate tip asymmetry and increase projection [44]. It is often used in revision surgeries (Fig. 12.8a, b).
3. Buttress graft: Sutured just above the shield graft to prevent its cephalic migration and obtain an aesthetic transition to the supratip [44] (Fig. 12.8c–e).
4. Tip onlay graft: It is sutured on the domes to increase projection and obtain better tip definition [45] (Fig. 12.9a–d). Tip grafts are camouflaged to prevent visibility due to shrink-wrapping of skin (Fig. 12.9d).

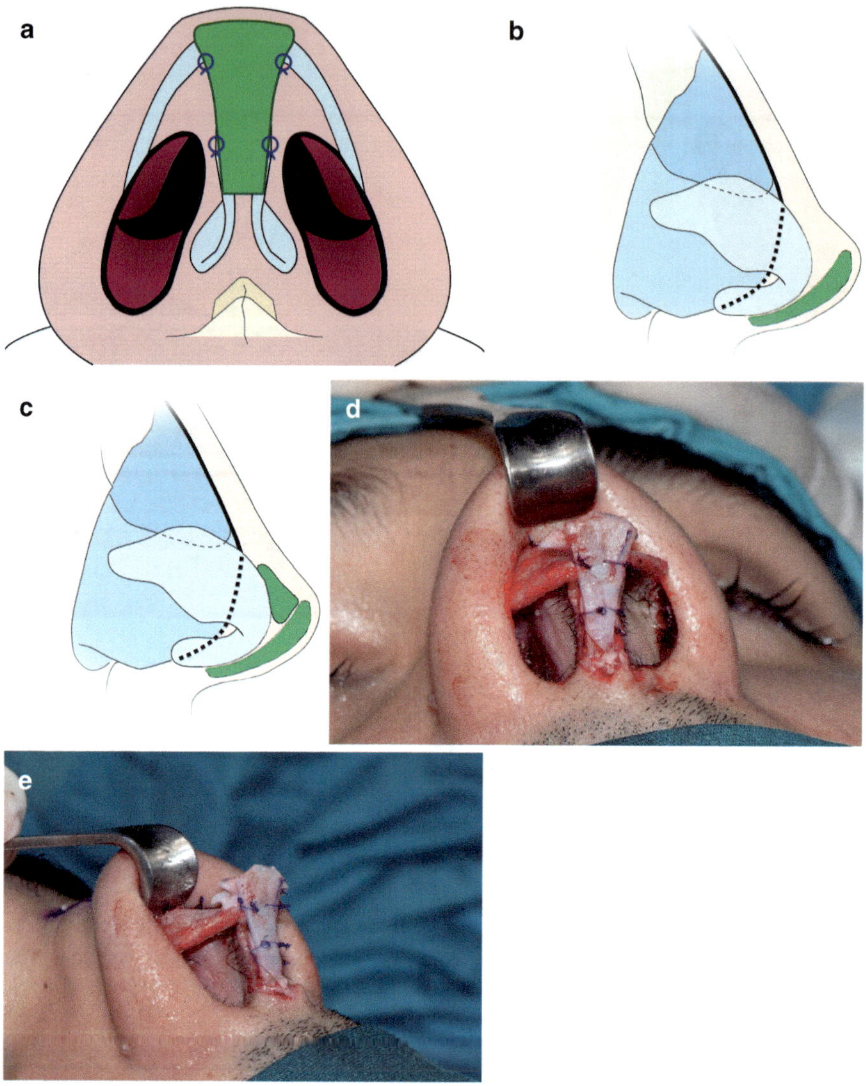

Fig. 12.8 Shield graft is a great tool to obtain a symmetric and defined tip in revision cases. It is possible to increase the projection as well. It is fixed to the medial crura and domes by sutures (**a**, **b**). A buttress graft is sutured just behind the shield graft to prevent its cephalic migration and obtain a smooth transition around the graft (**c**–**e**)

5. Lateral crural strut graft: It is sutured under the lateral crus to have a better shape, as a support if there is a need to repositioning or to reconstruct the lateral crura [46] (Fig. 12.10a, b).
6. Alar batten graft: They are described to support external and internal valves when there is an alar collapse or internal valve stenosis [35] (Fig. 12.10c). Their

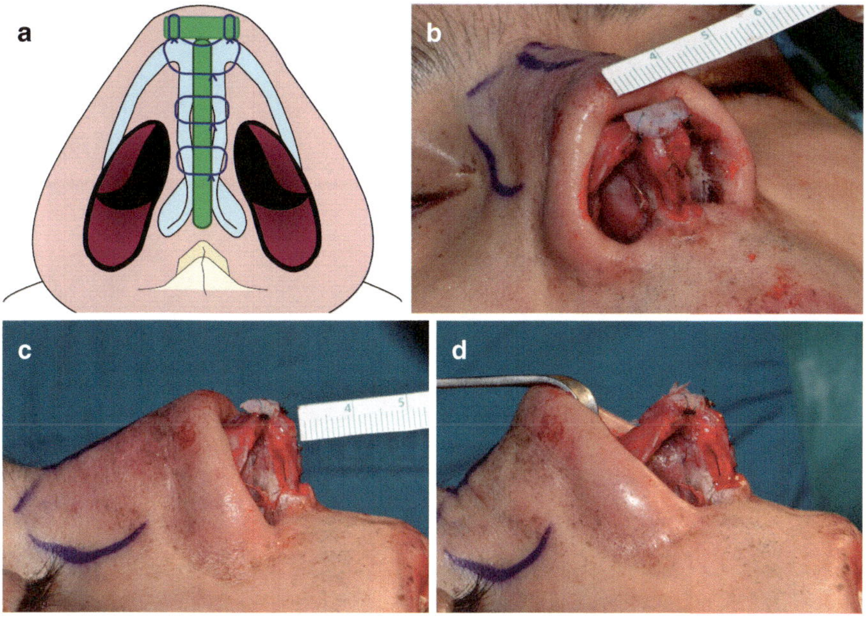

Fig. 12.9 Tip graft is great to increase the projection and create a better tip definition (**a–c**). To decrease visibility, camouflage is performed by cartilage chips (**d**)

use for internal valve problems is limited because the patient can see and palpate the graft in the long term that can become aesthetically unacceptable. However, they are helpful to support and reshape the alae.

7. Alar rim graft: Alar rim grafts are inserted in a pocket along the alar rim when there is an alar retraction, alar contour anomaly or alar collapse [47]. They can be used as a floating graft or sutured to the lateral crura as articulated grafts [36] (Fig. 12.10d, e).

   Cartilage dust and chips are helpful around the grafts to prevent visibility in the long-term (Fig. 12.10f, g).

12.5.2 Nasal Septum

During rhinoplasty, I use two approaches to the nasal septum. If I want to keep the membranous septum intact, I like using the hemitransfixion incision, otherwise the nasal septum is approached after dissecting or cutting the ligaments between the medial crura. I elevate the mucoperichondrium on the right side by keeping an intact area of mucoperichondrium at the upper half of the nasal septum. At this portion I like dissecting a pocket of 3–4 mm under the dorsum, which enables the placement of the spreader flaps or grafts much easier. A much limited dissection is performed on the left side. In traumatic or very badly deviated noses, a much wider dissection is performed.

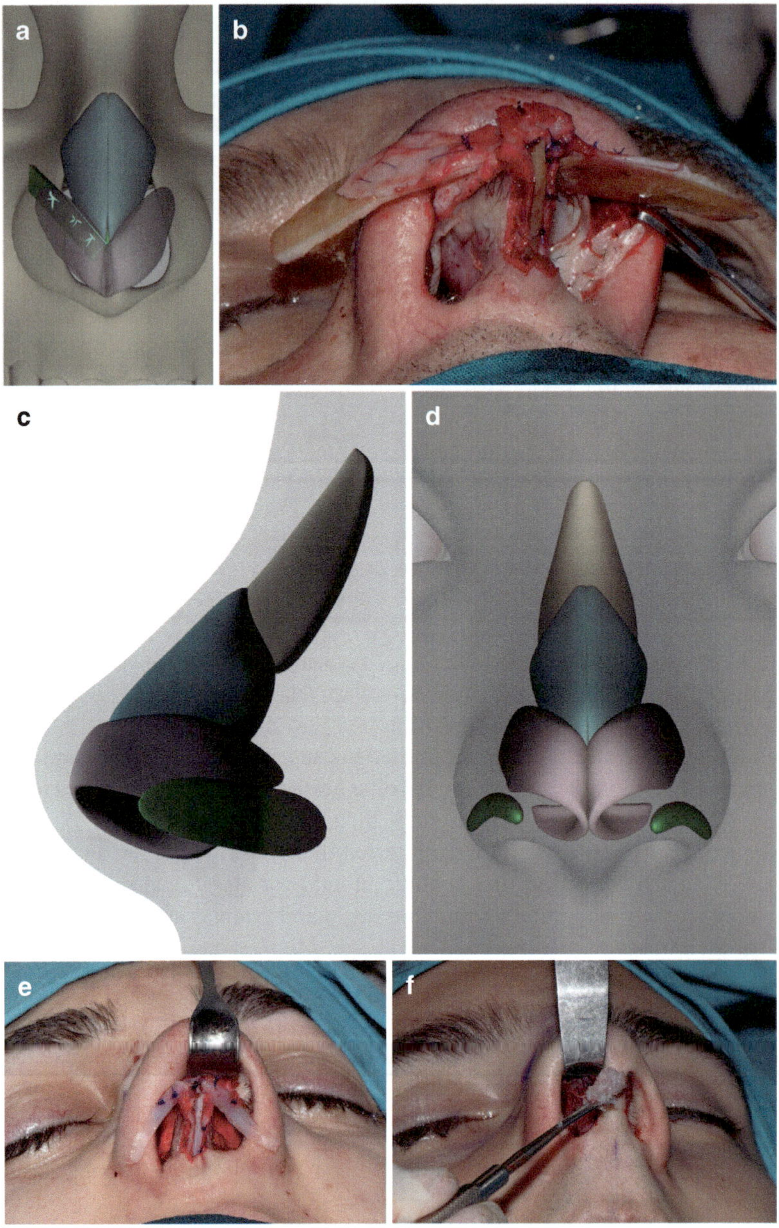

Fig. 12.10 Lateral crural strut graft is put under the lateral crus to reshape and support it (**a**). It is useful when repositioning of the lateral crura is required (**b**). Alar batten grafts are used to support the external valve and give a better shape to ala (**c**). Alar rim grafts are great in contouring the alar rim and support the external valve (**d**). They can be sutured to the dome as articulated rim graft to increase its effect (**e**). Cartilage dust (**f**) and chips (**g**) are my favorite camouflage material in revision cases and around the grafts

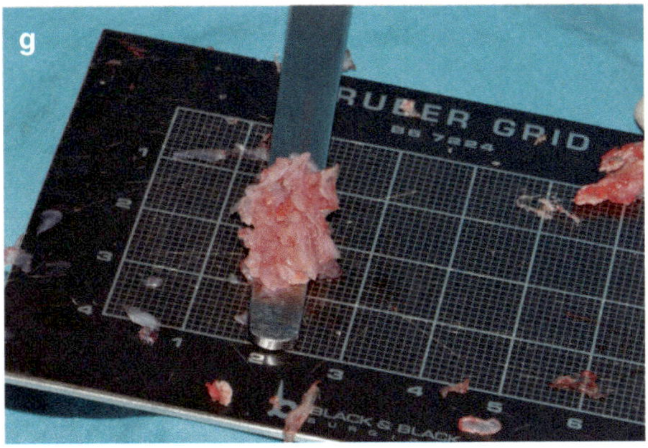

Fig. 12.10 (continued)

In cases where the L-strut framework is straight, an L-strut of 12–15 mm is kept in place while harvesting the rest of the cartilaginous septum. However, in cases where this framework is crooked, segmental septal reconstruction methods are used.

12.6 Segmental Septal Reconstruction

1. *Dorsal segment:* The deviations of the dorsal segment are seen in crooked noses such as C- shaped or S-Shaped deviations of the nose. The workhorse of the reconstruction of these deviations is the use of splinting spreader grafts, which are applied after cross-hatching of the concave side of the cartilage or partial resection of the deflected portion [48]. If the deviation is at the key area, the splinting should cover the upper third of the nose as well.
2. *Caudal segment:* The caudal segment of the nasal septum is a major support for the nasal tip. The main problems seen here are subluxation, concavity, retraction and fractures. There are two main approaches: splint the existing caudal segment by a batten or caudal septal extension graft (Fig. 12.11a, b) or replace it with a straighter caudal septal replacement graft [49] (Fig. 12.12a–c).
3. *L-Strut framework:* In case of severely crooked noses, the septal cartilage can be so badly deviated that an L-strut graft can be the best option to splint the L-strut framework (Fig. 12.11c–e). I have been mainly using the septal cartilage, on rare occasions ethmoid lamina and bony-cartilaginous grafts [50].
4. *Subtotal reconstruction:* In severely crooked noses, the L-strut framework can be affected by fractures. Here, most of the cartilaginous and bony septum is removed during surgery by leaving superior part of the dorsal segment adjacent to the key area intact. Because this small piece of cartilage is used as an anchoring cartilage for the spreader grafts. Later, the caudal septal replacement graft sutured to the

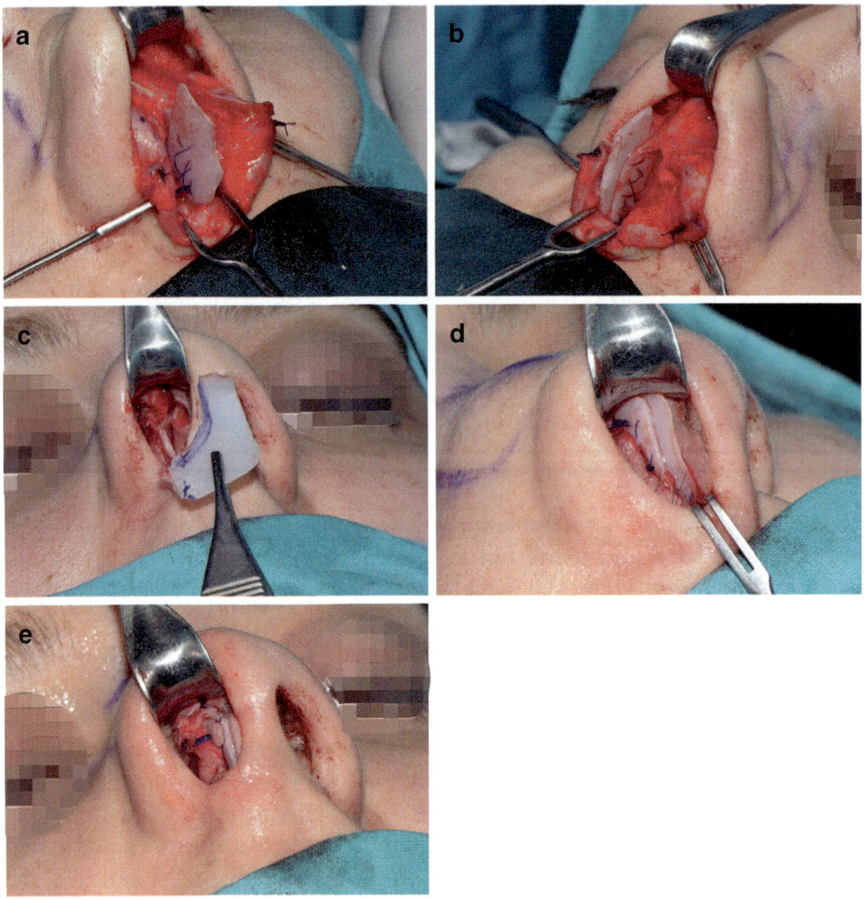

Fig. 12.11 Segmental septal reconstruction is my preferred way of dealing with crooked noses. If the caudal segment is deviated, a caudal septal extension graft is useful in splinting this deviation and acts as a columellar strut (**a**, **b**). If splinting of the dorsal and caudal segments is necessary, an L-strut graft is a great option and supported by a spreader graft contralaterally (**c**–**e**)

anterior nasal spine is connected with these two spreader grafts to create the new L-strut framework [51] (Fig. 12.13a–e). In case of cartilage deficiency such as revision cases, cartilage from the ear concha or rib can be used.

12.6.1 Revision Rhinoplasty

In my daily practice, the main reasons that patients seek for revision are nasal obstruction, dorsal irregularities, loss of tip projection and rotation and crookedness. Rarely, they complain from overrotated tips as well. In minor problems,

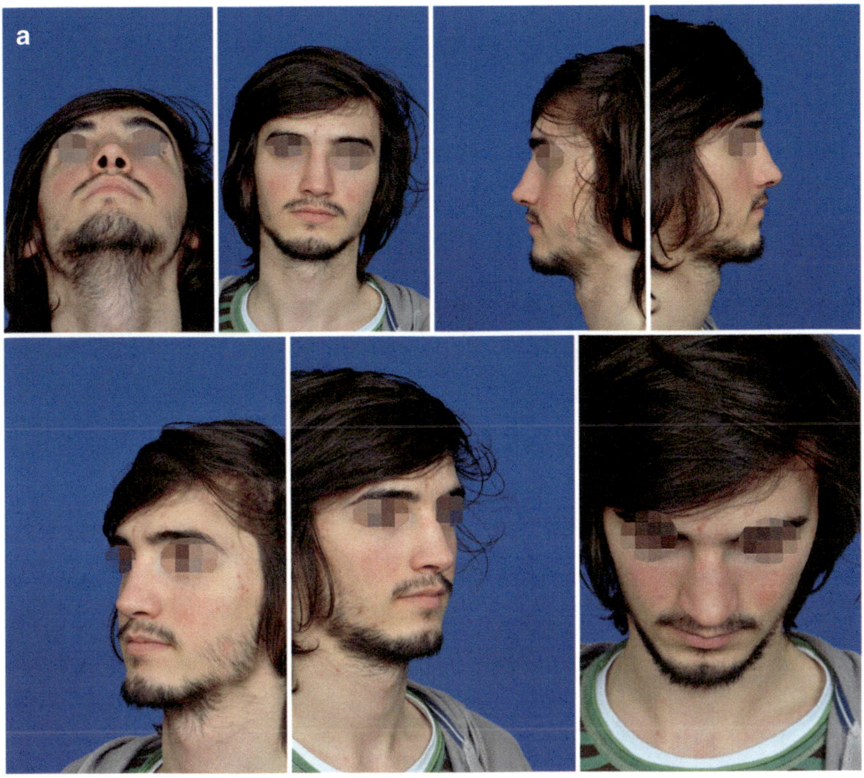

Fig. 12.12 A 22-year old young man with a crooked nose (**a**). As can be seen, the left nasal passage is totally blocked by septal deviation (**b1**). When the septal cartilage is exposed, three fracture lines proved that it was a traumatic deformity (**b2**). In these cases, it is better to remove all the fractured segments and apply a caudal septal replacement graft (**b3**, **4**). Then, it is supported by a splinting spreader graft (**b5**). A tongue-in-groove technique is issued to suture the medial crura to the caudal septal replacement graft (**b6**). A tip graft is issued to have a better tip definition (**b7**). The pictures taken 2 years after surgery show that the crookedness is corrected (**c**)

endonasal approach with small procedures can solve the problem. However, in major deformities, the operation starts with the reconstruction of the nasal septum after using the external approach. Conchal and tragal cartilage is sufficient in some cases. However, in the majority of the cases, the sixth or seventh rib is harvested. It is possible to obtain multiple grafts of various thicknesses and lengths by using the oblique split technique such as spreader grafts, caudal septal replacement or extension grafts, alar battens or lateral crural strut grafts, alar rim grafts, shield graft, dorsal onlay grafts, diced cartilage, cartilage chips and dust [52, 53] (Fig. 12.14a–c).

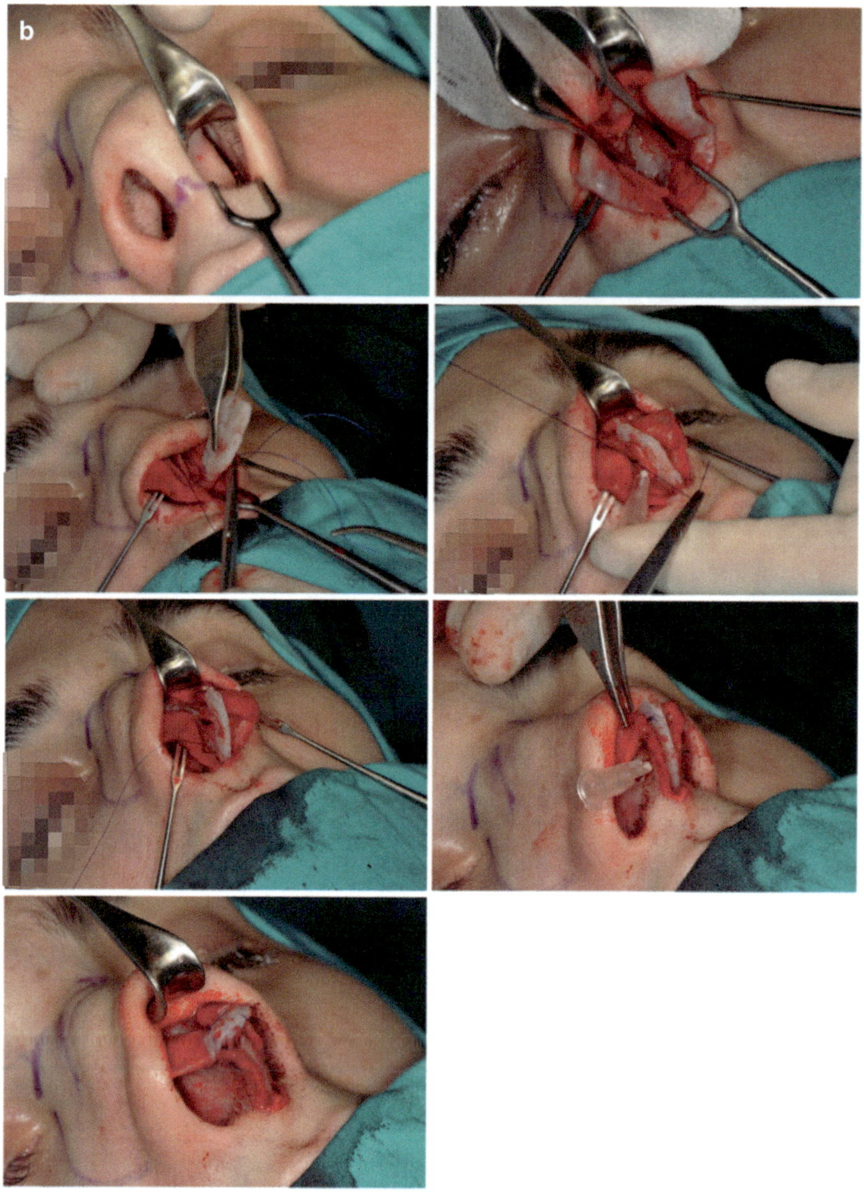

Fig. 12.12 (continued)

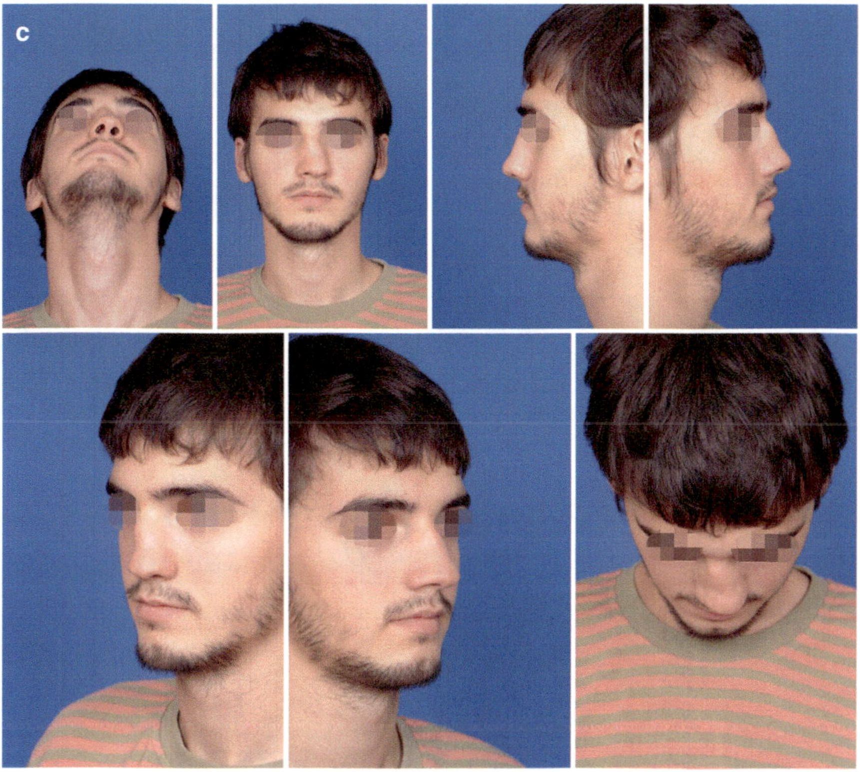

Fig. 12.12 (continued)

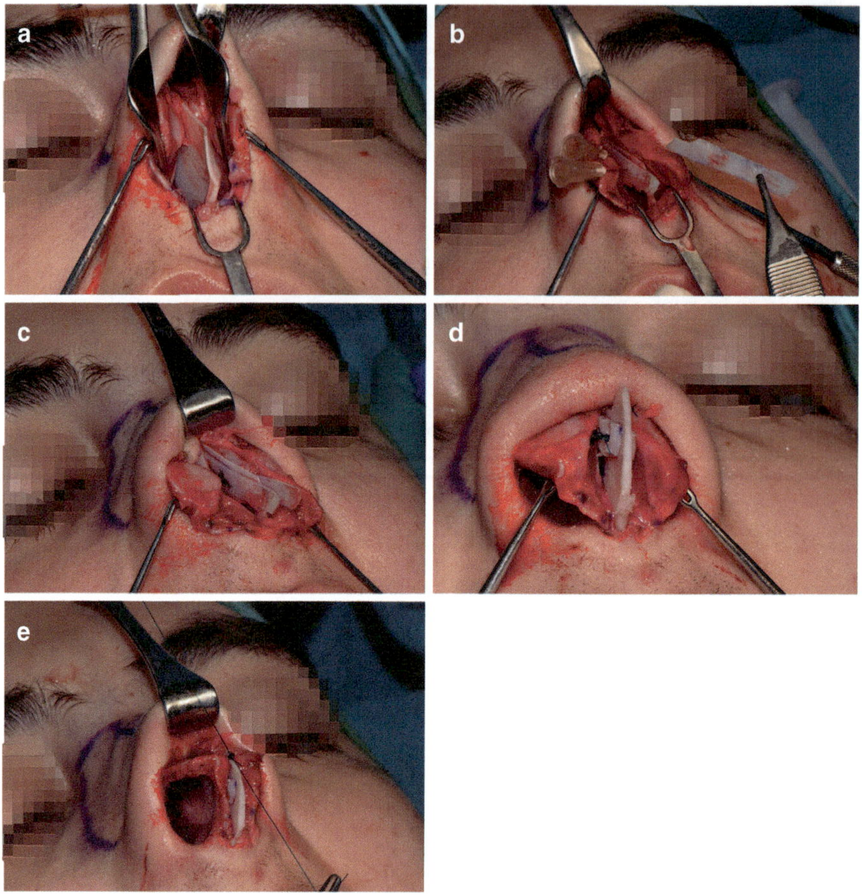

Fig. 12.13 Subtotal septal reconstruction is reserved for cases where the septal deviation is severe (**a**). The best way is to suture two splinting spreader grafts to the dorsal segment adjacent to the key area (**b**, **c**) and couple them to a caudal septal replacement graft (**d**, **e**)

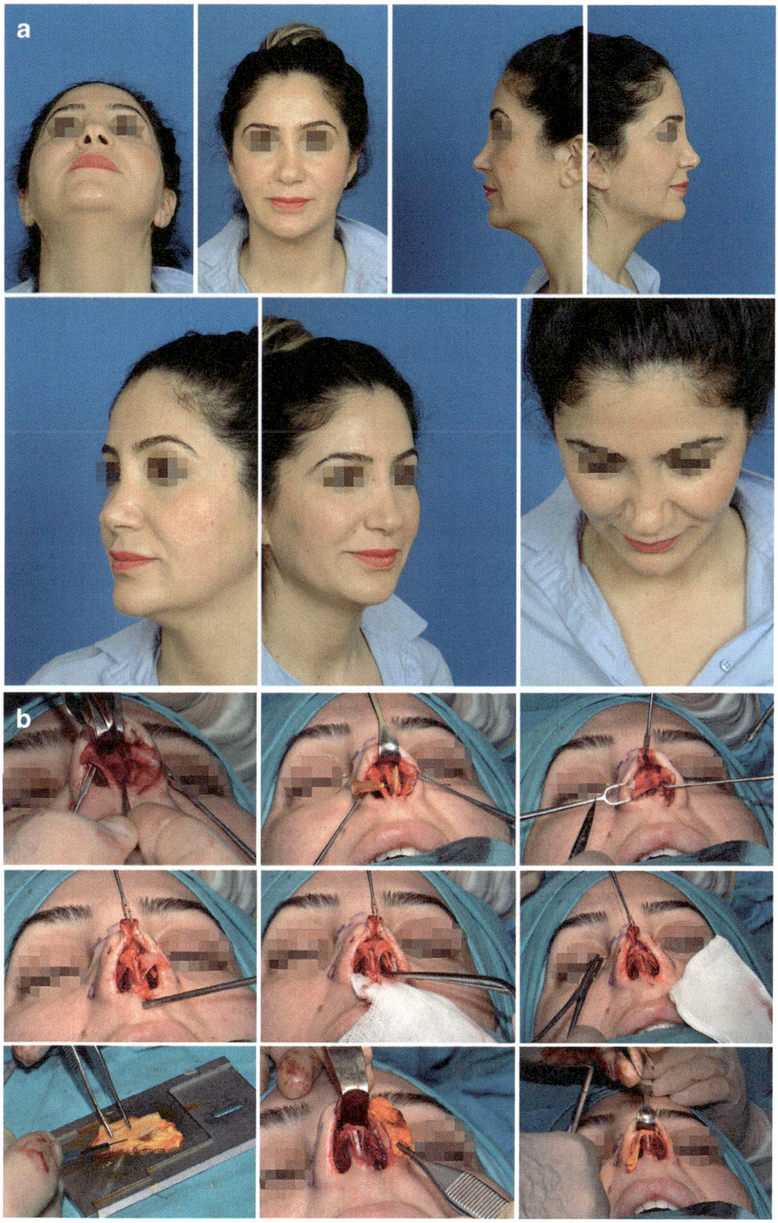

Fig. 12.14 This is a 35-year old woman who had 3 previous rhinoplasties and still cannot breathe through her nose and unhappy with the crooked nose (**a**). When the nasal septum was exposed, it was seen that there was not much septal cartilage left and the remaining caudal and dorsal septum was still crooked (**b1**). Cartilage grafts are obtained by oblique-split technique from the rib cartilage. Two splinting spreader grafts and one caudal septal extension graft are used to reconstruct the L-strut framework (**b2**). The lateral half of the lateral crura were resected in previous rhinoplasties (**b3, 4**). They were reconstructed by lateral crural strut grafts (**b5, 6**). The dorsal onlay graft was covered by the rectus abdominis fascia and inserted on the dorsum (**b7, 8**). The tip is covered by perichondrium (**b9**). It is possible to see the pictures taken 4 years after the surgery (**c**). It is not a perfect result and the patient should be aware that it is impossible to obtain a perfect result, especially in revision cases

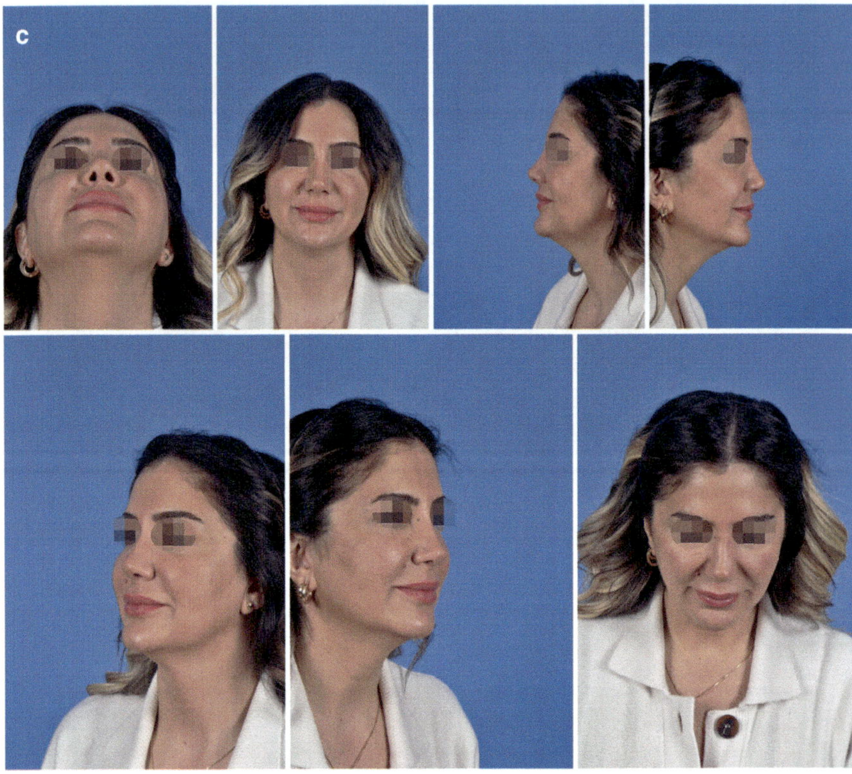

Fig. 12.14 (continued)

Disclosure No disclosures.

References

1. Gode S, Tiris FS, Akyildiz S, Apaydin F. Photogrammetric analysis of soft tissue facial profile in Turkish rhinoplasty population. Aesthet Plast Surg. 2011;35:1016–21.
2. Al-Qattan MM, Alsaeed AA, Al-Madani OK, Al-Amri NA, Al-Dahian NA. Anthropometry of the Saudi Arabian nose. J Craniofac Surg. 2012;23:821–4.
3. Bizrah MB. Rhinoplasty for middle eastern patients. Facial Plast Surg Clin North Am. 2002;10:381–96.
4. Rohrich RJ, Ghavami A. The middle eastern nose. In: Gunter JP, Rohrich RJ, Adams WP, editors. Dallas rhinoplasty: nasal surgery by the masters. 2nd ed. St. Louis: Quality Medical Publishing; 2007.
5. Rohrich RJ, Ghavami A. Rhinoplasty for middle eastern noses. Plast Reconstr Surg. 2009;123:1343–54.
6. Daniel RK. Middle eastern rhinoplasty in the United States: part I. Primary rhinoplasty. Plast Reconstr Surg. 2009;124:1630–9.
7. Azizzadeh B, Mashkevich G. Middle eastern rhinoplasty. Facial Plast Surg Clin North Am. 2010;18:201–6.

8. Gode S, Ozturk A, Sahin M, Berber V, Apaydin F. Turkish validation of the standardized cosmesis and health nasal outcomes survey. Facial Plast Surg. 2019;35(4):397–9.
9. Lekakis G, Picavet VA, Gabriëls L, Grietens J, Hellings PW. Body dysmorphic disorder in aesthetic rhinoplasty: validating a new screening tool. Laryngoscope. 2016;126(8):1739–45.
10. Abdelwahab M, Saltychev M, Elkholy NA, Elsisi H, Moubayed SP, Most SP. Arabic validation of the standardized cosmesis and health nasal outcome survey for Arabic-speaking rhinoplasty patients. Plast Reconstr Surg. 2019;143(3):673e–5e.
11. Apaydin F, Akyildiz S, Hecht DA, Toriumi DM. Rhinobase: a comprehensive database, facial analysis, and picture-archiving software for rhinoplasty. Arch Facial Plast Surg. 2009;11:209–11.
12. Cakir B, Oreroğlu AR, Doğan T, Akan M. A complete subperichondrial dissection technique for rhinoplasty with management of the nasal ligaments. Aesthet Surg J. 2012;32(5):564–74.
13. Cerkes N. Concurrent elevation of the upper lateral cartilage perichondrium and nasal bone periosteum for management of dorsum: the perichondro-periosteal flap. Aesthet Surg J. 2013;33(6):899–914.
14. Gerbault O, Daniel RK, Kosins AM. The role of piezoelectric instrumentation in rhinoplasty surgery. Aesthet Surg J. 2016;36(1):21–34.
15. Joseph J. Nasenplastik und sonstige Gesichtsplastik nebst einem Anhang über Mammaplastik. Leipzig: Verlag Curt Kabitzsch; 1931.
16. Sheen JH. Spreader graft: a method of reconstructing the roof of the middle nasal vault following rhinoplasty. Plast Reconstr Surg. 1984;73(2):230–9.
17. Constantian MB, Clardy RB. The relative importance of septal and nasal valvular surgery in correcting airway obstruction in primary and secondary rhinoplasty. Plast Reconstr Surg. 1996;98(1):38–54, discussion 55–58.
18. Seyhan A. Method for middle vault reconstruction in primary rhinoplasty: upper lateral cartilage bending. Plast Reconstr Surg. 1997;100(7):1941–3.
19. Oneal RM, Berkowitz RL. Upper lateral cartilage spreader flaps in rhinoplasty. Aesthet Surg J. 1998;18(5):370–1.
20. Toriumi DM. Management of the middle nasal vault. Oper Tech Plast Reconstr Surg. 1995;2:16–30.
21. Rohrich RJ, Hollier LH. Use of spreader grafts in the external approach to rhinoplasty. Clin Plast Surg. 1996;23(2):255–62.
22. Fomon S, Gilbert JG, Caron AL, Segal S. Collapsed ala: pathologic physiology and management. Arch Otolaryngol. 1950;51:465–84.
23. Saban Y, Daniel RK, Polselli R, Trapasso M, Palhazi P. Dorsal preservation: the push down technique reassessed. Aesthet Surg J 2018 17; 38(2): 117–131.
24. Apaydin F. Rebuilding the middle vault in rhinoplasty: a new classification of spreader flaps/grafts. Facial Plast Surg. 2016;32(6):638–45.
25. Byrd HS, Salomon J, Flood J. Correction of the crooked nose. Plast Reconstr Surg. 1998;102(6):2148–57.
26. Cerkes N. The crooked nose: principles of treatment. Aesthet Surg J. 2011;31(2):241–57.
27. Neves JC, Arancibia-Tagle D, Dewes W, Ferraz M. The segmental preservation rhinoplasty: the split Tetris concept. Facial Plast Surg. 2021;37(1):36–44.
28. Tellioglu AT, Cimen K. Turn-in folding of the cephalic portion of the lateral crus to support the alar rim in rhinoplasty. Aesthet Plast Surg. 2007;31(3):306–10.
29. Apaydin F. Lateral crural turn-in flap in functional rhinoplasty. Arch Facial Plast Surg. 2012;14(2):93–6.
30. Ozmen S, Eryilmaz T, Sencan A, Cukurluoglu O, Uygur S, Ayhan S, Atabay K. Sliding alar cartilage (SAC) flap: a new technique for nasal tip surgery. Ann Plast Surg. 2009;63(5):480–5. https://doi.org/10.1097/SAP.0b013e31819538a8. PMID: 19801923.
31. Taş S. Superior-based transposition flap: a novel technique in rhinoplasty. Aesthet Surg J. 2019;39(7):720–32.
32. Janis JE, Trussler A, Ghavami A, Marin V, Rohrich RJ, Gunter JP. Lower lateral crural turnover flap in open rhinoplasty. Plast Reconstr Surg. 2009;123(6):1830–41.

33. Kridel RW, Konior RJ. Controlled nasal tip rotation via the lateral crural overlay technique. Arch Otolaryngol Head Neck Surg. 1991;117(4):411–5.
34. Toriumi DM, Asher SA. Lateral crural repositioning for treatment of cephalic malposition. Facial Plast Surg Clin North Am. 2015;23(1):55–71.
35. Tardy ME, Garner ET. Inspiratory nasal obstruction secondary to alar and nasal valve collapse: technique for repair using autologous cartilage. Oper Tech Otolaryngol Head Neck Surg. 1990;1:215–8.
36. Ballin AC, Kim H, Chance E, Davis RE. The articulated alar rim graft: reengineering the conventional alar rim graft for improved contour and support. Facial Plast Surg. 2016;32(4):384–97.
37. Dosanjh AS, Hsu C, Gruber RP. The hemitransdomal suture for narrowing the nasal tip. Ann Plast Surg. 2010;64(6):708–12.
38. Daniel RK. Rhinoplasty: creating an aesthetic tip. A preliminary report. Plast Reconstr Surg. 1987;80(6):775–83.
39. Daniel RK. Rhinoplasty: a simplified, three-stitch, open tip suture techniques. Part I: primary rhinoplasty. Plast Reconstr Surg. 1999;103:1491–502.
40. Tardy ME Jr. Rhinoplasty tip ptosis: etiology and prevention. Laryngoscope. 1973;83(6):923–9.
41. Tardy ME Jr, Patt BS, Walter MA. Transdomal suture refinement of the nasal tip: long-term outcomes. Facial Plast Surg. 1993;9(4):275–84.
42. Tebbetts JB. Shaping and positioning the nasal tip without structural disruption: a new, systematic approach. Plast Reconstr Surg. 1994;94(1):61–77.
43. Rohrich RJ, Hoxworth RE, Kurkjian TJ. The role of the columellar strut in rhinoplasty: indications and rationale. Plast Reconstr Surg. 2012;129(1):118e–25e.
44. Johnson CM, Toriumi D. Open structure rhinoplasty. Philadelphia: Saunders; 1990.
45. Peck GC. The onlay graft for nasal tip projection. Plast Reconstr Surg. 1983;71(1):27–39.
46. Gunter JP, Friedman RM. Lateral crural strut graft: technique and clinical applications in rhinoplasty. Plast Reconstr Surg. 1997;99(4):943–52.
47. Guyuron B. Alar rim deformities. Plast Reconstr Surg. 2001;107(3):856–63.
48. Porter JP, Toriumi DM. Surgical techniques for management of the crooked nose. Aesthet Plast Surg. 2002;26(Suppl 1):S18.
49. Kim DW, Toriumi DM. Management of posttraumatic nasal deformities: the crooked nose and the saddle nose. Facial Plast Surg Clin North Am. 2004;12(1):111–32.
50. Apaydin F, Garcia RFF, Tas V. L-strut graft: a very versatile graft in the management of crooked and traumatic noses. Facial Plast Surg Aesthet Med. 2021;23(2):110–7.
51. Apaydin F. Segmental reconstruction for nasal septal deviation. Facial Plast Surg. 2013;29(6):455–63.
52. Taştan E, Yücel ÖT, Aydin E, Aydoğan F, Beriat K, Ulusoy MG. The oblique split method: a novel technique for carving costal cartilage grafts. JAMA Facial Plast Surg. 2013;15(3):198–203.
53. Apaydın F.. Oblique split technique: a game changer in costal cartilage sculpting. Plast Aesthet Res 2019 (2019): n. pag.

Further Readings

Al-Qattan MM, Alsaeed AA, Al-Madani OK, Al-Amri NA, Al-Dahian NA. Anthropometry of the Saudi Arabian nose. J Craniofac Surg. 2012;23:821–4.
Apaydin F. Rhinoplasty at the global crossroads. Arch Facial Plast Surg. 2009;11:421–3.
Apaydin F. Lateral crural turn-in flap in functional rhinoplasty. Arch Facial Plast Surg. 2012;14:93–6.
Apaydin F. Segmental reconstruction for nasal septal deviation. Facial Plast Surg. 2013a;29:455–63.
Apaydin F. Bone recycling in nasal septal reconstruction. Facial Plast Surg. 2013b;29:473–8.
Apaydin F, Akyildiz S, Hecht DA, Toriumi DM. Rhinobase: a comprehensive database, facial analysis, and picture-archiving software for rhinoplasty. Arch Facial Plast Surg. 2009;11:209–11.

Azizzadeh B, Mashkevich G. Middle eastern rhinoplasty. Facial Plast Surg Clin North Am. 2010;18:201–6.

Bafaqeeh SA, Al-Qattan MM. Open rhinoplasty: Columellar scar analysis in an Arabian population. Plast Reconstr Surg. 1998;102:1226–8.

Bizrah MB. Rhinoplasty for middle eastern patients. Facial Plast Surg Clin North Am. 2002;10(381–396):5.

Daniel RK. Middle eastern rhinoplasty in the United States: part I. Primary rhinoplasty. Plast Reconstr Surg. 2009;124:1630–9.

Foda HM. External rhinoplasty: a critical analysis of 500 cases. J Laryngol Otol. 2003;117:473–7.

Foda HM. External rhinoplasty for the Arabian nose: a columellar scar analysis. Aesthet Plast Surg. 2004;28:312–6.

Gode S, Tiris FS, Akyildiz S, Apaydin F. Photogrammetric analysis of soft tissue facial profile in Turkish rhinoplasty population. Aesthet Plast Surg. 2011;35:1016–21.

Guyuron B, DeLuca L, Lash R. Supratip deformity: a closer look. Plast Reconstr Surg. 2000;105:1140–51.

Hanasono MM, Kridel RW, Pastorek NJ, Glasgold MJ, Koch RJ. Correction of the soft tissue pollybeak using triamcinolone injection. Arch Facial Plast Surg. 2002;4:26–30.

http://en.wikipedia.org/wiki/Middle_East

http://www.guinnessworldrecords.com/longest-nose-on-a-living-person/

Kridel RW, Konior RJ, Shumrick KA, Wright WK. Advances in nasal tip surgery. The lateral crural steal. Arch Otolaryngol Head Neck Surg. 1989;115:1206–12.

Pedroza F. A 20-year review of the "new domes" technique for refining the drooping nasal tip. Arch Facial Plast Surg. 2002;4:157–63.

Rohrich RJ, Ghavami A. The Middle Eastern nose. In: Gunter JP, Rohrich RJ, Adams WP, editors. Dallas rhinoplasty: nasal surgery by the masters. 2nd ed. St. Louis: Quality Medical Publishing; 2007.

Rohrich RJ, Ghavami A. Rhinoplasty for middle eastern noses. Plast Reconstr Surg. 2009;123:1343–54.

Rohrich RJ, Muzaffar AR, Janis JE. Component dorsal hump reduction: the importance of maintaining dorsal aesthetic lines in rhinoplasty. Plast Reconstr Surg. 2004;114:1298–308.

Tardy ME Jr, Patt BS, Walter MA. Transdomal suture refinement of the nasal tip: long-term outcomes. Facial Plast Surg. 1993;9:275–84.

Toriumi DM, Becker DO. Rhinoplasty dissection manual. Philadelphia: Lippincott; 1999.

GPSR Compliance

The European Union's (EU) General Product Safety Regulation (GPSR) is a set of rules that requires consumer products to be safe and our obligations to ensure this.

If you have any concerns about our products, you can contact us on ProductSafety@springernature.com

In case Publisher is established outside the EU, the EU authorized representative is:

Springer Nature Customer Service Center GmbH
Europaplatz 3
69115 Heidelberg, Germany

Batch number: 10732044

Printed by Printforce, the Netherlands